the blood sugar repair plan

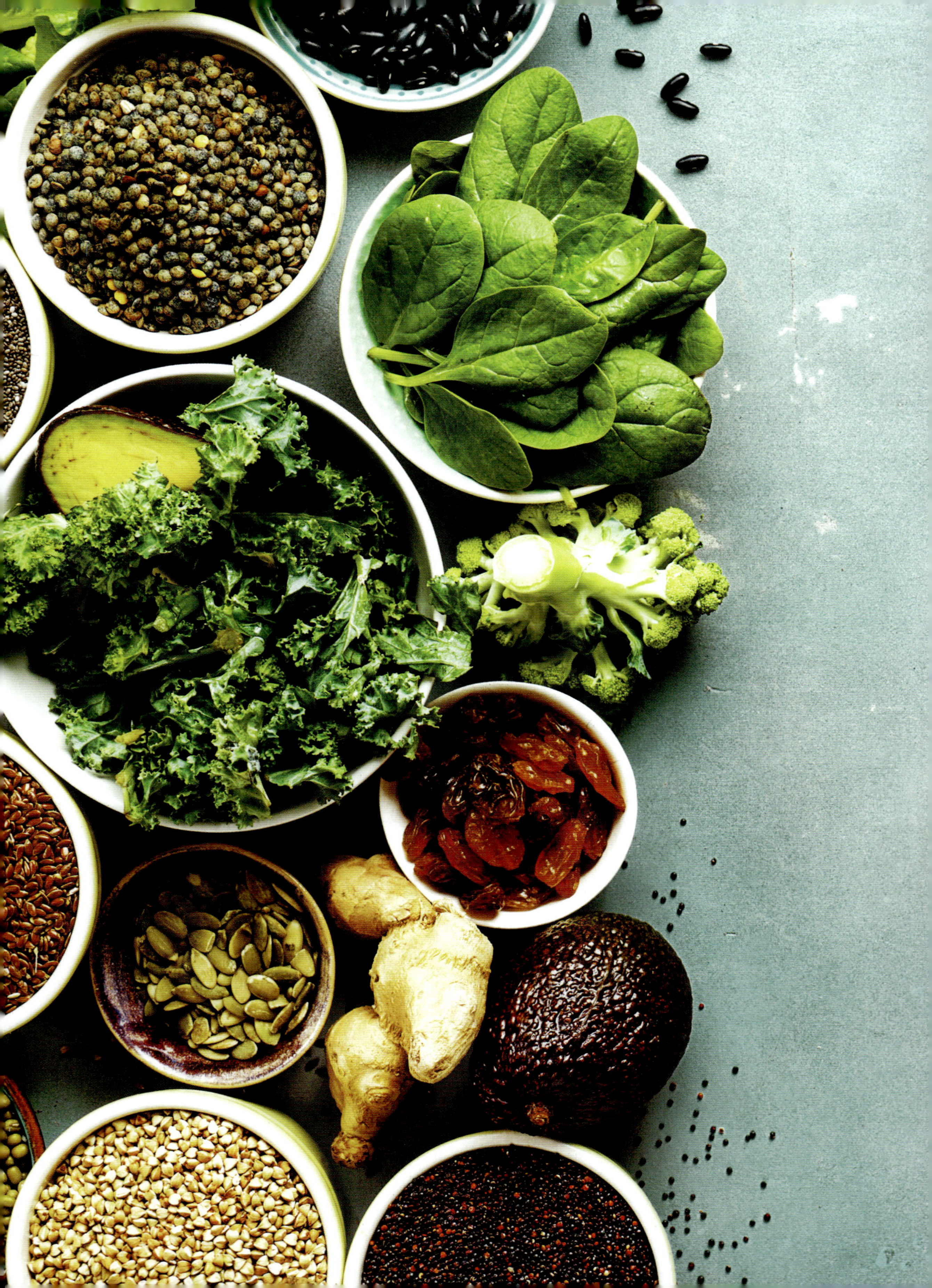

A PROGRAM FOR TYPE 2 DIABETES, INSULIN RESISTANCE, PREDIABETES AND OBESITY

the blood sugar repair plan

SARAH DI LORENZO
CLINICAL NUTRITIONIST

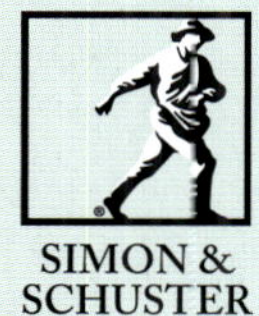

SIMON & SCHUSTER

New York · Amsterdam/Antwerp · London · Toronto · Sydney/Melbourne · New Delhi

THE BLOOD SUGAR REPAIR PLAN: A PROGRAM FOR TYPE 2 DIABETES, INSULIN
RESISTANCE, PREDIABETES AND OBESITY
First published in Australia in 2026 by
Simon & Schuster (Australia) Pty Limited
Level 4, 32 York St, Sydney NSW 2000
This edition published in 2026

10 9 8 7 6 5 4 3 2 1

New York Amsterdam/Antwerp London Toronto Sydney/Melbourne New Delhi
Visit our website at www.simonandschuster.com.au

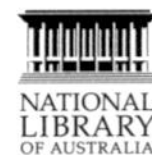

A catalogue record for this
book is available from the
National Library of Australia

ISBN: 9781761423925

Cover and internal design: Casey Schuurman
Back cover images: Lawrence Furzey Photography (left), Scott Ehler (right)
Recipe photography: Lawrence Furzey Photography
Food stylist: Fiona Sinclair
Printed and bound in China by Asia Pacific Offset Limited

NOTES TO READERS:
1. Throughout the book we use both the terms blood sugar and blood glucose. The terms are
   interchangeable and mean the same thing – the amount of sugar (glucose) found in your
   bloodstream.
2. The information in this book is for general purpose only. Although every effort has been made
   to ensure that the contents are accurate, it must not be treated as a substitute for qualified
   medical advice. Always consult a qualified medical practitioner. Neither the author nor the
   publisher can be held responsible for any loss or claim arising out of the use, or misuse, of the
   suggestions made or the failure to take advice.

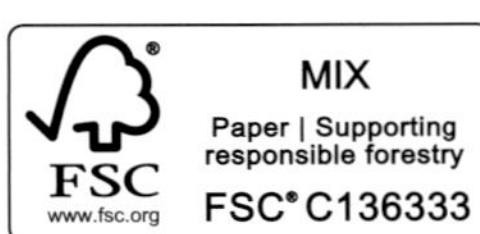

DEDICATION

I always dedicate my books to my three daughters: Charlotte,
Coco and Chloe. They are the loves of my life and support me
in everything I do. I feel so lucky to have been blessed with
such amazing daughters.

I also have to dedicate this book to all my patients who have
walked through my clinic doors with type 2 diabetes, insulin
resistance, obesity and prediabetes. It was you, your stories
and successes that inspired me to write this book.

I would also like to dedicate this book to my Facebook community:
The Sarah Di Lorenzo Community. I wanted to write this book
for all of you to continue to inspire and educate you. I love this
community so much. I started the community back in 2018
to get people who were doing my programs to start chatting
and support each other. This was four years before I was first
published. Now, the community has tens of thousands of people
and the foundation still stands strong – it's a community
about sharing, caring, supporting and being kind.

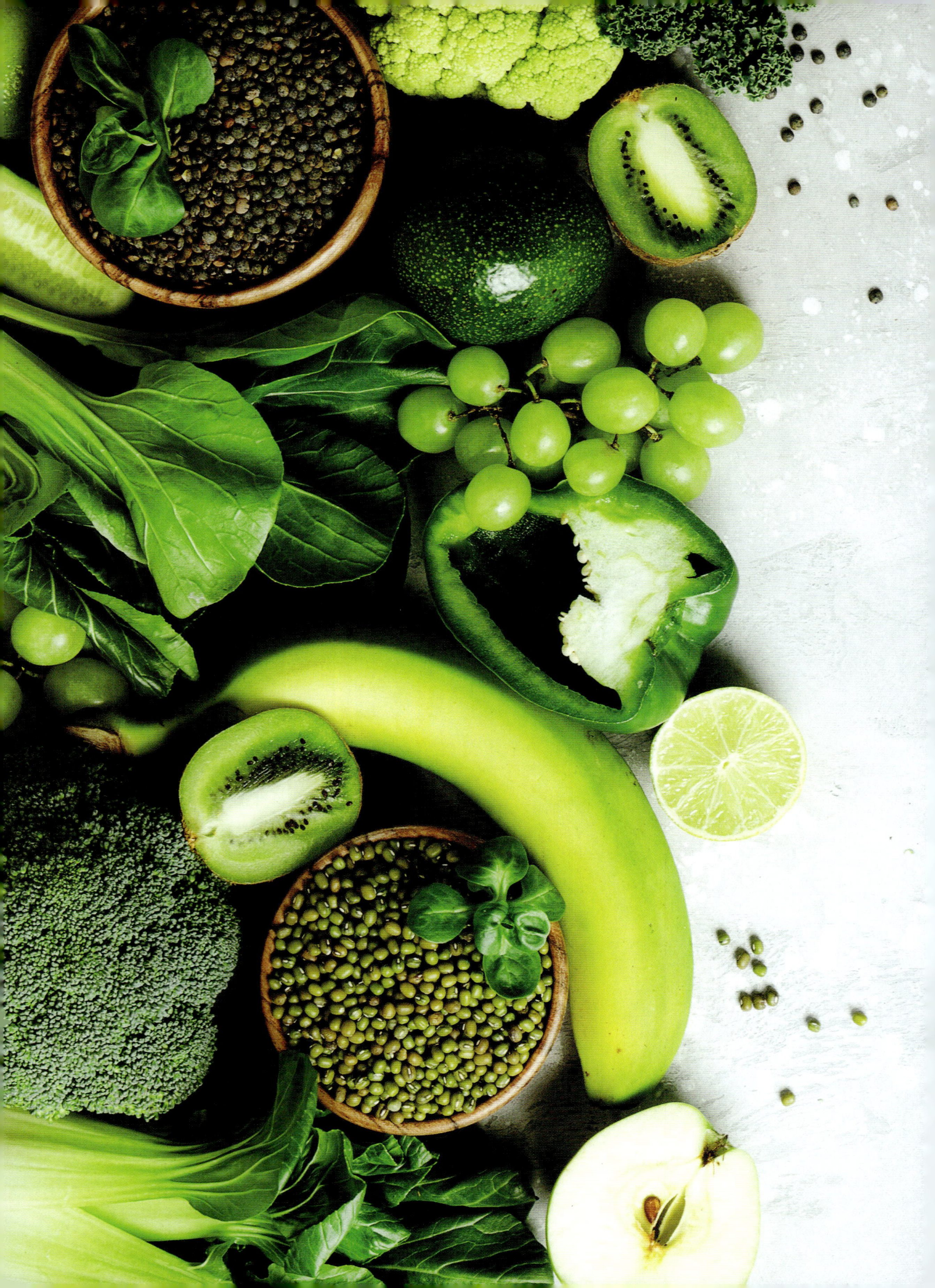

CONTENTS

FOREWORD

There comes a moment in medicine when we must acknowledge that our approach to a disease has been fundamentally backwards. For decades, we've treated diabetes as a chronic, progressive condition – something to be managed with an ever-increasing arsenal of medications but never truly reversed. We've told millions of patients that their diagnosis is a life sentence, that the best they can hope for is to slow the inevitable decline. This book challenges that narrative, and it does so with scientific rigour and compassionate practicality.

I have been a doctor for more than 46 years and have witnessed the devastating complications of poorly managed diabetes: the amputations, blindness, kidney failure, heart attacks. This work arrives at a critical time. The global pandemic of 'diabesity' shows no signs of slowing, yet here is a roadmap that offers genuine hope for reversal, not merely management.

The Blood Sugar Repair Plan doesn't promise a miracle cure or quick fix. Instead, Sarah Di Lorenzo provides what patients have been desperately seeking: a clear, evidence-based understanding of how diabetes develops at a cellular level, and a systematic program to address its root causes. This is not another fad diet dressed up as medical advice. This is a comprehensive intervention that respects the complexity of metabolic disease while making the science accessible to everyone.

What sets this book apart is the nine-week program at its heart. This isn't a vague suggestion to 'eat better and exercise more'. Sarah has created a structured, week-by-week protocol that addresses nutrition, movement, sleep, stress management and the psychological aspects of behaviour change. Each week builds on the last, allowing the body to adapt and heal progressively.

As one of Australia's premier nutritional experts, Sarah Di Lorenzo navigates the contentious landscape of dietary advice with remarkable balance, while providing clear, practical meal plans that real people can actually follow. She understands that sustainability matters more than perfection, and that the best diet is the one you can maintain long-term.

Perhaps most importantly, this book addresses the emotional dimensions of living with diabetes. The shame, frustration and sense of failure many patients experience are real obstacles to healing, and Sarah meets them with empathy and practical strategies. She recognises that changing ingrained habits requires support, self-compassion and belief that change is possible.

I must add a note of realism: not every person with type 2 diabetes will achieve complete reversal through lifestyle intervention alone. Disease duration, beta-cell dysfunction, genetic factors and other variables all play a role. Some individuals will still require medication, and that's acceptable. But this program offers you the opportunity to dramatically improve metabolic health, reduce medication burden and prevent complications. Even partial reversal represents a profound victory.

The evidence supporting lifestyle intervention for diabetes reversal has grown considerably in recent years. Large-scale studies have demonstrated that intensive lifestyle programs can achieve remission rates that exceed what medications alone can offer. Yet this has been slow to translate into clinical practice, in part because our healthcare system is better equipped to prescribe pills than support sustained behaviour change. This book helps bridge that gap, empowering patients to take charge of their own healing.

As you embark on this nine-week journey, I encourage you to approach it with patience and self-compassion. Healing is rarely linear. You will face setbacks and frustrations. But you will also have victories – the moment you realise your energy has returned, the day you check your blood sugar and see a number you haven't seen in years, the appointment where your doctor reduces your medication dose. These victories are worth fighting for.

The question is no longer whether type 2 diabetes can be reversed. The question is whether you're ready to begin. And if you've opened this book, you've already taken the first step.

Dr Ross Walker
Consultant cardiologist/Author/Media presenter

INTRODUCTION

There are many reasons why I wanted to write a book about blood sugar. As an author, the books I'm inspired to write come from me wanting to make changes on a much larger platform than my own clinic setting.

What inspires me are the day-to-day patients I've seen over the years – their stories, their journeys, and what has and hasn't worked for them before they come to see me. I see the confusion and frustration they feel. I see their success after we change their diet and lifestyle, and I want to share this with all of you.

I've had patients come to me with type 2 diabetes, morbid obesity, insulin resistance and prediabetes, who have tried everything and failed. They've been on diet after diet; they've tried fads and trends, supplements and medications, but the only thing changing is that they're going on more medication to treat their symptoms, not the underlying disease.

Many patients of this profile who have come to see me have already been to their doctor. They've been offered or prescribed GLP-1 medications – some aren't recommended to make dietary changes, but just start the medication. What really surprises me is that I've had many type 2 diabetic patients who have been taking these medications without any success. Many people felt completely frustrated and lost. The thing is, most of these people give up on taking GLP-1 injectable medications within two years, mainly due to side effects, cost or lack of success.

But the solution is so simple. These are diseases of the diet, so change the diet!

When I treat these people with diet and lifestyle changes, they start to see results very quickly. Many feel almost angry that they had to go down different treatment plans/paths with some taking a lot of medication before being put on the correct diet to treat the disease.

It was this frustration, anger and disappointment I saw in so many of my patients that made me decide to write this book.

I have thousands of patient success stories, both from my clinic and people purchasing my last nine bestselling books. You just need to look at the success of my weight-loss program The 10:10 Plan – so far this has got millions of kilograms of fat off people and shows them how to keep it off for life in a healthy way. My book *The Gut Repair Plan* has healed so many people's guts and shown them how to eat for optimal gut health.

And my incredibly successful book *The Liver Repair Plan* treats liver disease – some patients following the plan have achieved more in one month than with other methods over years, even decades. In 2025, I brought two of these patients onto Channel 7's *Sunrise* program, where I am the resident nutritionist, to chat about this very topic.

In writing this book, I wanted to return to awareness about understanding blood sugar. Many of my new weight-loss patients, who have been struggling to lose weight, have no idea they are insulin resistant. This is the first stage of disease progression; insulin resistance makes weight loss harder and most people have no idea they have it. Clients following my programs have seen results including lower cholesterol, lower inflammation, lower blood sugar levels, better sleep and better overall health. What I love about this is that I know my programs work. All you need to do is head to my Facebook community – The Sarah Di Lorenzo Community – and read the thousands of success stories.

I wanted to show people with type 2 diabetes how you can reverse the disease, and bring about remission. I want to inspire you to not just give in and accept managing your diabetes; rather, to know you can make changes that work. I also wanted to give you all the tools possible to treat the disease, not only from diet but also lifestyle choices.

This book is also for people with prediabetes, a condition you can have for years without any symptoms. I hope that if someone with prediabetes picks up this book, they get an 'ah-ha' moment and change their life before the disease progresses further into type 2 diabetes.

This book is also for those who want to lose weight. While the 9-week program is focused on managing blood sugar, it is also an incredible weight-loss program that I have carefully curated to treat the body holistically.

The 9-week program in this book is like no other. This is where the book really shines. The program is comprehensive and very successful. The 9 weeks are divided into three phases: Getting into ketosis, Adaptation and check-up, and Continued weight loss. Each week not only focuses on weight loss but also contains foods targeted specifically to treat the complications of diabetes with regard to skin health, immunity, mental health, eye health, heart and vascular system, inflammation, and gut health – all while losing weight. If you don't have diabetes, this is an added bonus to nourish the body along the way, which I love so much.

In the past, people with type 2 diabetes, insulin resistance, obesity and prediabetes were treated through measuring, medicating and managing blood glucose – their disease was treated with numbers. But think about it: if this this was the best way to treat these conditions, why are we now facing record rates of metabolic disease in every age group and country? Behind these numbers, so much more is going on in the human body, which is about how the body stores energy, metabolises food, heals and responds to stress. I will go through this in detail in the book.

The Blood Sugar Repair Plan is not another diet book; it is a plan to treat disease, educate, correct metabolic health, lose weight and give you your life back. Metabolic health is the way your body handles energy, processes what you eat, stores energy, and responds to hormones such as insulin and cortisol. It is so comprehensive for your overall health.

When your body is struggling, the signs are obvious: cravings, afternoon slumps/crashes, brain fog, high triglycerides, high blood pressure, poor sleep, belly fat and a constant draining feeling that your body isn't working how it should. Many people dismiss much of this as aging, genetics, menopause or just a busy life in general. I want people to pick up on these symptoms and not just accept them, but make the first step to get help and change the trajectory of their life.

The Blood Sugar Repair Plan is going to help you understand everything happening inside your body. It contains all you need to know about glucose, insulin, and signs and symptoms. I share all my tips that I give my clinic patients. This book will take you through what our pancreas is, how it functions, and how to keep or return it to optimal functioning. The book will teach you about whole-body communication, how insulin resistance is not just a problem of the pancreas and that type 2 diabetes has developed over time – it's not something you get overnight.

See this book as a wonderful opportunity to get on top of your health. It is practical, packed with lifestyle tips and changes, and full of brand-new, nutrient-dense recipes that are easy to make.

I am so proud of this book and can't wait to see all the success stories. It's never too late for anyone to give this program a go. Embracing *The Blood Sugar Repair Plan* will give you a complete understanding of your body, and a tool to confidently reclaim your health.

Good things come from putting in the effort. It's so worth it.

You could say writing these books is a 'calling', but the truth is, I just love seeing people healthy, happy and living their best lives – this is what drives me, and my purpose.

Sarah x

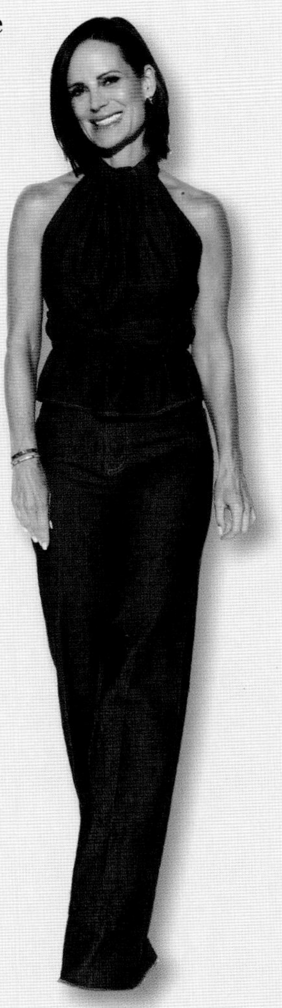

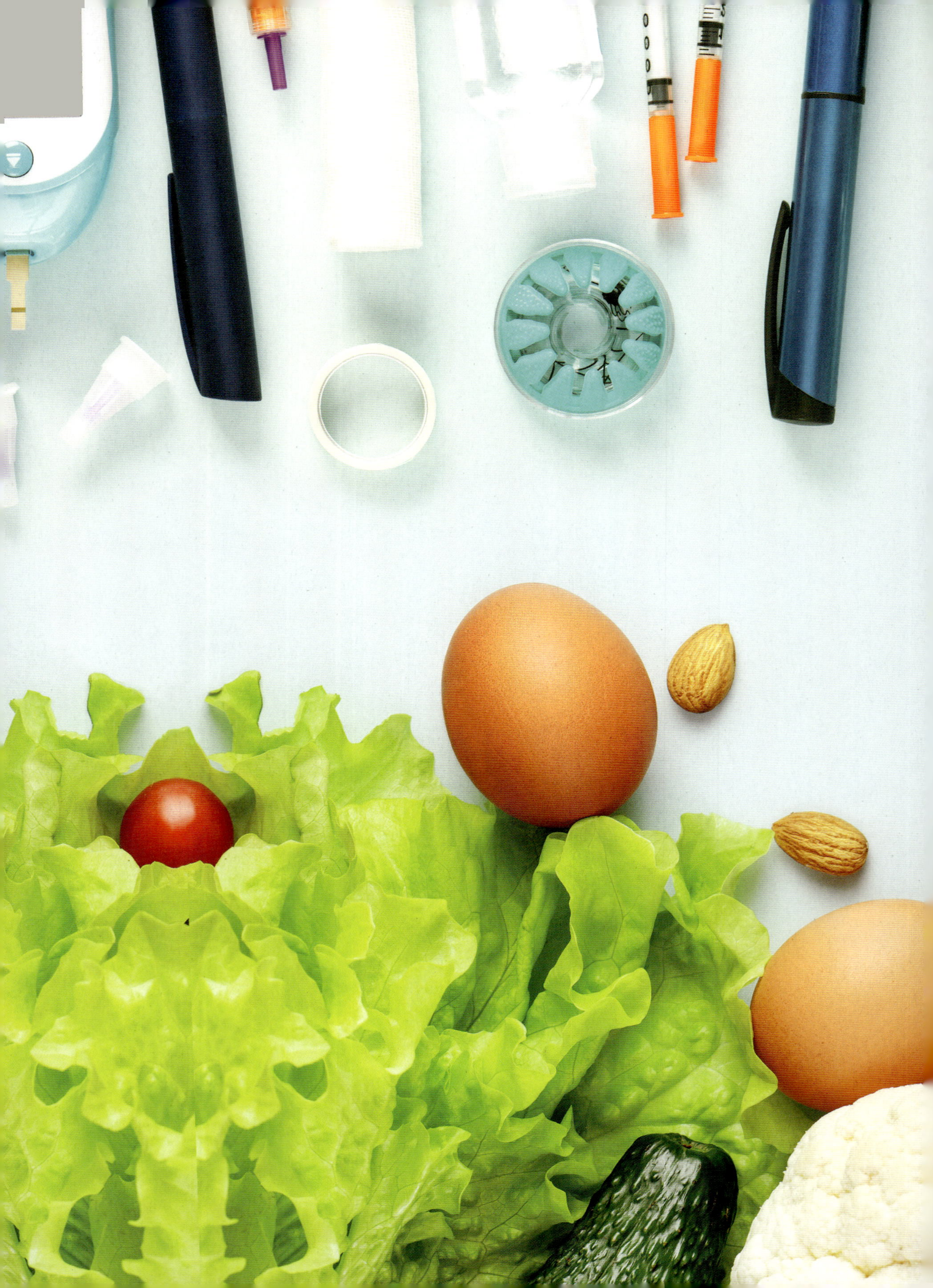

PART ONE

Everything you need to know about diabetes

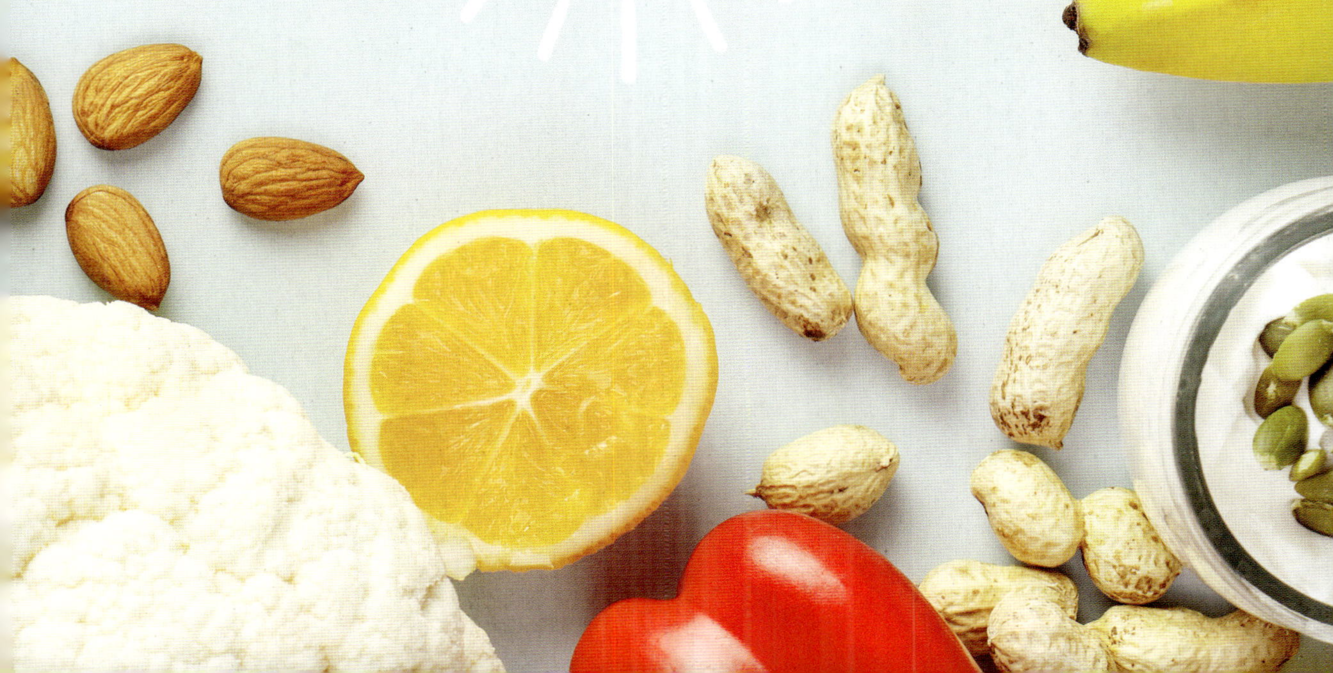

CHAPTER 1

Understanding type 2 diabetes

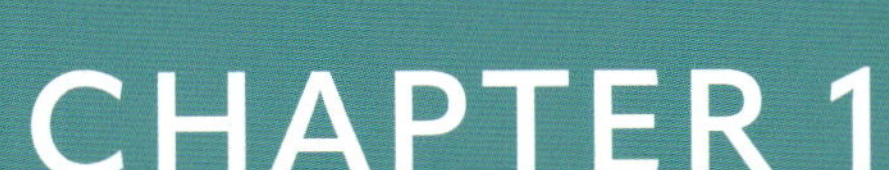
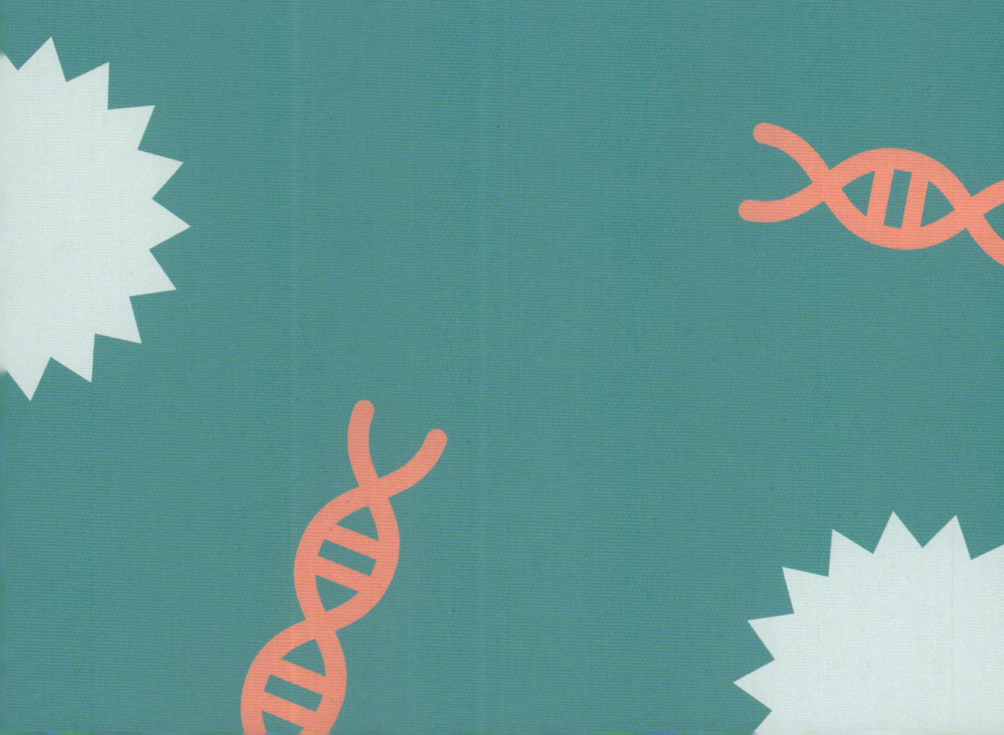
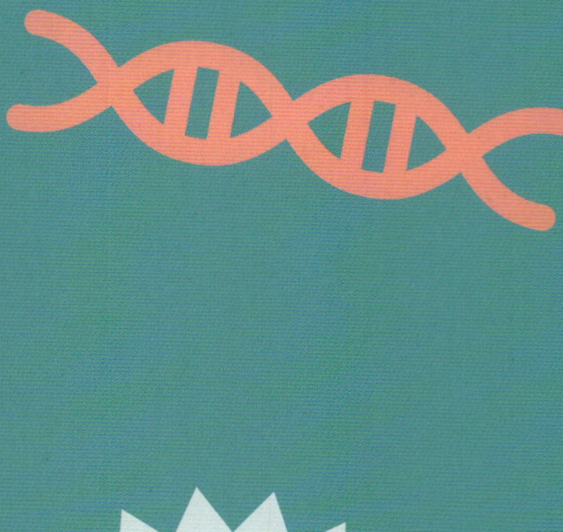
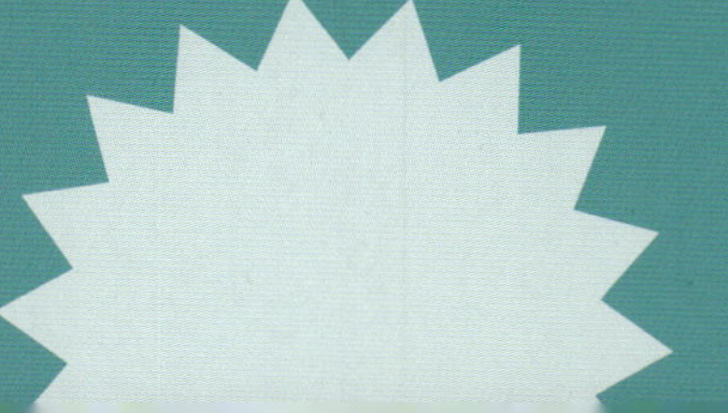

Diabetes creeps up on you with no real symptoms at all. You may notice that you are a little more fatigued than usual, you don't feel as great as you used to, you could be feeling more thirsty, maybe your vision isn't that great (but you put that down to aging), you're losing weight, possibly you're feeling nauseated, you've got itchy skin that you think may be a rash or skin infections (such as eczema or dermatitis). You may blame these symptoms on a busy life, overwork and feeling burnt out. This can go on for years.

You're finding that you're using the bathroom more. Trips or outings spark thoughts of where the public toilets are. You're noticing you could be weeing more at night and put this all down to an aging bladder. But you're also thirsty for water a lot more than usual without really feeling your thirst quenched.

Does this sound like you? Well, the chances are you have type 2 diabetes (T2D) or are prediabetic.

It would be fair to say that diabetes is a global problem, with the number of people with T2D increasing rapidly. The latest reports indicate that about 537 million people are currently living with diabetes; that is, 1 in 10 adults. If you look at the graphs, diabetes has quadrupled since 1985, and what horrifies me as a clinician is just how normalised type 2 diabetes, prediabetes and insulin resistance have become. Some of my patients talk to me about their diabetes like they've just brushed their teeth or visited the grocery store.

This inspired me to write this book. I want to change how people see diabetes and understand just how serious the disease really is, because what we are doing now is not slowing it down at all, it's doing the exact opposite. As part of my initial treatment, I tell my patients about the consequences of potential blindness, amputations, heart attacks, strokes, liver disease, diabetic myopathy, obesity, reduced life expectancy and quality of life to make them understand just how dangerous it is.

WHAT IS DIABETES?

To put it simply, diabetes is a chronic disease in which the body can't regulate the amount of sugar in the blood – the blood sugar (glucose) is too high. This high blood sugar is where diabetes starts. Not only will it accelerate your aging but it will increase your risk of heart disease. When blood sugar (glucose) builds up over time, the body will become prediabetic. Many people can live with prediabetes for up to 5 years without any symptoms.

Glucose is the primary source of energy in the body. While we get glucose from the foods we eat, our body can actually make glucose in a process called gluconeogenesis. Here, the liver turns glycogen into glucose in a process called glycogenolysis. Our liver can also manufacture glucose from amino acids, waste and fat, in a process called gluconeogenesis.

Insulin is a hormone made by the pancreas which escorts glucose into our cells to be used for energy. When you have diabetes, your body does not use insulin as it should. It does not make enough, or any, insulin. Glucose then stays in your blood and doesn't reach your cells. When your blood sugar is high, insulin can't do its job of moving glucose into the cells. Now, this isn't the fault of the insulin – it's because of the excess glucose in the blood and cells of your body. Type 2 diabetes results from that excess glucose in the cells.

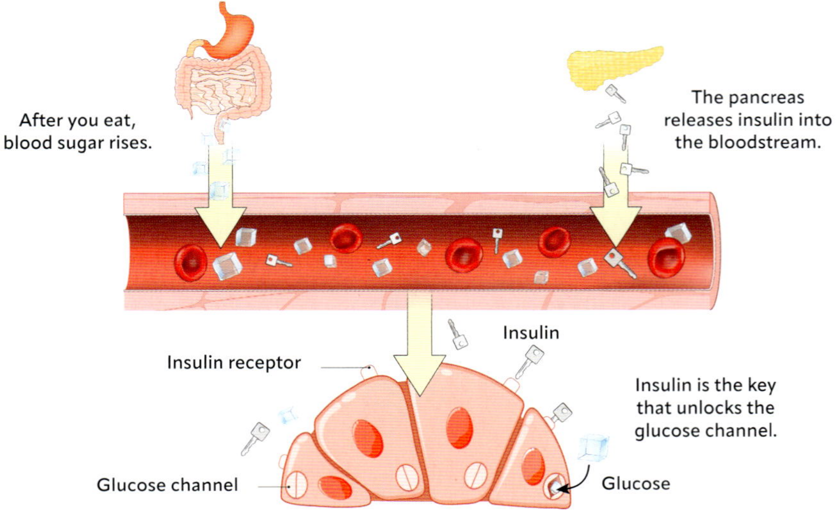

I often explain the idea to my patients like this: imagine glucose is in the blood and bonds to insulin. Insulin escorts glucose to the entrance of a cell (a receptor site). A traffic light is at the entrance. In a healthy body, the glucose gets a green light and enters the cell to be used for energy. When the cell is already full of glucose, the amber light will flash. The red light appears when there is no more room for glucose to enter, hence insulin resistance.

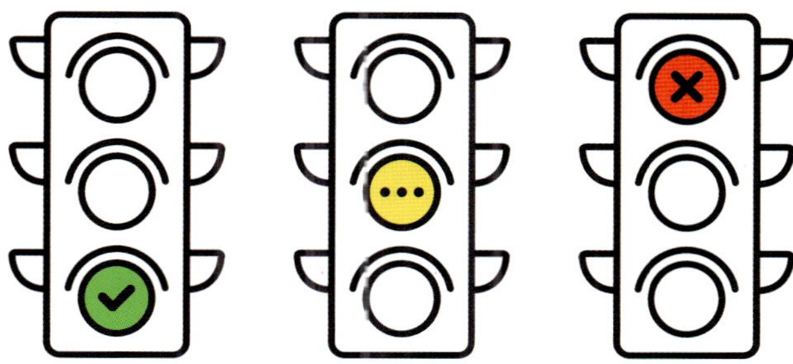

When this is all happening, the body responds to the crisis by making more insulin. This is like a band-aid solution; the problem of the excess sugar is still there. No matter how much insulin the pancreas makes, the body can't force more glucose into cells. It becomes a cycle, but eventually the blood sugar will spike because there will be a point at which insulin will be outdone by the blood sugar. This is type 2 diabetes.

90% of people with diabetes globally have type 2 diabetes.

Type 2 diabetes (or T2D for short) has an enormous societal and economic consequence. Between 1980 and 2020, the number of people with type 2 diabetes has risen from 108 million to 537 million. Then factor in obesity: in 1980, 100 million were obese globally; today, 764 million people are obese. Diet plays a huge role in your risk of T2D. The thing about type 2 diabetes is that it increases your risk for blindness, kidney disease, fatty liver disease, cancer, infections and cardiovascular diseases, and it has a massive impact on our healthcare systems.

38% of US teenagers are prediabetic – a sobering statistic.

Today, the term 'diabetes' most commonly refers to diabetes mellitus. Diabetes mellitus is itself an overarching term for several different diseases involving problems with processing sugars that have been consumed, or glucose metabolism.

HISTORY OF DIABETES

We have been aware of diabetes for thousands of years. We can trace its history way back to the ancient Egyptians where it was described in the Ebers papyrus in 1550 BCE.

Ayurvedic physicians in the fifth and sixth centuries BCE noted the taste of diabetic urine being sweet and named the condition *madhumeha*, which means 'honey urine'.

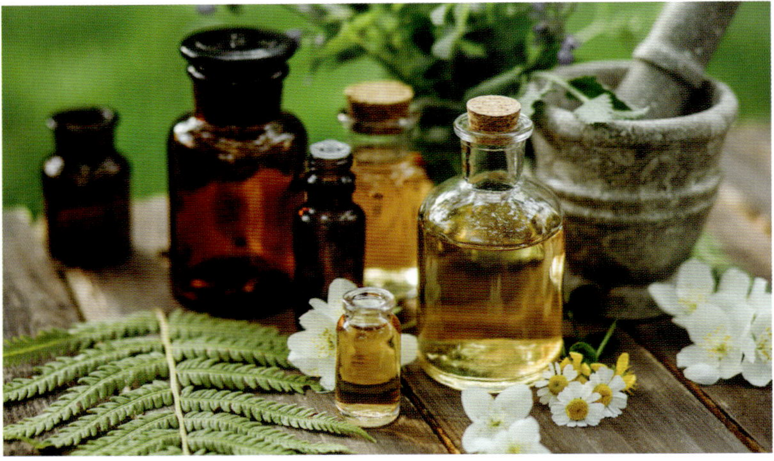

The term diabetes is the shortened version of its full name, *diabetes mellitus*, derived from the Greek word *diabetes*, meaning 'siphon' and the Latin word *mellitus*, meaning 'sweet'. This is because excess sugar passes out of the body through the urine, making it sweet. This sweetness had been written about by the ancient Greeks, Chinese, Egyptians, Indians and Persians. Diabetes was known in the 17th century as the 'pissing evil'. Byzantine writers from around that time had also documented descriptions of the disease.

Ancient Greek writers in the Hippocratic Corpus made statements referring to excessive and watery urine. Hippocrates believed that the slumbering (fatigue) and thirst that results from high blood sugar was linked to problems with digestion, and the weakness resulted from low blood sugar because the body was missing a meal.

The treatment plan of the Greek physicians was to exercise, preferably on horseback, to alleviate excess urinating. Other forms of therapy were to drink wine and overfeed to compensate for loss of fluid weight, or a starvation diet. One thing we do know from the history of treatment in both ancient times and the Middle Ages was that if you had diabetes, it was fatal.

It was thought that diabetes was a disease of the kidneys until 1674, when Thomas Willis suggested it may be a disease of the blood. The involvement of the pancreas was discovered in 1889. It was not until the 20th century that insulin was discovered, named after the islet cells of the pancreas, named islets of Langerhans (the Latin for island is *insula*). Think about the thousands of years of people suffering from diabetes and not knowing the pathophysiology – that it is the result of a lack of insulin.

In 1919, the treatment for diabetes was strict dieting or complete starvation. The discovery of insulin in 1921 by Frederick Grant Banting and Charles Herbert Best was a game changer. The Canadian researchers worked out how to isolate insulin from the pancreas and refine it. The first injection of insulin was to a 14-year-old boy in Canada dying from type 1 diabetes, who was in a state of diabetic ketoacidosis. It saved his life.

An effective treatment for diabetes became available in 1922, with Best and Banting winning the Nobel Prize in Physiology that year. This incredible breakthrough gave millions of people diagnosed with diabetes the incredible gift of life.

In 1936, Sir Harold Percival Himsworth discovered the difference between type 1 and type 2 diabetes. Biosynthetic human insulin, which is identical in its structure to human insulin, was created and mass produced in 1982.

Today, insulin comes in many varieties, from regular human insulin identical to the insulin produced by our pancreas to long-acting and ultra-rapid insulin. People with diabetes now have the freedom to choose what is best for them and their lifestyle.

HOW DID THIS ANCIENT DISEASE BECOME TODAY'S EPIDEMIC?

If you look back over the last 75 years, you can see the rise of heart disease around 1950, particularly myocardial infarction (heart attack). The health advice of the time was to avoid dietary fats. Fat was the bad guy; it was completely demonised.

Back then, fats were believed to increase cholesterol. Incredibly heart-healthy foods such as avocado, olive oil and nuts were avoided. This paved the way for the low-fat food industry, which meant people then ate more carbs. You'd see 'fat free' and 'low fat' everywhere, and people really did believe these products would make them thin. Well, this could not be further from the truth.

The low-fat movement brought with it artificial sweeteners to make the food taste good (when the fat gets removed so does the flavour). Today, research shows that artificial sweeteners are linked to weight gain because they do not hit the reward centre in the brain that signals satiety.

If you are around my age (I am 52 as I write this), you may recall the old food pyramid. This had a huge emphasis on refined and complex carbohydrates, which made up about 60% of the daily recommended food intake. The food pyramid is very different today, that's for sure!

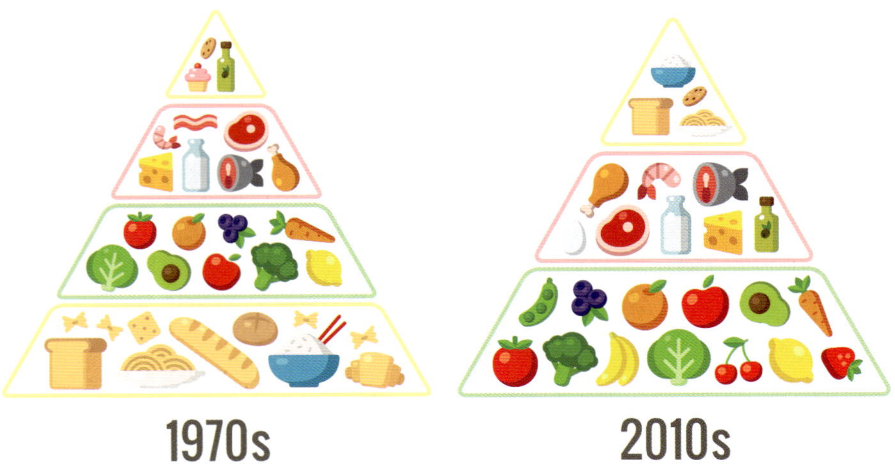

Did you know that marketing people created the food pyramid?

The predominance of the low-fat, high-carb diet, along with an increased consumption of processed and discretionary foods, set the perfect stage for the quadrupling of type 2 diabetes in the past 40 years. It aligns with the obesity epidemic, which has been fuelling the type 2 diabetes epidemic. Our aging population and sedentary lifestyles have also had an impact. In 2026, we now see a new food pyramid in the USA with an emphasis on protein, healthy fats, fruit and vegetables – something I have been recommending for years.

DIET AND DIABETES

We don't just eat too much refined rice and wheat and excess processed meats, we eat more – you just need to look at portions and plate sizes. In the 1950s, a typical dinner plate was much smaller than today, on average about 23 cm in diameter. Today, modern standard dinner plates are more commonly 27–30 cm, meaning plate size has increased about 15% to 30% since the mid-20th century. Bigger plates mean we can load much more food onto them, which tempts us to overeat.

We're also not getting enough dietary fibre in our diets, due to all the processed foods and lack of fruit and vegetables. The modern diet also lacks good fats and contains too much sugar and junk foods, including sugary beverages.

23 cm

**Dinner plate size
in the 1950s**

32 cm

**Dinner plate
size today**

Here is some food for thought. In 2025, the anti-diabetic drugs market in Australia had a revenue of A$975 million. It is projected to grow at about a rate of 7.13% annually to reach A$1.33 billion by 2029. The USA has an even bigger market, with US$40.82 billion (A$61.55 billion) expected revenue in 2025. And the growth and demand just continue to increase. Makes you wonder how different those numbers might look if more people were supported to manage type 2 diabetes at its root cause, with evidence-based nutrition and lifestyle changes, not just prescriptions.

MEDICATIONS – BAND-AID FIXES

Regardless of all the prescriptions you can get, such as metformin or injections, if you don't change the way you eat, the core problem of energy and glucose overflow and excessive glucose is still in the body. Medications can be life-saving and important but on their own they are just mopping up the excess rather than turning off the tap. This is not the solution. As insulin resistance worsens, your body needs more insulin for the same effect. This usually means escalating doses and more medications. Excess glucose and energy are continually stored away, especially as fat in the liver, around the organs and in existing fat cells, so while your glucose reading are looking better, the underlying metabolic stress is still there. Without targeting diet, movement, sleep and weight, this pattern is unsustainable and the chronic disease simply progresses.

What do you think happens to the body?

You start to gain weight. Because the cells are resistant to glucose, insulin stores all the excess glucose as fat. Insulin is the fat locker! The thing is, while you are gaining weight, your appetite is also increasing because cells such as those in your muscles need energy, so they are messaging the brain to eat.

Think of the impact of this on the human body over years and years.

It impacts the entire body system. Why do you think people with diabetes go blind? The glucose has reached there. What about the liver? It becomes fatty and too damaged to heal itself. All that glucose begins ulcerating legs, and diabetic neuropathy (or damaged nerves) is because of excess glucose. Doctors refer to these as complications of diabetes, almost insinuating that it's not as bad as it may seem. The good news is that when diabetes is reversed, these 'complications' go away and the body will return to normal.

Type 2 diabetes is a disease caused by diet. To treat it, your diet needs to change. Medication cannot help with diet. Disease needs to be treated from the core of the issue, not with band-aids.

METFORMIN

One of the body's biggest regulators of blood glucose is skeletal muscle. Metformin is the most common diabetic medication sold globally and can be very helpful for lowering glucose but is not a perfect treatment. Research suggests metformin may upregulate myostatin, a hormone that puts the brakes on muscle growth. This could contribute to muscle loss under some conditions. So it's not a perfect treatment – there are trade-offs, especially if we don't protect muscle with adequate protein and resistance training. Just something to think about. I will go into this more later in the book.

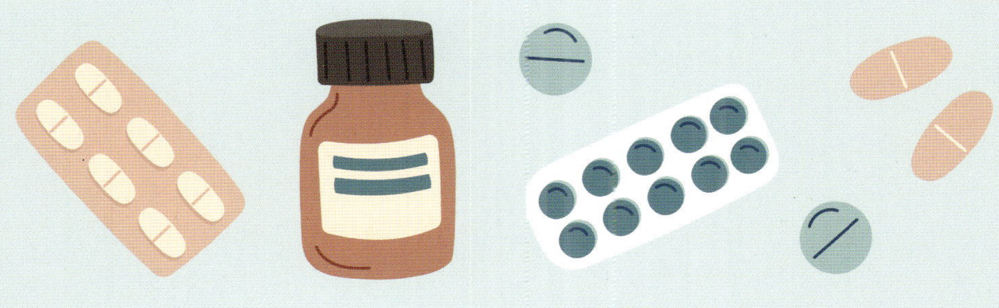

CAUSES OF DIABETES

Regardless of the type of diabetes, the cause is having too much sugar or glucose in the bloodstream. The reason why the blood glucose levels are high depends on what type of diabetes you have.

- **The pancreas cannot work properly.** The pancreas gradually struggles to keep up with the high demand for insulin. Excess fat stored in the liver and pancreas is strongly linked to the loss of beta cell function. Reducing this ectopic fat is key to helping restore insulin production and avoiding the progression to type 2 diabetes.

- **Insulin resistance is where cells in our liver, muscles and fat stop responding to insulin.** Remember the red traffic light? This is type 2 diabetes, which results from having a poor diet, unhealthy lifestyle and obesity, as well as genetics, hormones and in some cases medications. For more on this, see Chapter 6: **Insulin and insulin resistance**.

- **Autoimmune issues can cause type 1 diabetes.** Type 1 diabetes is an autoimmune condition where the immune system attacks the insulin-producing cells in the pancreas. It is driven by a mix of genetic susceptibility and environmental triggers, such as certain viral infections. Other forms of diabetes can be caused or unmasked by pregnancy, pancreatic damage, in rare cases genetic mutations, or medications such as corticosteroids and HIV/AIDS medications – but these are not classic type 1.

- **Diabetes can run in families.** Many children can be born with the genes that increase their risk of type 1 diabetes, but most will never develop the disease. In genetically susceptible people, viral infections and other environmental factors can trigger the autoimmune process that leads to type 1 diabetes. Type 2 diabetes also has a strong genetic link; children of type 2 diabetic parents are more inclined to get type 2 diabetes, but they can reduce or delay this risk with diet and lifestyle changes.

For more, see Chapter 3: **Causes of type 2 diabetes**.

THE DIFFERENT TYPES OF FAT

Fat comes in different forms in the body, each with accompanying risks for those who are insulin resistant or have diabetes. Here is where in the body we store fat:

- **Subcutaneous fat.** This is fat under the skin, often in the thighs, bum and the back of the arms.

- **Visceral fat.** Deep inside the abdomen, visceral fat is found around organs such as the liver, heart and intestines. This is dangerous fat.

- **Ectopic fat.** This is fat stored in tissues not usually designed for fat storage, including the liver, pancreas and even heart.

The location matters – visceral and ectopic fat are closely linked to an increased risk for conditions such as type 2 diabetes, heart disease and inflammation, whereas subcutaneous fat stored in the hips and thighs is generally less harmful.

Genetics, hormones, age and lifestyle determine each person's pattern of fat storage. Something exciting to know when we start a weight-loss journey is that visceral fat tends to decrease at a higher rate. This is inspiring!

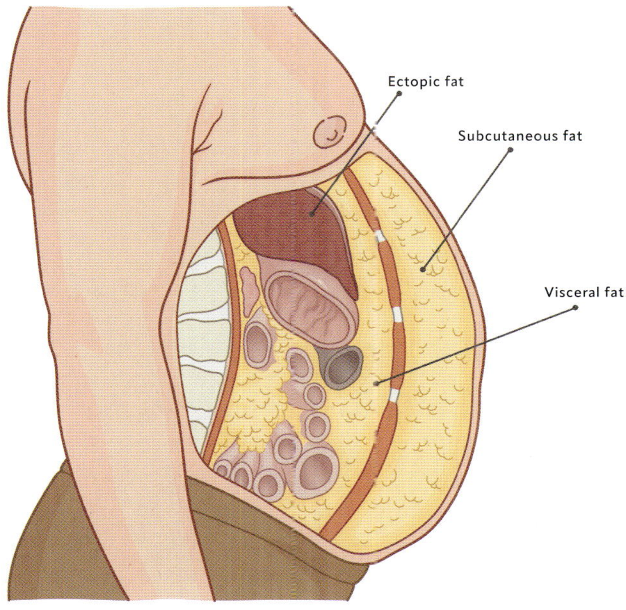

SUBCUTANEOUS FAT

Subcutaneous fat occurs under the skin – it's what you see on the thighs, bum, hips and arms. When your glucose intake exceeds your energy needs, insulin will convert excess glucose into fatty acids that are then stored as fat (or triglycerides). Your subcutaneous fat buffers the excess energy but once its storage capacity is exceeded the overflow goes around the organs as visceral fat. This process is driving today's epidemics of obesity, T2D and metabolic disease.

VISCERAL FAT

This type of fat is more metabolically active and keeps driving insulin resistance. It drains via the portal vein to the liver and causes fat build-up in the liver. Visceral fat directly impairs the body's ability to regulate blood sugar, making it the hidden culprit behind the rise in metabolic disease.

Why is visceral fat so dangerous?

It's much more metabolically active and harmful than subcutaneous fat, making it a major target for lifestyle change and disease prevention. Also known as adipose tissue, it is inflammatory and a state of disease. Visceral fat:

- wraps around vital organs (heart, liver, intestines, kidneys), increasing risk for organ dysfunction

- releases toxic chemicals and hormones (cytokines, inflammatory proteins) that trigger widespread inflammation

- raises blood pressure by producing hormones (e.g. angiotensin precursor) that constrict blood vessels

- promotes insulin resistance, making blood sugar harder to control and raising the risk for type 2 diabetes

- elevates cholesterol and triglycerides while lowering 'good' high-density lipoprotein (HDL) cholesterol, contributing to heart disease

- increases your risk for stroke, heart attack and atherosclerosis

- is associated with metabolic syndrome, which combines high blood pressure, high blood glucose, excess body fat and abnormal cholesterol levels

- is linked to certain cancers (breast, colorectal, liver) since it can stimulate uncontrolled cell growth

- increases your risk for dementia and Alzheimer's disease due to inflammatory pathways and the impact on blood vessels in the brain

- contributes to asthma, sleep apnoea, fatty liver and other organ diseases

- can be present even in people with a 'normal' body mass index (BMI), making waist size a critical risk measure.

The good news is that when you lose weight, visceral fat is the first to go!

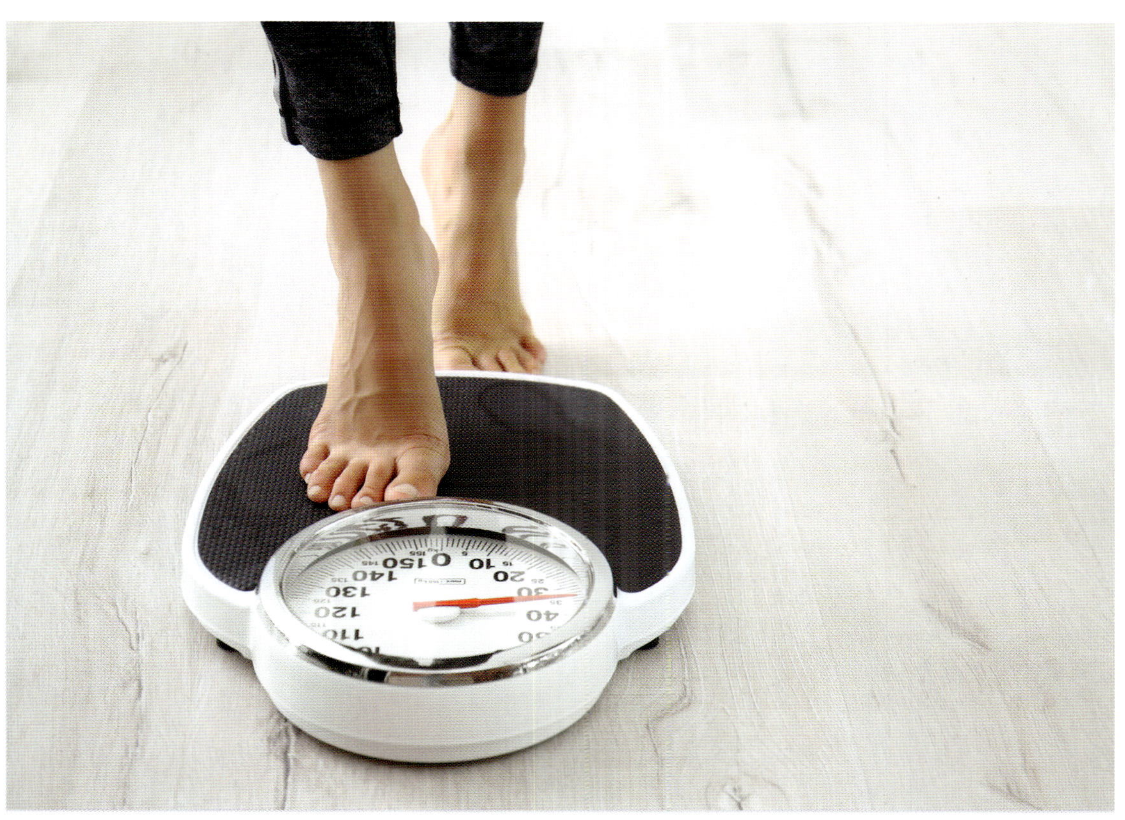

ECTOPIC FAT

Fat (lipid) droplets stored within cells (e.g. in the liver, muscles and pancreas) is called intracellular fat. In a healthy person, fat within cells is used for energy production and as building blocks for cell structure. Intracellular fat is stored as triglycerides, which can be broken down when the body needs fuel.

But when the body's capacity to store fat has been exceeded, fat begins to build up in the liver, heart, pancreas, skeletal muscle and even the blood vessels, which do not normally store much fat. This called ectopic fat, meaning 'fat in the wrong place'.

Ectopic fat build-up is clearly linked to insulin resistance, type 2 diabetes and metabolic diseases. It impairs normal cell function and can trigger inflammation or organ dysfunction. It can even enter the brain, affecting cognitive function.

But again, ectopic fat can be reversed with diet, weight loss, lifestyle changes and exercise.

SKINNY FAT

You don't have to be overweight to get diabetes. Diabetes can also happen to individuals who are not overweight but may have a high amount of fat, something I call 'skinny fat'. Skinny fat is formally known as MONW – metabolically obese, normal weight.

About 80% of people with type 2 diabetes are overweight or obese, but another 10% are skinny fat. People who are skinny fat are at high risk of metabolic syndrome as well as type 2 diabetes. Genes, age, build, muscle definition and your hormones can impact your body fat percentage.

1 in 10 people with type 2 diabetes aren't overweight but have too much visceral fat.

Other risks for being skinny fat are high blood pressure, poor diet and lifestyle, stress, family history, high cholesterol and triglycerides as well polycystic ovary syndrome (PCOS). The thing is that people with visceral fat don't realise how bad it is for their health. A good approach is to look at body composition rather than the scale, using a body composition test or DEXA scan.

PERSONAL FAT THRESHOLD

This is the idea that each individual has a genetically determined capacity to store fat safely in the subcutaneous fat. When you exceed your own threshold, any extra fat spills over into organs not designed for fat storage, such as the liver, pancreas or muscle. Imagine wagyu beef!

This ectopic fat disrupts how your organs function, damages insulin signalling and causes inflammation, leading to increased blood glucose, insulin resistance and type 2 diabetes. This can happen even if your BMI is in the 'normal' range. If you have a low personal fat threshold, you can develop diabetes even if you're not overweight, while others with a lot more subcutaneous fat may remain metabolically healthier for much longer.

The good news? When your weight drops below your threshold, you can start to reverse type 2 diabetes. Losing weight will reduce the ectopic fat in the pancreas and liver, and restore insulin production and sensitivity.

Genetics, ethnicity, sex, hormones, and lifestyle influence your personal fat threshold.

Everyone's risk for diabetes and metabolic disease doesn't depend just on body weight or BMI, but on your individual capacity to store fat safely and avoid overflow into critical organs. Now you can understand why thin people can develop metabolic disease and why weight loss can benefit health even in people who aren't overweight or obese.

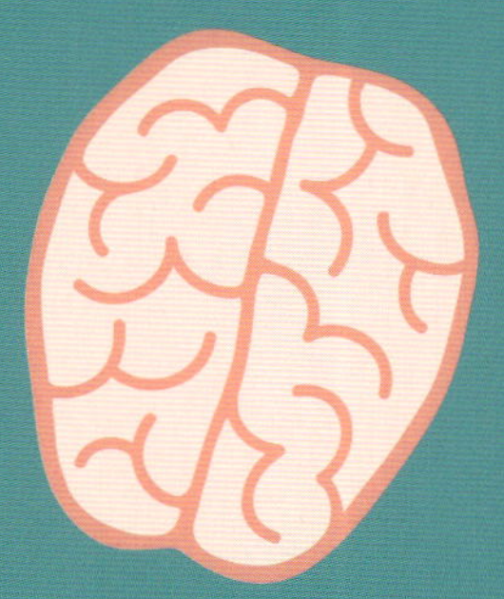

CHAPTER 2

Different types of diabetes

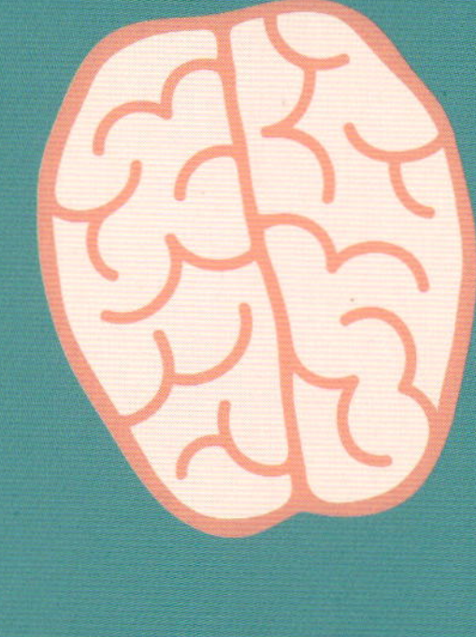

TYPE 1 DIABETES

This type of diabetes can occur at any age, but is most commonly diagnosed in children, teens and young adults, with the majority diagnosed between 10 and 14 years old. The incidence of type 1 diabetes has been increasing. Unlike type 2, type 1 is an autoimmune disease. The body's own immune system damages the cells that secrete insulin, which results in an insulin dependency.

1 in 10 people with diabetes have type 1.

With type 1 diabetes, the body makes little or no insulin because an autoimmune reaction has damaged the insulin-producing cells in the pancreas. Recall that insulin is a hormone that moves glucose from the blood into the cells to be used for energy; if there is no insulin, the glucose sits in the blood causing hyperglycaemia (high blood sugar).

There is no cure. You treat T1D with an insulin pump or injections. Unlike T2D, where the onset is gradual without obvious symptoms, with T1D the symptoms include increased thirst, frequent urination, rapid weight loss, hunger and fatigue. At the outset, many people will present with diabetic ketoacidosis (DKA).

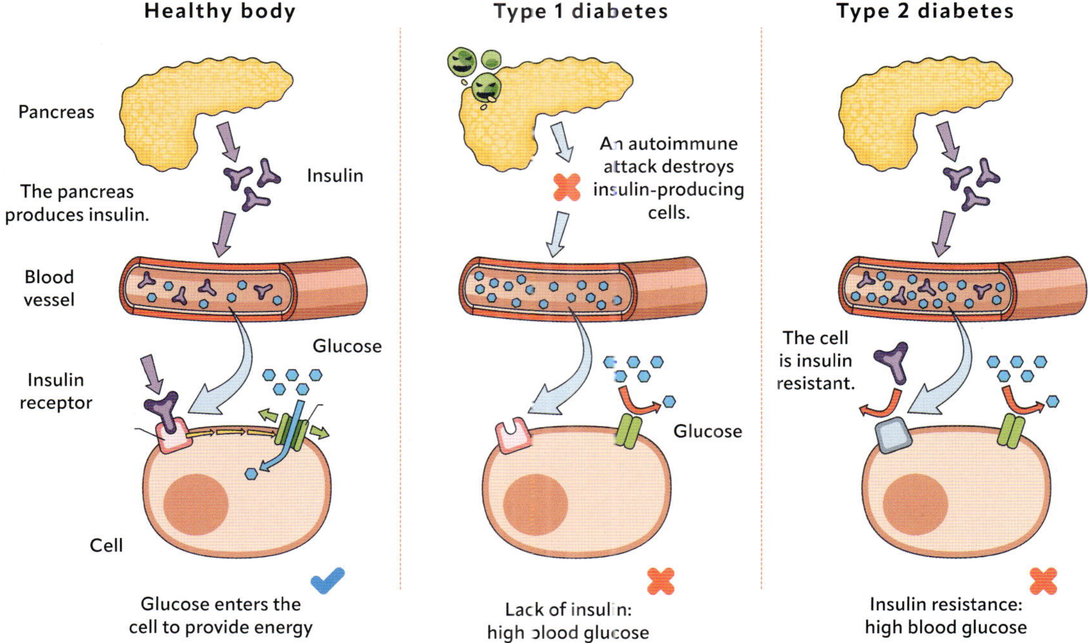

DKA is a medical emergency. You can determine DKA by someone being unconscious or, if still conscious, they seem really confused. Other symptoms include a funny-smelling breath like nail polish remover, stomach pain, fast heart rate, and vomiting or nausea. They could also be dehydrated or have really red cheeks.

WHAT ARE THE SYMPTOMS FOR TYPE 1?

A simple strategy to remember the symptoms of type 1 diabetes is that they all start with 'T':

- **Thirst** – feeling thirsty and hungry all the time
- **Tired** – feeling weak and tired all the time
- **Toilet** – noticing significantly more trips to the toilet
- **Thinner** – weight loss without trying to lose weight.

In some cases, people may have blurred vision. Most people will feel like this for a few weeks before they seek medical help.

ENDING THE STIGMA AROUND DIABETES

I remember when my younger sister Catherine worked in a company that manufactured insulin pumps for type 1 diabetics. We'd chat about how different type 1 and type 2 diabetes are. She told me how all the type 1 diabetics she met in her work could never understand why people would allow themselves to get type 2 diabetes and then live with it, not trying to reverse the disease with dietary changes instead of living on medication.

The type 1s felt their diabetes was something they could never get away from. The type 1s also suggested over the years that type 1 should be renamed to get away from the stigma of type 2 diabetes. Catherine and I would have many conversations about this. I feel it's time for a name change for type 1 and type 2 diabetes to clearly differentiate the diseases.

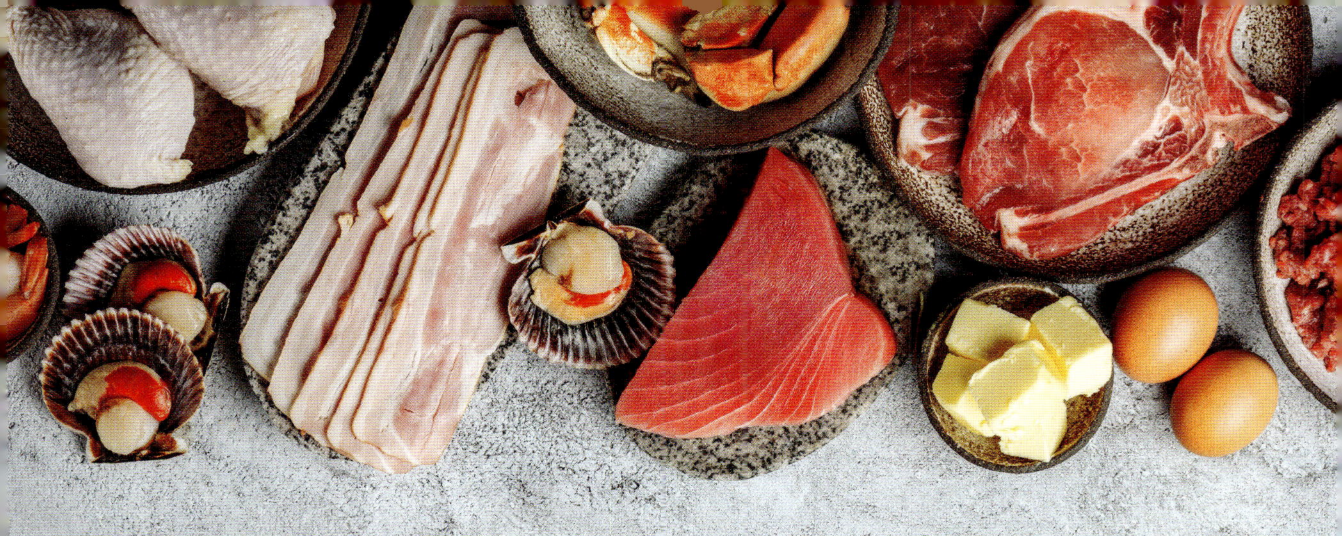

WHAT CAUSES TYPE 1 DIABETES?

The truth is, no one really knows the precise cause of type 1 diabetes. It is not fully understood. In most cases, it is an autoimmune condition where the body's immune system mistakenly attacks the insulin-producing cells in the pancreas. Genetics provide a strong predisposition; type 1 diabetes can run in families but environmental triggers, such as certain infections, are also thought to be involved. Many people with a genetic risk never fully develop the disease.

If you feel this could be you, ask your doctor for the following tests: finger-prick blood glucose test and urine sample to test for ketones and glucose. Once diagnosed, you need to really understand this diagnosis. You should be with a team to help support you in the adjustment process to your new way of life, forever. Knowing which resources are available and working with a healthcare professional or team are essential to get your healthcare plan in place. I tell my patients: think of it like a job or project where you're learning something completely new and need to behave like a student.

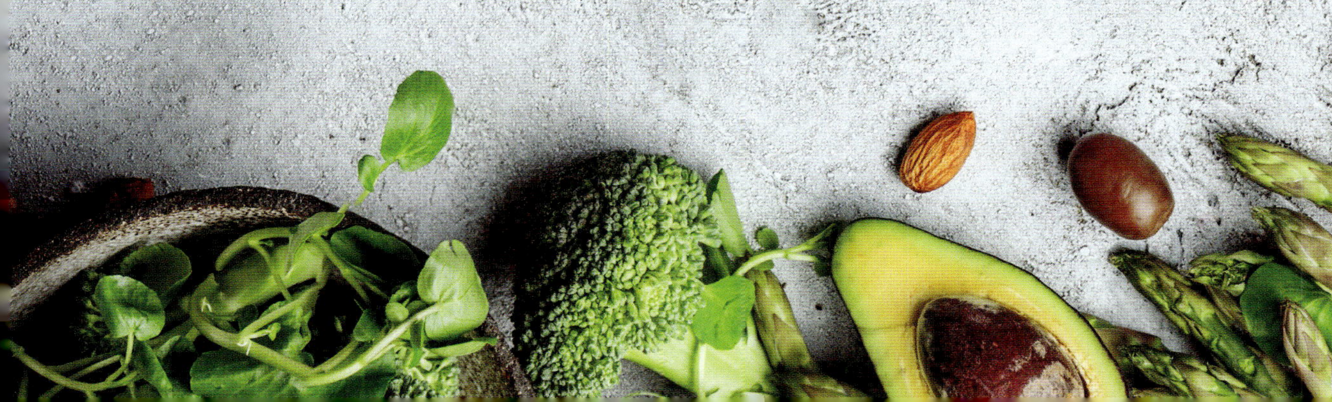

TREATING TYPE 1 DIABETES

Before the discovery of insulin, the diet for a type 1 diabetic was practically the carnivore diet: fatty meat. Fat does not need insulin to tell it what to do. The body creates ketones that can happily feed the brain. The discovery and commercial production of insulin meant that someone with type 1 could eat whatever they wanted because they were covered by taking insulin. Many type 1s have constant blood sugar fluctuations; when they learn to eat a low-carb diet, not only does their insulin dose plummet but they don't have the constant fluctuations. Another example of why diet is everything!

Today, type 1 diabetes is treated with insulin, which helps control blood sugar. This is often done with a pen but now many prefer a pump. I tell my type 1 patients that even though they are getting treatment, a healthy diet and exercise are amazing at controlling blood sugar levels. When your blood sugar is managed well, you can significantly lower any risk of complications. Staying on top of your health is really important.

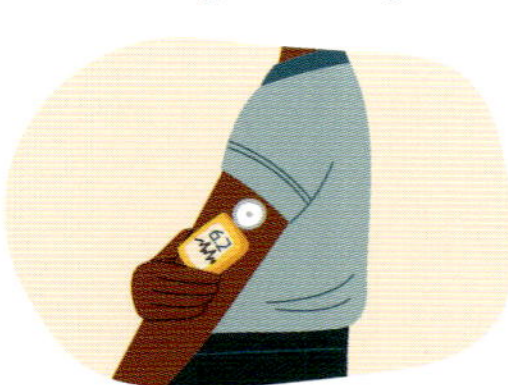

Monitoring of blood glucose

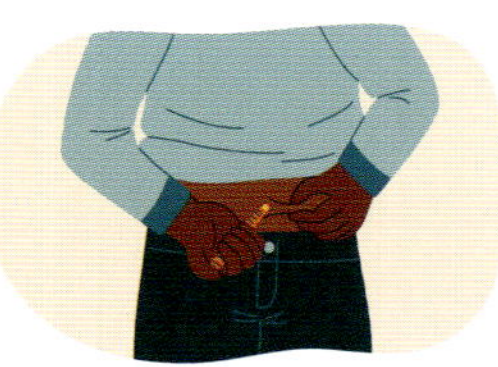

Insulin injection

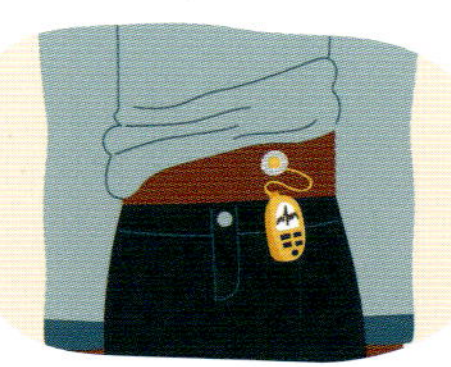

Insulin pump

The first port of call for type 1 diabetes is to align with healthcare professionals such as a specialist diabetes educator to help guide you, especially in the early stages. Next, educate yourself on blood glucose and the condition. A healthy diet is so important, as is daily exercise, even just a walk. Regular check-ups include blood tests, kidney health, blood pressure, and having your feet and eyes checked.

Type 1 diabetes does have complications. The most common are heart disease and stroke, along with peripheral vascular disease (the narrowing of arteries in legs and feet), nerve problems, food problems, eye health issues and kidney disease. Plus, people with type 1 have a higher incidence of depression.

Staying on top of your treatment plan is so important. With type 1, you can develop diabetic ketoacidosis (DKA) if you get an infection or miss your insulin injections. DKA is really serious. When someone is in this state, they can seem really confused or, in the worst case, be unconscious. If you are ever in this situation, the first thing you need to do is call emergency services. DKA happens when the body burns fat instead of glucose-producing ketones.

There is a difference between a regular ketogenic diet for someone doing weight loss and a diabetic going into ketoacidosis. In a regular person, the body makes ketones but not enough to make your blood too acidic, so ketosis is not dangerous – the body still has enough insulin and is functioning normally. But in diabetic ketoacidosis, the ketones build up way too fast and the blood becomes acidic. When this happens, it can be fatal.

Unfortunately, type 1 diabetes can't be prevented, no matter how healthy your diet and lifestyle are. But some interesting evidence has shown that breastfeeding can reduce a child's risk by 15%. This is because breastmilk plays a role in developing a baby's gut microbiome and immune system. Early-childhood nutrition can also help lower the risk: a healthy diet full of whole real foods, and have the infants enjoy vegetables first before introducing fruit. When I did this with my babies, I found they loved pumpkin, broccoli and carrots the most. I also made sure they were eating from all food groups, including nuts such as nut butter, by age one. For mothers who cannot breastfeed, I always recommend they give their babies probiotics for the first three years of life.

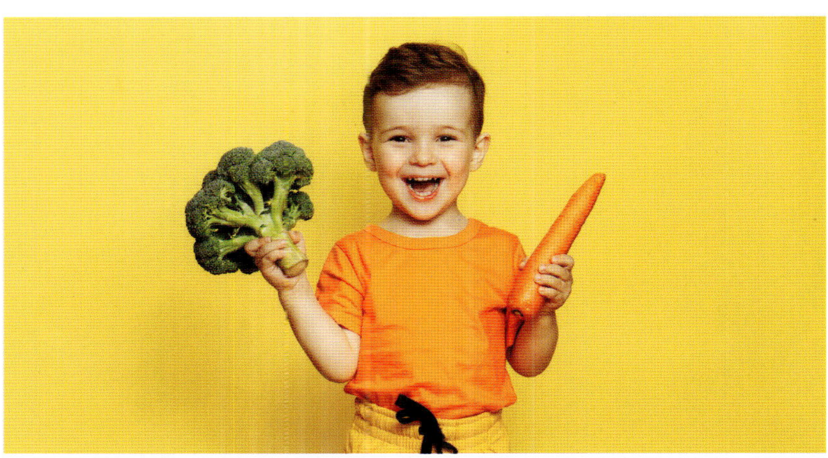

PREDIABETES

This is the stage before type 2 diabetes. Basically, your blood sugar levels are higher than normal but not high enough for you to be diagnosed with type 2 diabetes. But it's not to be dismissed, which many people do. It's your warning sign to get on top of your health and make changes to your diet, lifestyle and exercise. People can be prediabetic for many years and not know – about 80% don't know they're prediabetic. The evidence clearly shows that making lifestyle changes can decrease your risk of prediabetes progressing to diabetes for up to 10 years.

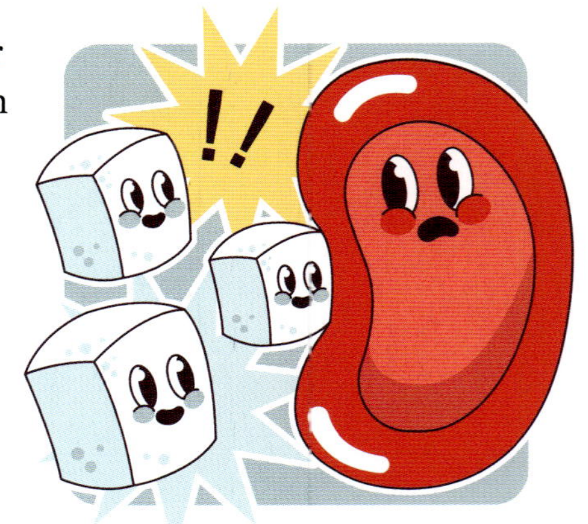

Prediabetes can lead to other health conditions such as stroke and heart disease. Prediabetes can also be referred to as impaired glucose tolerance (IGT), meaning you have higher than normal blood sugar after a meal, or impaired fasting glucose (IFG), meaning you have higher than normal blood sugar first thing in the morning before you eat, and your haemoglobin A1C (HbA1C) level is between 5.7% and 6.4%.

The thing about prediabetes is it has no obvious symptoms. Some people have dark, thick patches of skin, but these are also linked to PCOS. You may have seen people with this patchy skin around their elbows, knees, neck, armpits and the backs of their hands, around their knuckles. Skin tags are another telltale sign. If you are prediabetic and start to feel the symptoms associated with diabetes – such as frequent urination, blurry vision, cuts that won't heal, feeling tired all the time and really thirsty – then you should see your doctor and seek the help of a nutritionist.

The cause is the same as for type 2 diabetes: primarily insulin resistance. Factors that increase your risk of insulin resistance include:

- sedentary lifestyle
- obesity or excess body fat, especially visceral fat
- genetics
- poor diet full of fatty, refined, processed high-carbohydrate foods

- medications such as steroids
- hypothyroidism
- chronic stress
- poor sleep
- Cushing syndrome.

WHAT INCREASES YOUR PREDIABETES RISK

- Smoking
- A family history of diabetes
- Not exercising much
- Gestational diabetes
- Sleep apnoea
- PCOS
- Being over 45

The more risk factors you have, the higher the risk. Some risks you can't change, such as family history, but you can definitely start exercising, change your lifestyle and stop smoking.

Like type 2 diabetes, prediabetes comes with complications such as heart attack, kidney issues, eye issues, stroke and nerve damage. Prediabetes can be reversed – I have done it so many times in my clinic. But some of these complications can't be reversed.

THE IMPORTANCE OF ANNUAL CHECK-UPS

I tell all my patients to do a full check-up and blood test every year. I personally do mine on my birthday as a gift to myself for staying on top of my health. When you do them regularly, even though your results may not be in the out-of-range sections, you can start to see trends. You'll watch things slowly changing, which will help you get on top of your health quicker. Ask for a fasting glucose blood test, which you need to do first thing in the morning on an empty stomach.

TREATING PREDIABETES

In my clinic, I reverse prediabetes with a healthy diet plan and appropriate lifestyle changes like exercising. It starts with a good healthy diet, full of nutrient-dense wholefoods. Other changes include getting to a healthy weight, not adding sugar to beverages and avoiding processed foods.

If you have a lot of stress, consider getting your own blood pressure machine at home and start tracking it. This also helps to avoid white-coat hypertension. This is where your blood pressure elevates in a clinical setting but is fine when you're at home. I've seen it many times as a practitioner – people can be prescribed unnecessary blood pressure medications when they have white-coat hypertension, which is so dangerous.

Sleep is everything! Focus on getting good-quality sleep, and make sure you don't have any sleep disorders you are unaware of, such as sleep apnoea.

For most people with prediabetes, if they see their doctor they'll generally be prescribed metformin or other antidiabetic medications. But as I have said before, prediabetes is a disease of the diet. Treat it by changing the cause – your diet.

If you do get a diagnosis of prediabetes, education is key. I tell my patients to learn all you can about the condition, tell all your loved ones or close friends. Processing your diagnosis can feel overwhelming. Take things day by day; small changes are still changes. Work alongside a healthcare provider.

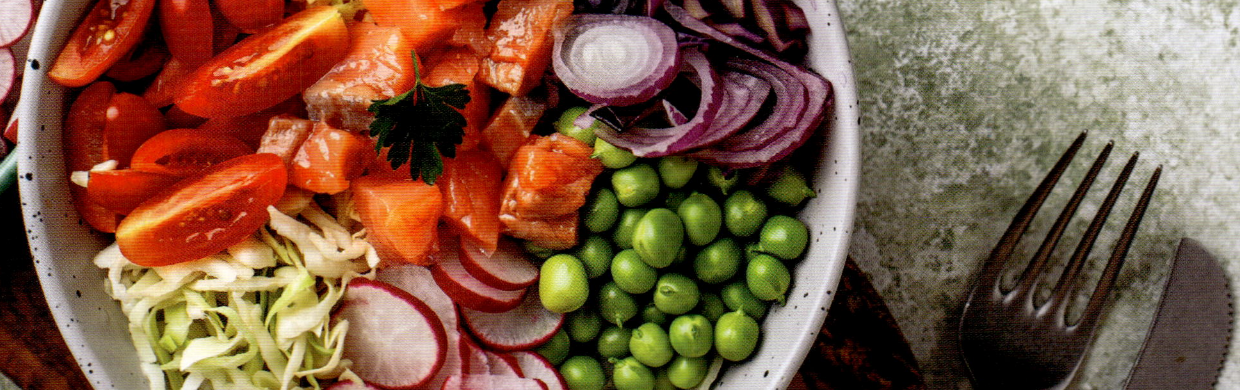

TYPE 2 DIABETES

T2D is where your body does not make enough insulin and the cells in your body don't respond to insulin, leading to insulin resistance. Type 2 makes up 90% of the diabetic population. It mainly affects adults but now, sadly, we are seeing it in children too.

CHILDREN WITH TYPE 2 DIABETES

Type 2 diabetes in children is increasing in countries such as the USA, Australia, Canada, New Zealand, UK, Hong Kong (China), Japan, Bangladesh and Libya. The average age of diagnosis is about 12–14 years, but children as young as 3 years have been diagnosed. More girls than boys have T2D and the diagnosis is always associated with obesity, family history and physical inactivity. Many of these children were exposed to diabetes while in utero from a mother with either type 2 diabetes or gestational diabetes. Currently, about 1.85 million young people under 20 are living with type 2 diabetes globally. This aligns closely with the ongoing rise in childhood obesity, sedentary lifestyle and poor diet.

Youth-onset type 2 diabetes is considered a growing crisis. We can now see it across all ethnic groups, with particularly high rates among Aboriginal and Torres Strait Islander youth. In 2022, almost 28% of Australians aged 5–17 were overweight or obese. This is, of course, where diabetes starts – with poor diet and weight gain. Parents and carers are so important in this journey because they are the ones purchasing and cooking children's food.

Nearly 50% of people with T2D also have micronutrient deficiencies, women more so than men – approximately 48.6% for women and 42.5% for men. A meta-analysis of studies published between 1998 and 2023 estimated mineral deficiencies in T2D patients. The research found 45.30% of all patients with T2D had micronutrient deficiencies, and among those with diabetic complications, 40% were deficient. Interestingly, vitamin D deficiency had the highest prevalence, at 60.45%.

60% of people with type 2 diabetes are deficient in vitamin D.

It is no secret that I have been campaigning for years to raise awareness of vitamin D deficiency, I need to be the vitamin D ambassador! But in all seriousness, almost 9 out of 10 people I see in my clinic are vitamin D deficient. It is not until I explain to them that vitamin D is not only important for our bones but also gives us energy, helps us maintain weight, and lowers our incidence of falls and risk of depression that they start to pay attention.

Another mineral I will forever campaign for is magnesium. About 80% of people don't get enough magnesium. Almost 42% of people with T2D have magnesium deficiency, followed by iron and vitamin B12. So when it comes to treating T2D, the focus is not only on food and nutrition, but also micronutrient deficiencies and your overall nutrition.

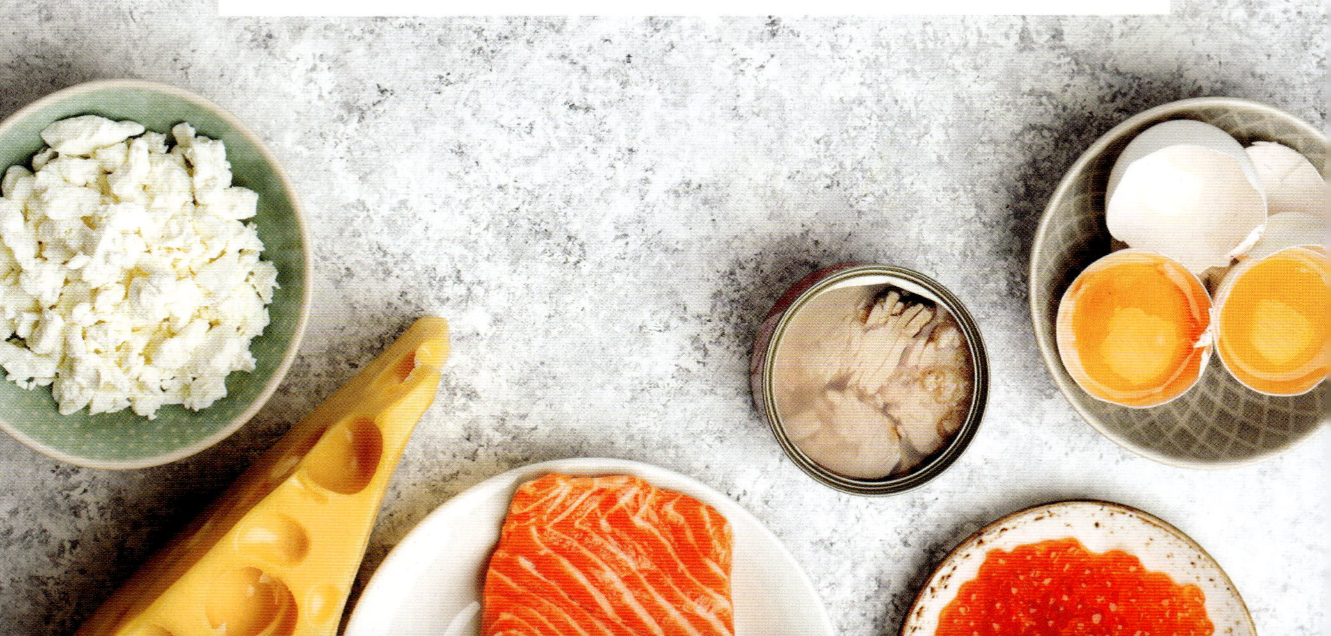

WHAT CAUSES TYPE 2 DIABETES?

Too much glucose circulating in your bloodstream causes diabetes, regardless of the type. However, T2D is also caused by insulin resistance, which is when the cells in our liver, muscles and fat don't respond as they should to insulin. We'll go into the causes of type 2 diabetes in more detail in the following chapters.

Here are some of the most obvious symptoms of T2D.

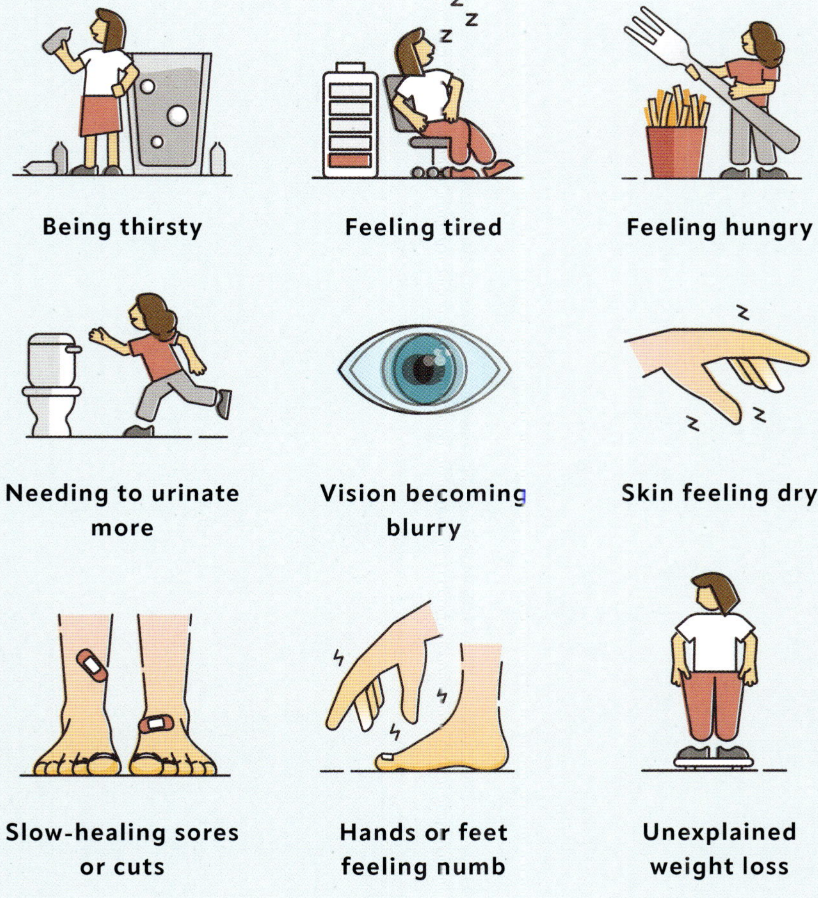

Women may also get a lot more urinary tract infections (UTIs) or vaginal yeast infections with T2D, which is often confused with postmenopausal UTIs.

WHAT ARE THE RISK FACTORS?

The key risk factors for T2D are:

- family history

- being over 45

- being overweight or obese

- nationality (Pacific Islander, Black, Aboriginal and Torres Strait Islander people)

- gestational diabetes

- sedentary lifestyle

- high cholesterol

- high blood pressure

- PCOS.

GESTATIONAL DIABETES

This type of diabetes impacts about 8% of pregnant women, but once the baby is born the mother's blood sugar levels return to normal. Women who experience gestational diabetes are at a higher risk of T2D.

Women are at higher risk if they are older than 40, are obese or overweight, have PCOS, or have had gestational diabetes with previous pregnancies. Nationality also plays a role, with Polynesian, Melanesian, Aboriginal and Torres Strait Islander women at greater risk.

It's not just the mother who gets affected, but the baby. The baby can accumulate excessive fat while growing in the womb if the mother has gestational diabetes. Once the baby is born, they can experience a drop in blood glucose.

When I was having babies, I had a few pregnancies around the same time as my neighbour. During her first pregnancy, she did not know she had gestational diabetes for most of it. Her babies were big, she was unwell and by the time she found out it was well into the pregnancy. So it's important to keep on top of your testing during pregnancy.

Gestational diabetes develops because of insulin. Either the insulin is not working or there is not enough insulin produced. The placenta produces hormones for the baby to grow; however, sometimes these hormones can stop the mother's insulin from working, causing insulin resistance. And true to insulin resistance, the pancreas cells make more insulin to manage the blood glucose and then type 2 diabetes develops.

Gestational diabetes is usually picked up in the second trimester, at around 26 weeks.

It can happen to women who have no risk factors.

The signs to look out for are being thirsty all the time, feeling tired and urinating a lot. Now, these symptoms are common for a healthy pregnant woman too. I recall being thirsty, my baby putting pressure on my bladder, and of course I was tired because I was working and juggling motherhood. So again, make sure you get regular testing if you are pregnant.

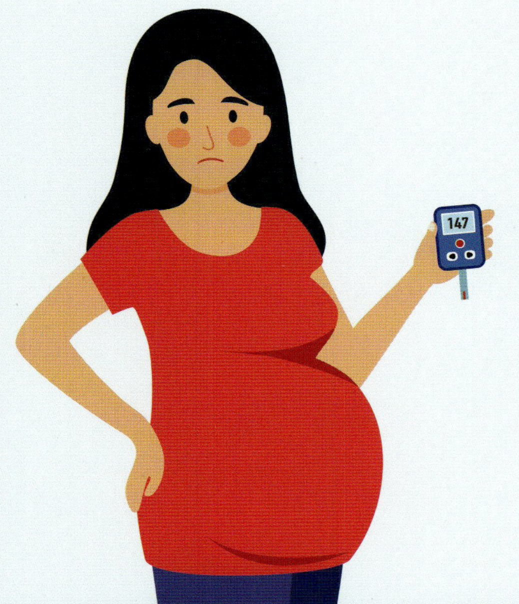

GLUCOSE TOLERANCE TEST

The pathology test for gestational diabetes is called the oral glucose tolerance test. It is done via a blood test and glucose drink. You have to fast overnight or for 10 hours, have the first blood test, then drink a sugary beverage that contains 75 grams of glucose. You wait and get a second blood test 2 hours after the drink to see whether your blood glucose has returned to baseline or remains elevated.

If diagnosed, you should seek the help of a healthcare professional, clinical nutritionist, doctor, dietician or diabetes specialist. The condition needs to be managed well, with blood sugar monitoring, a healthy diet, exercise and education about insulin.

Your diet needs to be full of vegetables, lean proteins, calcium-rich foods and low-carb fruit. You must avoid sugary drinks, fried takeaway foods, refined carbohydrates and foods with added sugar.

Once your baby is born, their blood sugar levels will be measured and monitored. Research shows these babies have a higher risk of T2D later in life.

Once you have had gestational diabetes, the chances are you will have it in subsequent pregnancies. The best way to reduce your risk is to eat healthily, exercise daily, have regular blood tests and be consistent with your eating plan.

TYPE 3 DIABETES

What is type 3 diabetes? This is an unofficial term used to describe Alzheimer's disease or dementia, which is thought to be linked to insulin resistance in the brain.

The theory is that, just as insulin resistance impairs the body's ability to manage blood sugar in type 2 diabetes, a similar process happens in the brain, where neurons are less able to respond to insulin. This impairs their metabolism, increases stress and inflammation, and could contribute to neurodegeneration – such as memory loss, confusion and cognitive decline.

Type 3 diabetes is not an officially recognised medical diagnosis; rather, it's a term used in research and some public discussions to highlight the link between diabetes, insulin resistance and Alzheimer's disease.

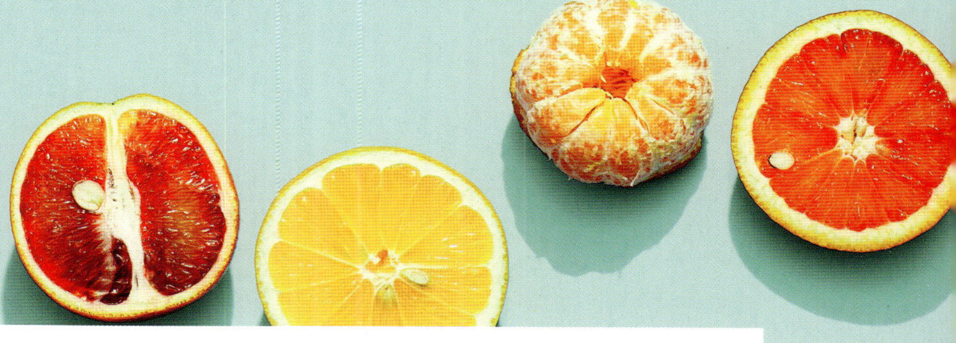

TYPE 3C DIABETES

We don't hear much about this type of diabetes. Type 3c develops when the pancreas is damaged, affecting its ability to produce insulin. This can be from conditions such as cystic fibrosis, chronic pancreatitis or having a part or all of the pancreas removed in a pancreatectomy. The pancreas has two main functions: exocrine, which produces enzymes that help with digestion, and endocrine, which sends out hormones such as insulin and glucagon to control blood glucose. People with Type 3c can lack the pancreatic enzymes needed for digestion; this is called exocrine pancreatic insufficiency.

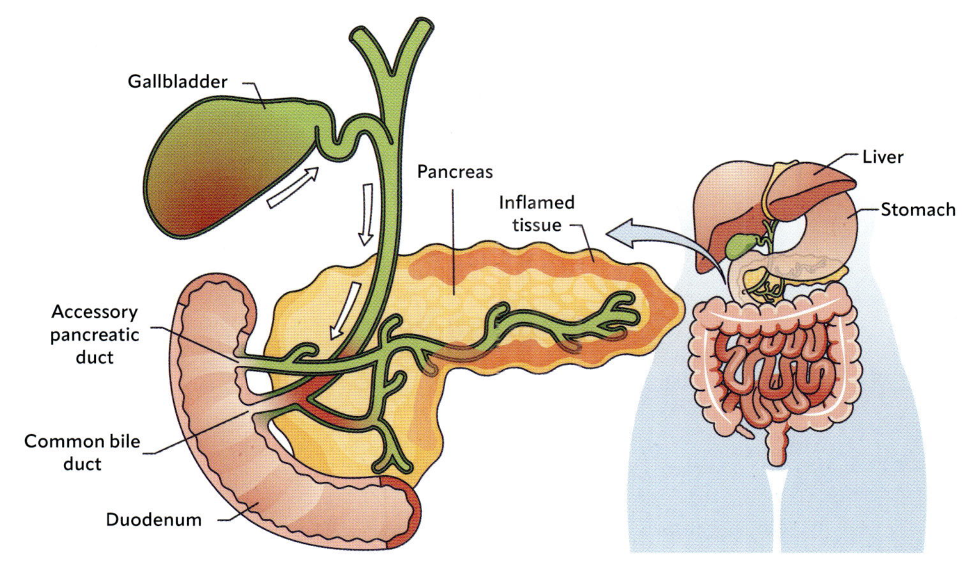

The symptoms of type 3c include:

- blurry vision
- slow healing
- thrush
- feeling thirsty
- dry mouth
- frequent urination
- unexplained weight loss
- skin infections
- numbness or tingling in hands or feet
- bloating, gas and abdominal pain
- fatty stools (pale colour and shocking smell)
- diarrhoea and constipation.

Type 3c is rare, probably about 1% of the diabetic population, and is not well known. In many cases, it's misdiagnosed as having gut issues.

The treatment plan is with healthy meals and regular exercise, blood sugar monitoring, and a healthy lifestyle. It is also managed with oral diabetic medication or insulin. Make sure you have your healthcare team around you to help understand and navigate this condition.

To try and help reduce the risk of type 3c diabetes, you should avoid or strictly limit alcohol consumption, stop smoking, and manage very high triglyceride levels because these factors drive pancreatic damage and chronic pancreatitis. In inherited conditions such as cystic fibrosis, however, you can't prevent the underlying disease. Early, aggressive treatment can help delay or reduce diabetes risk. Once type 3c diabetes is present, the long-term complications look similar to other forms of diabetes, including heart attack, stroke, atherosclerosis and coronary artery disease, as well nerve damage, retinopathy and foot problems.

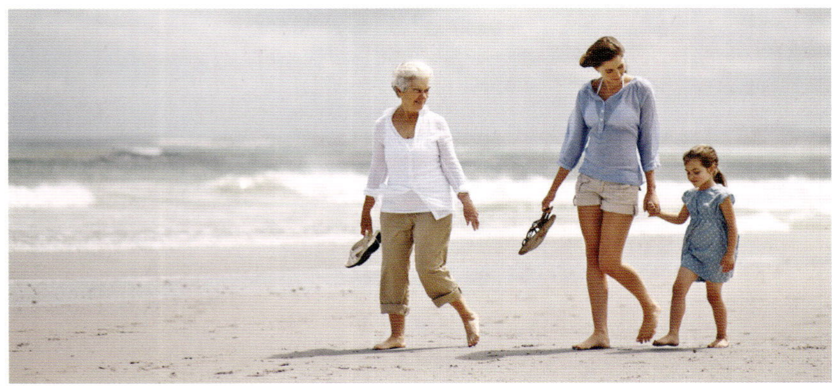

TYPE 4 DIABETES

The term 'type 4 diabetes' is not yet an official diagnosis in standard medical classifications, but it's being used in research to describe age-related insulin resistance in older people who are lean but don't fit the classic type 2 overweight or obese presentation.

It is similar to type 2 diabetes, with symptoms including frequent urination, fatigue, blurred vision, infections and thirst. Long term, if blood glucose remains poorly controlled, complications are a greater risk of heart disease, stroke, kidney disease, foot problems, nerve damage and eye disease.

Because type 4 diabetes is not formally defined, it doesn't have unique treatment protocols; rather, it is best managed similarly to T2D but tailored to older normal-weight people. You need to manage blood pressure, blood glucose and lipids, plus get good nutrition and enough exercise, with a focus on muscle mass and resistance training. Medications may also be needed.

TYPE 5 DIABETES

This is a newly recognised form of diabetes, officially acknowledged in 2025 by the International Diabetes Federation. Also known as malnutrition-related diabetes, it primarily affects lean, undernourished young people living in low- and middle-income countries across Asia and Africa. Type 5 diabetes results from chronic undernutrition during childhood or adolescence in individuals with a BMI lower than 18.5. Chronic nutrient deficiency impairs pancreatic development and leads to severe insulin deficiency.

Type 5 diabetes has similar symptoms to other diabetes types, including increased thirst, urination, fatigue, weight loss and slow wound healing. It can be managed with oral medication rather than insulin injections.

Recognising type 5 diabetes brings hope for better care and research.

CHAPTER 3

Causes of type 2 diabetes

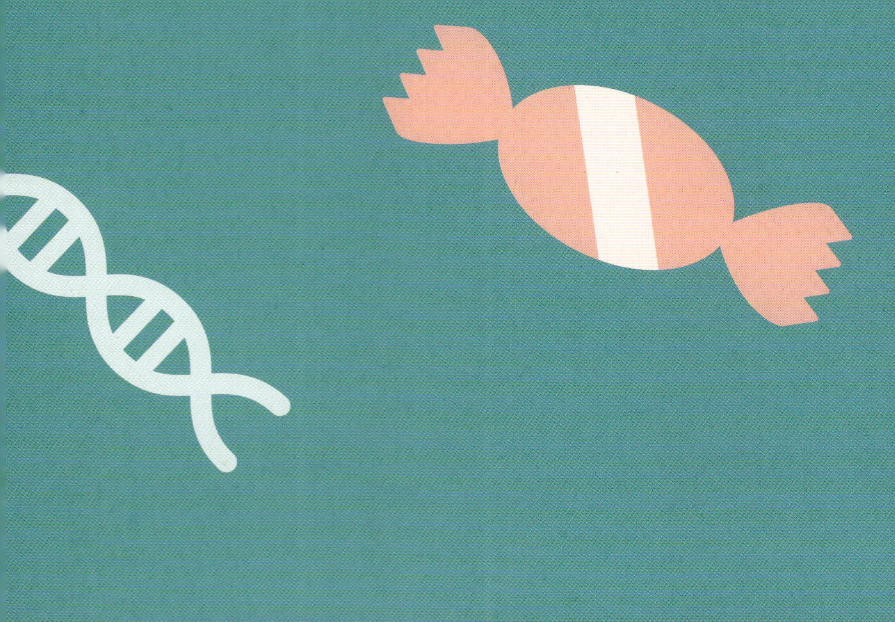
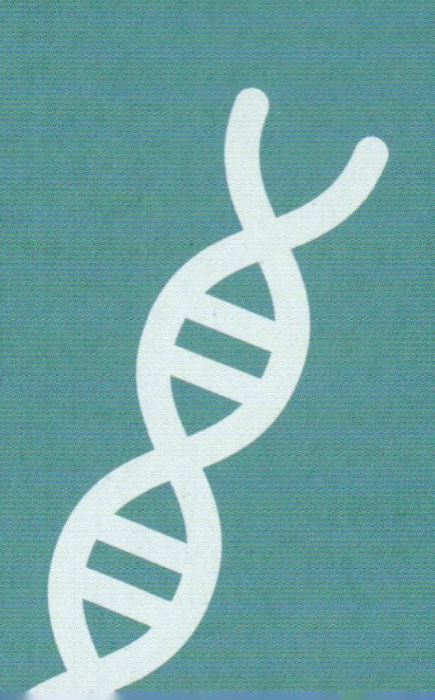

When someone is healthy and their system is working properly, the glucose in the blood is sent to the cells chaperoned by insulin and then released into your cells to be used as energy. In type 2 diabetes, either the body is not making enough insulin or the insulin produced does not work properly, known as insulin resistance. This causes glucose to build up in your blood and not be utilised for energy in the cells.

The biggest risk factor is being obese or overweight. Another is having a large waist circumference; that is, storing fat in the abdominal cavity, or visceral fat. Men's waists need to be less than 101 cm in circumference, and women's less than 88 cm. Excess fat that surrounds the liver and pancreas is linked to T2D.

Even if you're not overweight, having low muscle mass but high visceral fat means greater insulin resistance.

FOODS THAT CAUSE T2D

A poor diet and food choices not only leads to obesity and other diseases but also T2D. These are the main risky foods:

- soft drinks, sugary drinks, cordials and fruit juice concentrates

- refined carbohydrates such as white rice and white bread

- sugary and refined cereals

- processed meats such as sausages and ham

- processed foods and ultra-processed foods.

However, some foods can lower your risk of developing T2D. For more on this, see Chapter 9: **Why nutrition matters.**

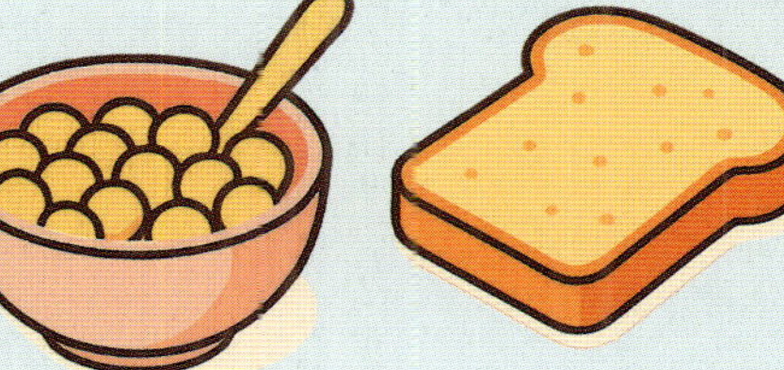

GENETICS

T2D is a complex metabolic disorder influenced by so many factors. While it's predominantly a disease of the diet, genetics can also play a role. There's not just one gene linked to T2D; rather, the condition is linked to hundreds of genes and the number is increasing all the time. Genes involved in insulin and glucose production, insulin secretion, glucose transport and pancreatic function are linked to increased risk.

Research shows you have a two to six times higher risk of developing T2D if a family member, such as a parent or sibling, has it. But the thing with families is that they often also share the same behaviours, eating habits and level of physical activity. Even with a strong genetic risk, your behaviour and environment are extremely important. Many people with a higher risk profile never go on to develop type 2 diabetes. Ultimately, the disease will only develop from poor diet, excess weight, aging, inactivity and poor lifestyle choices, regardless of genetics.

THE MICROBIOME

The gut microbiota have an important role in T2D. People with T2D often have lower levels of butyrate (a by-product of gut bacteria that is amazing for our health), allowing bacteria such as *Faecalibacterium* and *Roseburia* to flourish.

Recent research suggests that an imbalanced gut microbiome (dysbiosis) may contribute to insulin resistance and inflammation – both key factors in the development of T2D. The study found that people with T2D have lower levels of beneficial bacteria called *Akkermansia muciniphila*, which help regulate glucose metabolism.

Improving the gut microbiome can thus potentially be a therapeutic target for people with T2D. Research is currently investigating probiotic interventions to help prevent or manage T2D.

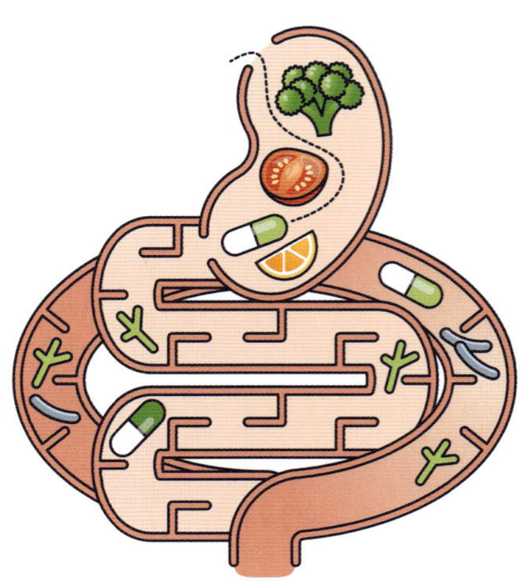

SLEEP

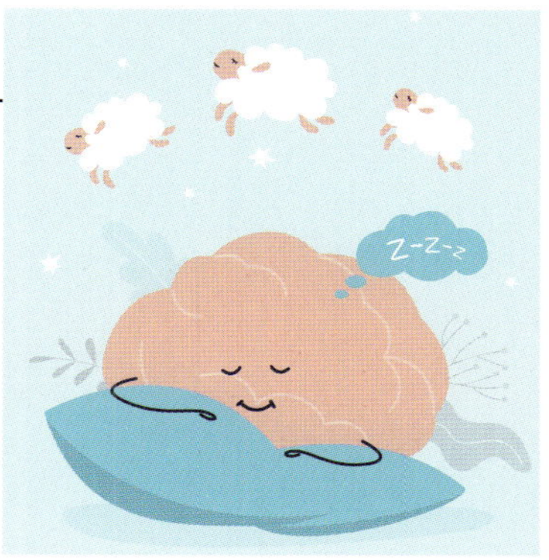

Poor sleep, especially for those of you who are shift workers, has been linked to higher levels of blood sugar and insulin resistance. Recent research found if you sleep less than 6 hours a night, your risk of developing T2D increases by 30%. When sleep patterns are irregular, it impacts your circadian rhythm, which can imbalance hormones and impact glucose metabolism. For more on sleep, see Chapter 11: **Lifestyle – what it means for type 2 diabetes**.

ARTIFICIAL SWEETENERS

Some artificial sweeteners, such as aspartame and saccharin, may negatively impact gut bacteria, potentially increasing the risk of metabolic disorders. Artificial sweeteners are also linked to weight gain because they do not hit the reward centre in the brain for satiety – because your appetite isn't suppressed, you consume more calories. For more on the dangers of artificial sweeteners, see Chapter 9: **Why nutrition matters**.

ENVIRONMENTAL CHEMICALS

Certain environment chemicals are endocrine disrupting, such as BPA (bisphenol A) and phthalates, found in plastics and pesticides. These may interfere with insulin production and glucose metabolism. A recent review found that people with a high exposure to PFAS (perfluoroalkyl substances), which is used in non-stick cookware, food packaging and fire-fighting chemicals, had a higher risk of developing insulin resistance and diabetes.

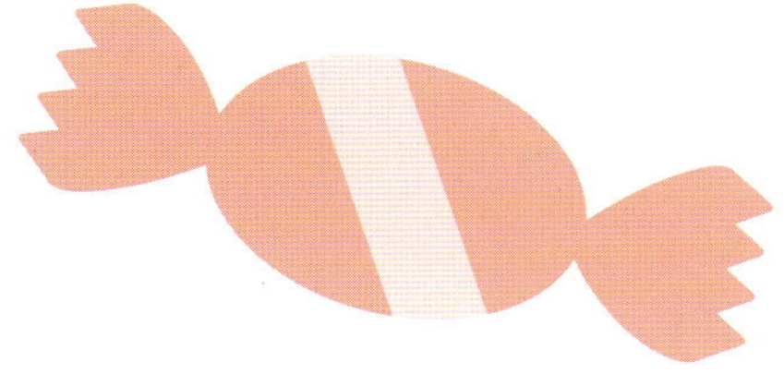

CHAPTER 4

Everything you need to know about glucose

Most people have a general idea that glucose is a word for sugar and it can be found in the foods and beverages we consume, or measured in a blood test. But what is it really? How is it stored in our body, how much is too much and how can we manage it? I get asked these questions a lot. In this chapter, I'm going to break down glucose for you so you can understand its impact on our health, its relationship with diabetes, different types of glucose, signs you could have elevated blood glucose, how it is tested and how to manage it.

WHAT IS GLUCOSE?

Glucose is a simple type of carbohydrate called a sugar, or monosaccharide, that is the main source of energy for our bodies, fuelling our organs, brains and muscles. Nature intended us to consume glucose because it occurs naturally in plants, where the sugars are coupled with fibres so the release of glucose is slow and stable.

FUNCTION OF CARBS

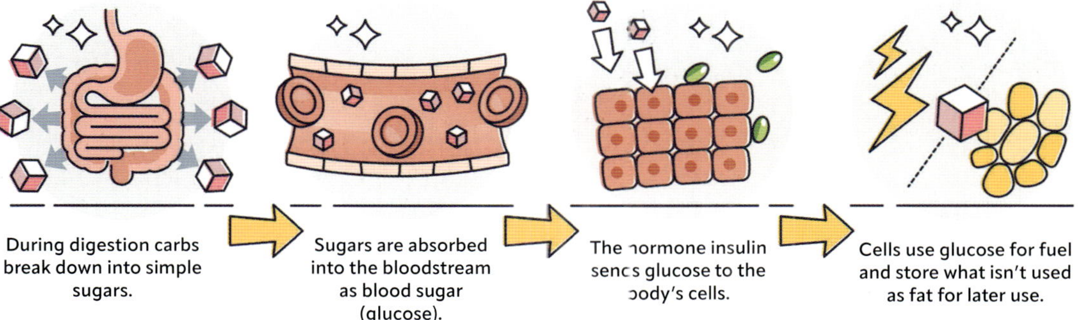

Glucose comes from all different types of carbohydrates in food. We find it in fruit, pasta, sugar and bread as well as many other foods. Think of it as the body's primary energy source. The body can also get fuel from fat and protein, but glucose is the primary source.

Now have a think about the Western diet today. What did you or people you know have for breakfast this morning? In my clinic, so many people at the start of a treatment plan tell me their breakfast is usually a bowl of cereal, pancakes, toast with a sweet spread such as jam, coffee with milk and sugar, and some juice. Think about all the advertising we are surrounded by with breakfast options – it's all about the sweet, sugary options. But what this will do is cause a blood sugar spike and then crash about two hours later. The person will be hungry again, looking for a sweet mid-morning treat like some biscuits.

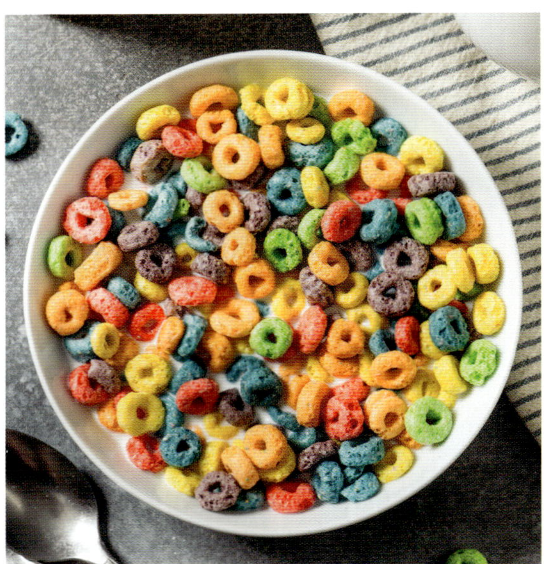 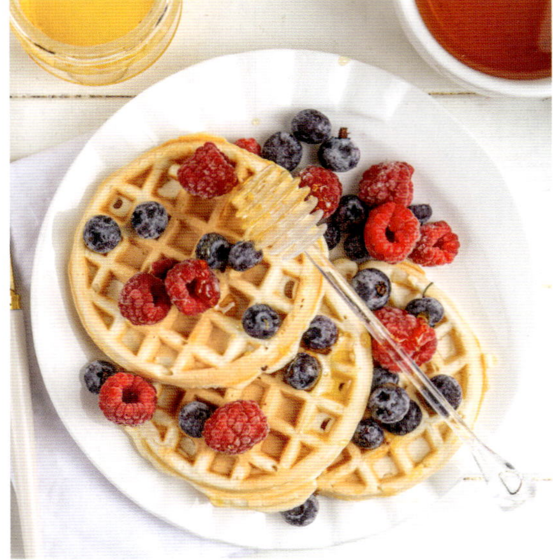

Our body stores glucose as glycogen in our liver and muscles for later use. Glycogen stored in the muscles also retains water. Glucose can also be stored as fat in the form of a triglyceride in fat cells. This occurs when the body has more glucose than it can use with its current energy output. Our liver plays an important role in both glycogen storage and the conversion of excess glucose to fat. When the diet contains too much sugar, this can lead to fatty liver disease.

The glucose pathway looks like this:

- We eat carbohydrates and the body starts processing glucose, with enzymes breaking it down.

- The body releases insulin from the pancreas, which helps cells take up glucose from the bloodstream to use as energy. Insulin manages the elevated blood glucose by moving glucose into your cells.

- The body stores excess glucose as glycogen, a complex carbohydrate, in the muscles and liver.

- When the glycogen stores are full, the body converts the remaining glucose into fatty acids, which are stored as triglycerides in fat cells, also known as adipose tissue.

Glucose is important to our everyday functioning. It powers the brain and supports the muscles to move, in general and when exercising.

We can have too much or too little blood glucose. Both high and low blood glucose will affect how your body functions every day:

- **Hyperglycaemia.** High blood glucose, which leads to energy crashing, diabetes and weight gain.

- **Hypoglycaemia.** Low blood glucose, in which you can get cravings, feel light-headed or dizzy, and be tired or fatigued.

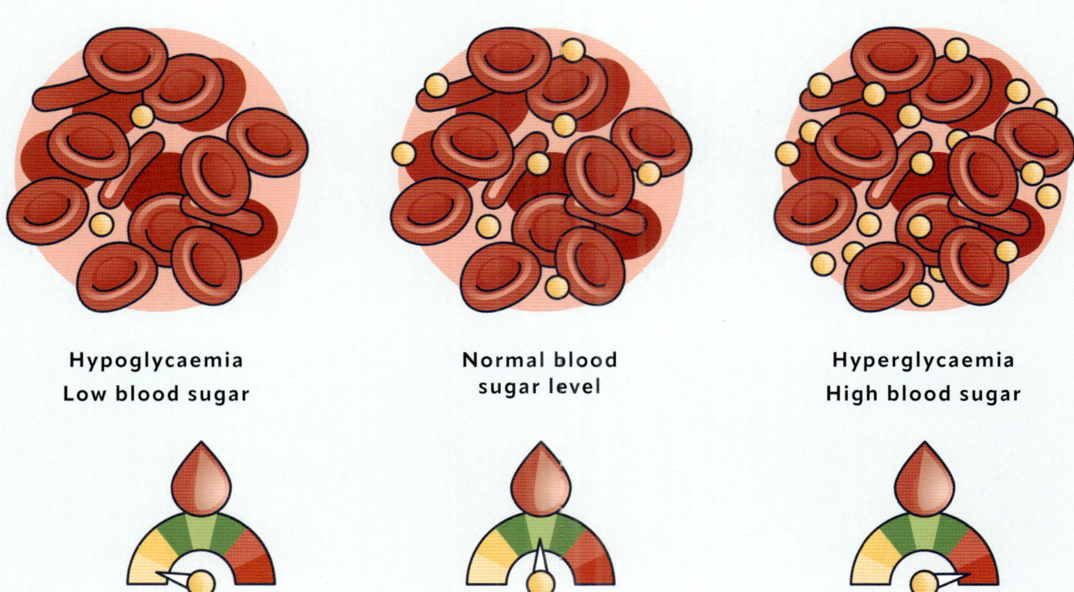

SOURCES OF GLUCOSE

SIMPLE CARBOHYDRATES	COMPLEX CARBOHYDRATES	LACTOSE
Honey	Fruit	Butter
Lollies	Grains	Buttermilk
Pasta	Nuts	Cheese
Soft drinks	Oats	Milk
Sweets	Vegetables	Yoghurt
Table sugar	Whole grains	
White bread		
White rice		

I only ever recommend eating complex carbohydrates because the body takes longer to digest them, so they are healthier and a consistent source of energy. My exceptions to this are honey and maple syrup, which are my preferred choice of sweeteners, followed by stevia. Complex carbohydrates are essential for people living with diabetes, because they cause the blood sugar to spike less than simple carbohydrates.

When blood sugar levels are not managed over time, the impact can be permanent and have severe side effects. The body stops responding to insulin and glucose is no longer able to enter the cells, resulting in them having no energy. Our cells respond by signalling for ketones. These are created in the liver from fat cells, or triglycerides.

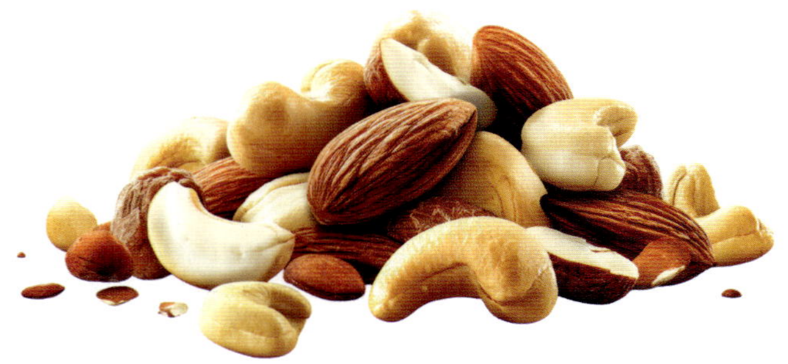

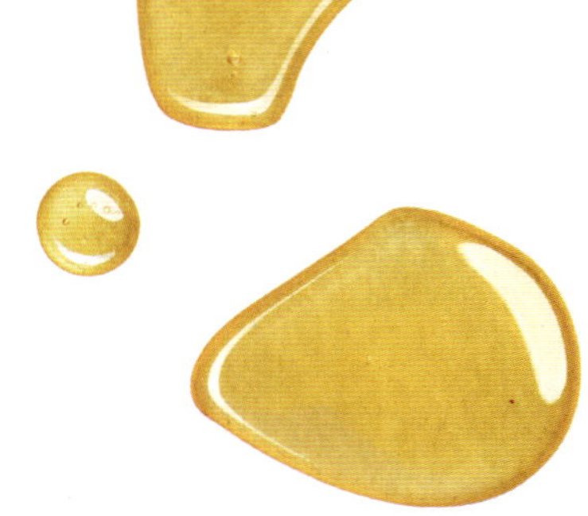

TELLTALE SIGNS OF DYSREGULATED BLOOD GLUCOSE

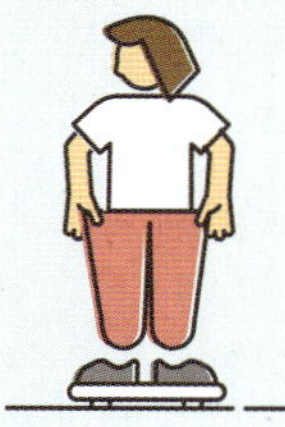

WEIGHT

- Needing to lose weight
- Waist circumference greater than 88 cm for women and 101 cm for men

CRAVINGS

- Feeling hungry all day
- Always feeling the need to eat
- Do you get hangry?
- Sweet tooth or sweet cravings
- Needing coffee all day

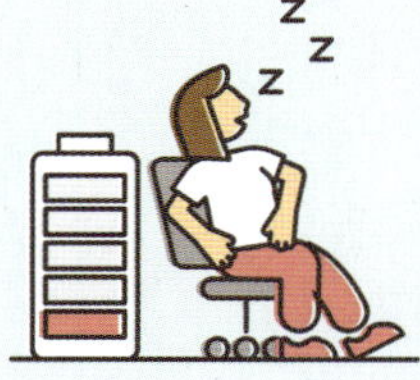

ENERGY

- Moody/anxious/depressed
- Tired all the time
- Light-headed
- Mid-morning slump
- Mid-afternoon slump
- Brain fog
- Energy crashes
- Trouble with sleep

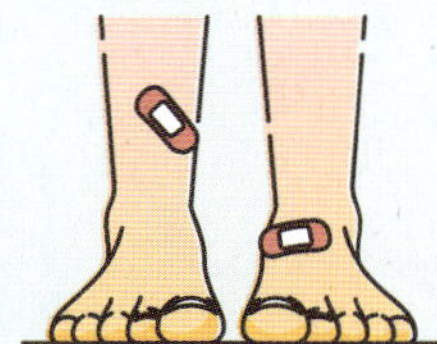

SKIN

- Acne
- Skin conditions
- Wounds that won't heal

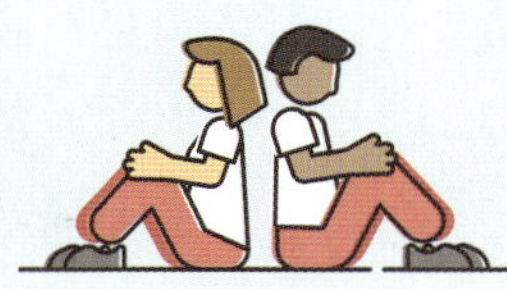

MEDICAL

- Poor immunity
- Waking with heart palpitations
- Heart disease
- Fatty liver – MAFLD (formerly NAFLD)
- Type 2 diabetes

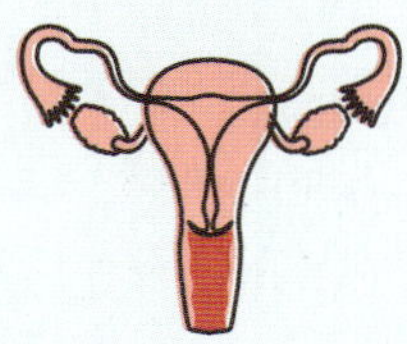

HORMONAL HEALTH

- Insulin resistance
- Infertility
- PMS
- PCOS

HOW GLUCOSE SPIKES AFFECT US

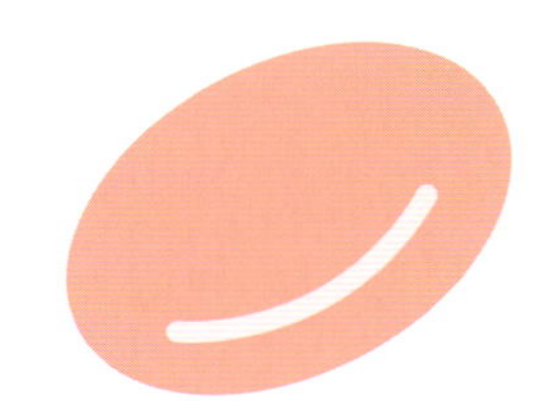

When we consume too much glucose, both our cells and our blood are full of glucose. The mitochondria (membrane-bound organelles that are the powerhouse of the cell) generate most of the chemical energy needed to power the cell's biochemical reactions. The mitochondria are like a little battery working away inside our cells. Over a long period of time, eating food that causes the sugar spikes and lows impacts the functioning of our mitochondria, leading to fatigue.

Glucose spikes can be a different experience for each person. Most get sugar and food cravings but others experience fatigue and brain fog, or feel anxious, dizzy and moody.

The higher our blood sugar spikes, the harder the crash and sugar cravings.

Feeling hungry all the time is linked to high insulin levels. When we eat, insulin steps in to store the excess glucose as fat. This increases our hunger hormone ghrelin. It becomes a cycle – the more weight we gain, the hungrier we become. Think about a time in your life when you have eaten way too much food, and thought to yourself: *I am not going to eat again for ages, I'm so full.* But then you wake up starving. This cycle is so unfair!

SPIKE AND CRASH CYCLE

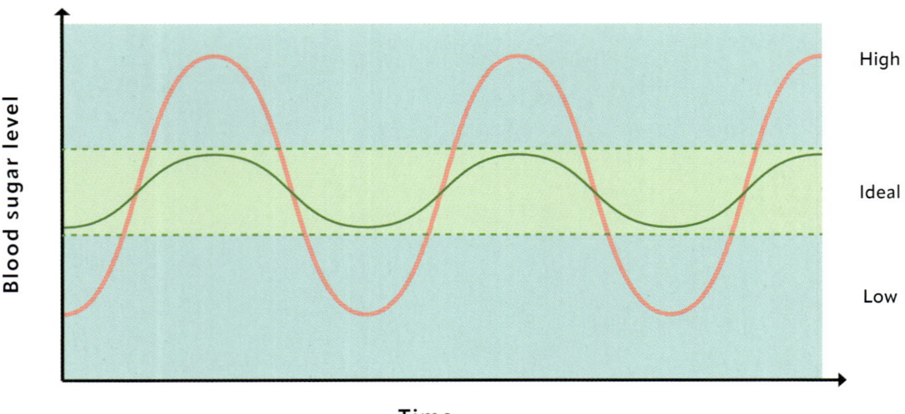

Eating out and celebrating with food is part of life. I always tell my patients to not cave into the next day's hunger; rather, have a lower calorie day. Focus on protein, vegetables and fruit, and avoid sugary foods. Start the day with some exercise and hydrate yourself. This is where education is key. So many people cave into their hunger hormones, but you can manage them and be in control of them.

When I see patients who complain about being tired all the time, I first ask about their diet. Many of us have a sweet tooth and it's so hard to control. If you're struggling with sugar cravings, here is what I tell my patients:

If you go sugar free for at least 1 month, your taste buds will change. Foods such as fruit will taste super sweet.

I have a sweet tooth. I love the dopamine hit I get from chocolate but understand why I crave it, and it's the way it makes me feel. Fruit is where I get my sweet fix. Choosing high-fibre fruits such as berries is a perfect solution. Try to have ½ cup berries every day. Grapes are also amazing!

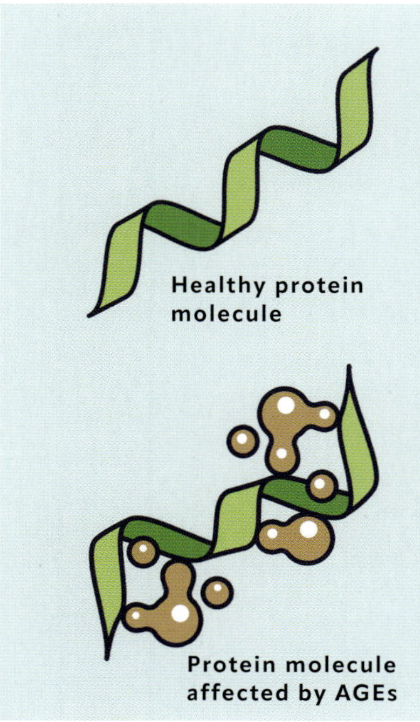

WHAT IS GLYCATION?

Glycation is when sugar in the body attaches to other molecules, leading to dysfunction, disease and inflammation. It occurs when blood glucose is high for long periods of time and is spontaneous.

Advanced glycation end products (AGEs) are unstable; they stiffen tissue, and trigger inflammation and oxidative stress. They damage proteins in the eyes, nerves, skin, blood vessels and other tissue, driving diabetes complications and cardiovascular disease.

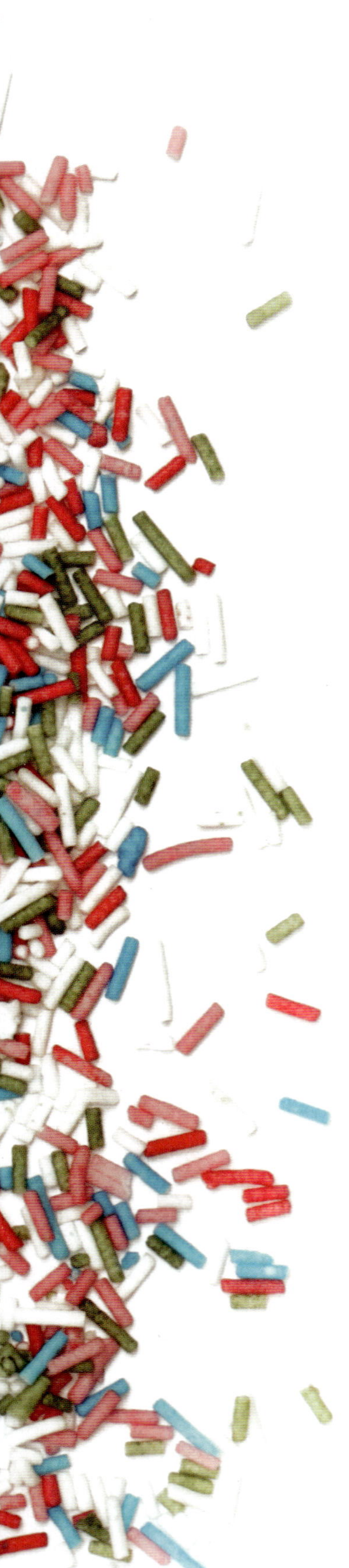

SLEEP

Dysregulated glucose impacts our sleep quality. I always encourage my patients to eat their dinner at 5–6 pm at the latest. I know this can be hard for many with work, but where there is a will there is a way. Pack your dinner and take it to work. When we eat late at night, the accompanying glucose spike is linked to insomnia. Research suggests that the body is less able to use insulin effectively at night. Night-time eating leads to weight gain and chronic disease. The solution is to flatten the glucose curve: eat earlier and avoid carbohydrates at dinner. Also, make sure you do regular exercise, avoid alcohol, limit caffeine after lunchtime, ensure your room is comfortable, sleep with the window open, shower before bed, no screens in the bedroom and consider supplementing with magnesium.

I am obsessed with getting a good night's sleep!

IMMUNITY

Glucose spikes affect our immune system. After a spike, you're more susceptible to infections and inflammation. Excess sugar binds to immune proteins, altering their structure and function. Your white blood cells, or neutrophils, can work less effectively when blood glucose is high because they struggle to move towards and engulf pathogens.

High blood glucose can trigger inflammatory responses throughout the body, damaging immunity and disrupting immune signalling. It can also interfere with the communication between immune cells and prevent them from coordinating effectively, weakening immunity. It compromises the complement system (part of our innate immune system that helps antibodies and immune cells clear pathogens), further reducing the body's ability to fight infections.

STRESS

I always talk to my daughters about this, especially when they have exams coming up. If you're looking for something sweet as a pick-me-up, think again. The glucose spike can impact your brain's power, memory and cognitive functioning. Optimal mental performance needs the right fuel: low-glycaemic index (GI) foods, lean proteins and wholefoods. Nothing is worse than a big sugary breakfast at 8 am, only to crash at 10 am and be desperate for more sugar. Imagine doing an exam, writing a book, being at work or even just doing your daily routine feeling like this! It all comes down to flattening that glucose curve.

DEMENTIA RISK

Diseases such as dementia and Alzheimer's disease are linked to glucose spikes. In fact, as I mentioned earlier, Alzheimer's is now being called type 3 diabetes, or diabetes of the brain. If you have T2D, you have a four times higher risk of developing Alzheimer's disease.

CHRONIC INFLAMMATION

Constantly elevated blood glucose has long-term health consequences. Skin conditions such as eczema, acne and psoriasis are driven by inflammation, which is caused by glucose spikes. For many, changing the diet can improve these conditions. Arthritis is also linked to inflammation. If you have a long-term history of glucose spikes, chances are you have a higher risk of arthritis.

When it comes to aging, the inflammation from ongoing glucose spikes will speed up the aging process. This is known as 'inflammaging'. This not only impacts us on the inside but on the outside, with more wrinkles and saggy skin.

HEART DISEASE

The inflammation from elevated blood glucose is linked to an increased risk of heart disease – it damages the lining of blood vessels and accelerates atherosclerosis, which is the build-up of plaque in the arteries. There is some research showing that postprandial (after-meal) glucose spikes can be a predictor of heart disease.

When you get your blood tests, always make sure your healthcare provider is testing for an inflammation marker called C-reactive protein. I also suggest to my patients to look for trends even if levels are still within the 'healthy' range.

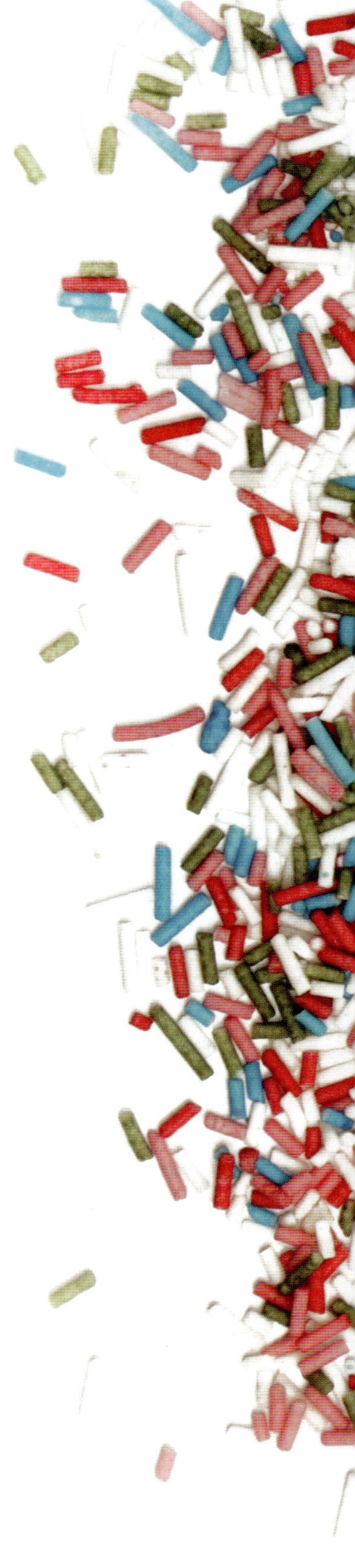

INFERTILITY AND PCOS

There is a link between regular glucose spikes, high insulin levels and infertility. PCOS, the leading cause of infertility among women, is linked to too much insulin. When I treat this condition in my clinic, one of my non-negotiables is doing a minimum of 40 minutes a day of exercise to help with the elevated blood sugar. The weight struggle for these women is very real. It's much harder to shift the weight when there is too much insulin and they are struggling to burn fat.

BLOOD SUGAR AND MENOPAUSE

Women going through menopause need to understand the impact of glucose spikes on their menopause. As hormones drop in menopause, many women experience symptoms such as insomnia, flushes, anxiety, weight gain, moodiness, night sweats and reduced libido. In my clinical experience, women who avoid refined, sugary and processed foods generally have a much better menopause experience. Women with a poor diet and high glucose and insulin levels, however, have more menopause symptoms. This is backed by research.

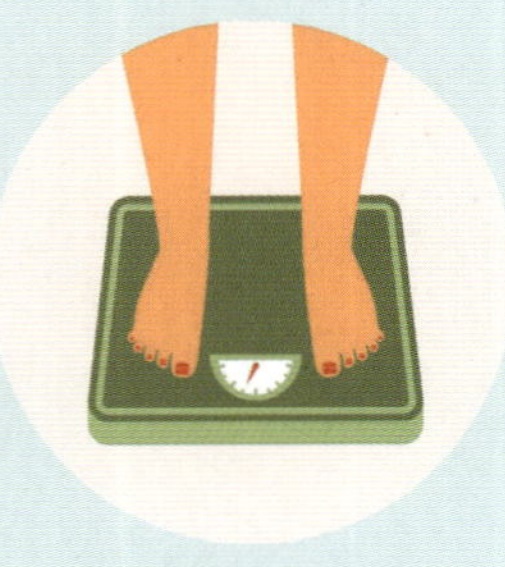

Weight gain

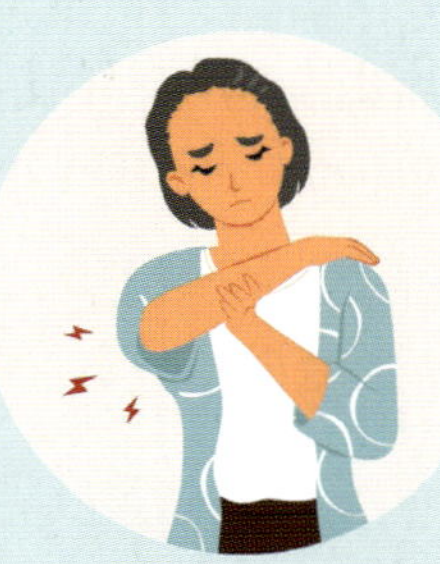

Joint pain

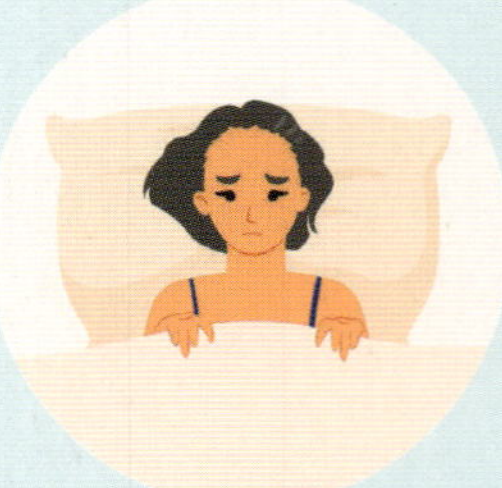

Insomnia

LIVER DISEASE

MASLD (metabolic dysfunction–associated steatotic liver disease) and glucose spikes are connected. They exacerbate each other. MASLD is associated with insulin resistance. As fat builds up in the liver, its ability to regulate blood glucose is impaired, leading to higher insulin levels.

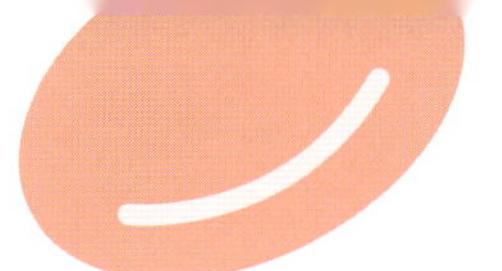

GLUCOSE AND TYPE 2 DIABETES

There is a direct relationship between T2D and glucose. Patients with T2D have insulin resistance, so their bodies don't respond to insulin the way they should. Because their bodies produce less insulin, blood glucose levels are high, leading to hyperglycaemia. When blood glucose is consistently high, the consequences include kidney disease, heart disease, stroke, vision problems (retinopathy), nerve damage (neuropathy) and non-healing wounds. The symptoms of T2D are hard to pick up in the early stages, so everyone should do regular check-ups from age 45, even if you have no risk factors.

I have treated many patients with T2D and insulin resistance. It is challenging in the beginning, but it's so wonderful to see their weight come off and symptoms dissipate. Once the symptoms start to clear, their bodies begin to function normally again. As a practitioner, it's so rewarding. You can do it; you just need consistency, commitment to the program and to take things day by day.

Managing glucose when you have T2D is so important. Many of my T2D patients wear a continuous blood glucose monitor in the early stages of the program, which I highly recommend for avoiding hypoglycaemia, or extremely low blood glucose.

The key to managing glucose when you have T2D:

- Eat low-GI foods and lean proteins.
- Avoid all processed, refined foods.
- Eat lots of fibre, protein and good fats, which slow down the absorption of glucose.
- Exercise regularly; this lowers blood glucose and improves insulin sensitivity.

For all my patients, the aim is getting to a healthy goal weight.

This is essential. My aim is to get them to at least within 10% of their healthy weight and teach them all about understanding glucose.

TESTING YOUR GLUCOSE LEVELS

You can test your blood glucose with a blood test, or blood glucose meter. It is very easy to use, and even if you're not a diabetic you can get one cheaply from your local chemist over the counter. You simply prick your fingertip with a needle, drop the blood onto a testing strip and place the strip into a meter. The meter will measure how much glucose is in your blood at that very moment.

You can also use a continuous blood glucose monitor (CGM), which is a tiny sensor placed under the skin, and a sensor disc or pod adheres on top. It is placed on the back of your upper arm, and continually measures blood glucose levels and sends the data to a smartphone app. The app will alert you if your levels are too low or too high. This is great because you can get continuous readings and manage your diabetes really well. It does require a prescription and is more expensive.

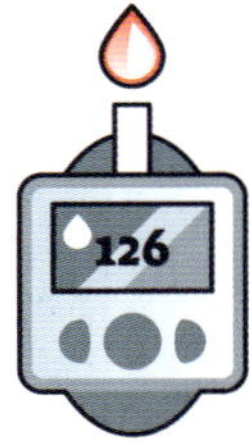

Blood glucose meter

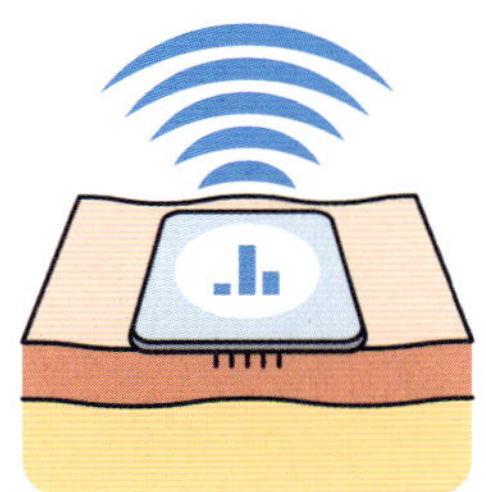

Continuous blood glucose monitor

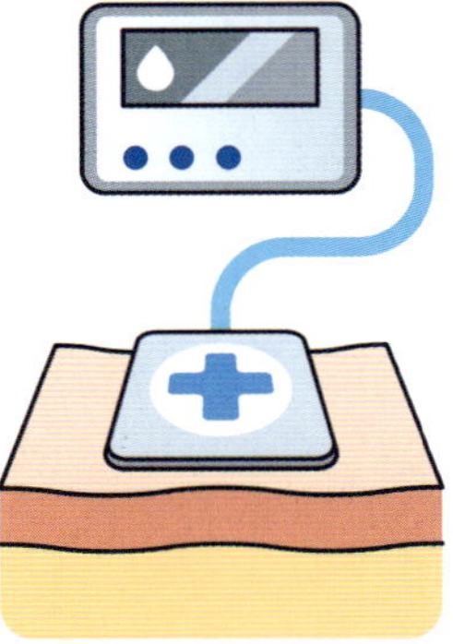

Insulin pump system

BLOOD TESTS

HbA1c TEST	This measures your average blood glucose level over 3 months; it provides a good overview.
FASTING GLUCOSE TEST	This measures blood glucose after fasting overnight.
ORAL GLUCOSE TOLERANCE TEST	This compares your blood glucose after drinking a sugary drink to your fasting blood glucose.
RANDOM BLOOD GLUCOSE TEST	This takes blood at any time during the day without fasting.

HOW OFTEN SHOULD YOU TEST?

How often you should check your blood glucose is completely individual. It depends on your current health status and health goals. If you're healthy, I suggest an annual blood test that includes fasting glucose, not random. If you have health issues, then staying on top of glucose levels is really important, especially for diabetics.

You should test your blood glucose levels:

- before and after meals
- before and after exercise, especially after really intense exercise
- before bed
- if starting new medications
- when travelling.

For people with T2D who are not insulin dependent, a glucose monitor can warn you of any changes so you can address it before anything serious happens. You need to be diligent with maintaining healthy blood glucose levels to keep your body functioning properly.

The test for haemoglobin A1c (HbA1c for short, also called glycated haemoglobin) is a blood test that shows the average blood glucose level over the past 2–3 months. It reflects how much glucose has attached to haemoglobin (the protein in red blood cells that carries oxygen).

As a general guideline, the target for HbA1c is less than 7% (53 mmol/mol). Factors such as age, health condition and type of diabetes can impact your HbA1C.

GLUCOSE LEVEL TARGETS

	TARGET BLOOD GLUCOSE LEVELS (BGLs)	
	BEFORE MEALS	2 HOURS AFTER STARTING MEALS
TYPE 1 DIABETES	4.0–7.0 mmol/L	5.0–10.0 mmol/L
TYPE 2 DIABETES	4.0–7.0 mmol/L	5.0–10.0 mmol/L

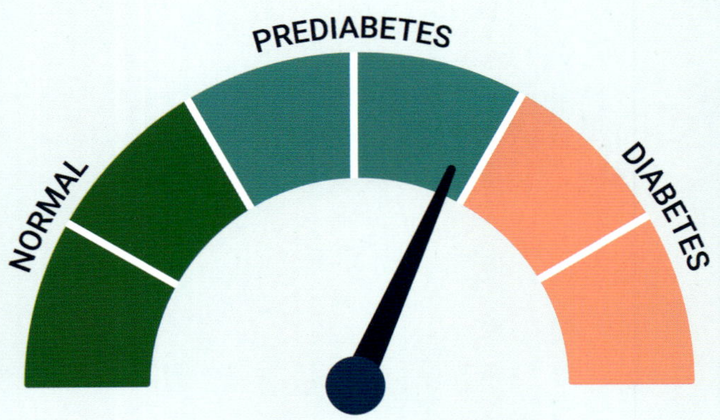

GLUCOSE LEVELS CHART

	HbA1c (%)	Fasting plasma glucose mmol/L	Oral glucose tolerance test mmol/L
DIABETES	6.5 or more	7 or more	11.1 or more
PREDIABETES	5.7–6.4	5.56–7	7.77–11
HEALTHY	5.6 or less	3.89–5.5	7.72 or less

Notes: HbA1c = haemoglobin A1C; mmol/L = millimoles per litre.

WHAT IMPACTS YOUR BLOOD GLUCOSE LEVELS?

Blood glucose levels can be impacted by more than food. Other factors include sunburn, caffeine, skipping breakfast, taking some medications, stress, illness and dehydration.

If you leave your blood glucose levels unregulated, it has a negative impact on your body over time. Potential complications include peripheral neuropathy, heart disease, skin infections, blindness, diabetic ketoacidosis, joint and extremity pain, depression, coma, severe dehydration, and hyperglycaemic hyperosmolar syndrome.

A danger with low blood glucose episodes is hypoglycaemia unawareness. This is where you stop noticing the signs until they drop too low. It can be extremely serious, resulting in a coma or loss of consciousness, or even death.

THE DAWN PHENOMENON

This is a surge of hormones between 4 and 8 a.m., causing a spike in blood glucose. The dawn phenomenon is common in people with diabetes. It's linked to a natural increase in hormones that signal the liver to release glucose. The body releases hormones such as cortisol and growth hormone in the morning as a signal for the liver to release stored glucose so we have energy to wake up.

When someone has diabetes, the pancreas may not produce enough insulin to respond to the rise in blood glucose, leading to elevated blood glucose levels in the morning. Other factors include poor sleep quality, high blood glucose before bed and insufficient insulin. The symptoms of the dawn phenomenon are thirst, hunger, headache, irritability, blurry vision and frequent urination. It can be diagnosed with a continuous glucose monitor.

You can manage the dawn phenomenon by adjusting your insulin use, using insulin with a longer duration or peak of action, avoiding carbohydrates before bed, and doing exercise in the evening.

HOW DIFFERENT FOODS IMPACT BLOOD GLUCOSE LEVELS

Blood glucose levels rise and fall depending on what food and drinks you consume. Some foods spike blood glucose and others give you a steady release of blood glucose over time. Knowing the difference in these foods is really important for your energy levels, overall health and managing diabetes if you have it.

UNDERSTANDING THE GLYCAEMIC INDEX

The glycaemic index is a way of ranking foods that contain carbohydrate based on how quickly they are digested and how blood glucose levels increase over a 2-hour period.

- **High GI foods.** Simple carbohydrates that break down quickly, such as white bread and potatoes, have a high GI. They are high-carb, low-fibre, and lack protein and good fats. This means they elevate blood glucose levels very quickly, leading to a spike then a crash.

- **Low-GI foods.** Complex carbohydrates that break down slowly, such as oats, have a low GI, meaning that the glucose response is slow and flat. Low-GI foods contain protein, healthy fats and fibre that prolong digestion due to their slow breakdown. These foods cause a slow and gradual rise in blood glucose, and can help you feel full for longer.

LOW GI (LESS THAN 55)	MEDIUM GI (55 TO 70)	HIGH GI (GREATER THAN 70)
Leafy greens (spinach, kale, broccoli), lean proteins (chicken, fish, tofu, eggs), healthy fats (avocados, nuts, olive oil), high-fibre fruit (berries, apples, pears), legumes (lentils, beans, chickpeas), quinoa	Orange juice, honey, basmati rice, whole grains (brown rice, wholewheat bread, wholemeal bread)	Potatoes, white bread, short-grain rice, sugary cereals, processed meals and snacks, fruit juice and soft drinks, lollies and sugary snacks, cakes and biscuits, ice cream, fast food

FLATTENING THE GLUCOSE CURVE

The glucose curve is a visual pattern or graph that shows how your blood glucose levels rise and fall over time in response to eating, physical activity, sleep or stress. It indicates how the body regulates and processes sugar.

After we eat, our blood glucose will rise and peak, then return to baseline as insulin helps the body process and store glucose. The curve traces these changes. The goal is to have a gradual rise and return rather than spikes and drops. A flatter, more stable curve is associated with better metabolic health.

Conversely, large spikes and crashes indicate insulin resistance, prediabetes or diabetes. The glucose curve helps us understand our metabolic health and can identify impaired glucose metabolism or insulin resistance.

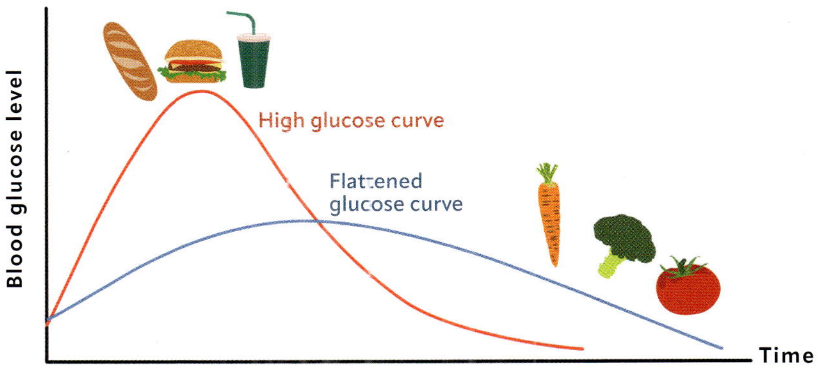

HIGH VERSUS FLATTENED GLUCOSE CURVE

HIGH GLUCOSE CURVE	FLATTENED GLUCOSE CURVE
Breakfast at 7 a.m. – sugary cereal or white bread with margarine and jam	Breakfast at 7 a.m. – eggs with avocado, spinach, tomato and mushroom on wholegrain toast
Spike then crash at 9 a.m.	Very mild rise
Cravings at 10 a.m.	Good amount of energy until 12 p.m.

After a meal, your blood glucose naturally goes up as your body digests carbs. Then insulin is released to take that glucose into your cells, which brings your blood glucose back down, returning to normal.

Healthy normal blood glucose levels:

- fasted = 5.6 mmol/L

- 1 hour after meal = less than 10 mmol/L

- 2 hours after meal = less than 8.6 mmol/L

- 3 hours after meal = less than 7.8 mmol/L.

WHY SHOULD WE FLATTEN OUR BLOOD GLUCOSE CURVE?

For starters, frequent glucose fluctuations indicate an increased risk of organ damage, blood vessel damage and poor long-term health outcomes.

- **Prevent high blood pressure (hypertension).** Research indicates that elevated blood glucose when fasting is a risk factor for high blood pressure over time. When blood glucose is chronically elevated, the blood vessels can get stiff and narrow, known as atherosclerosis), which directly contributes to high blood pressure.

- **Take care of our blood vessels.** Large swings in glucose can damage blood vessels, leading to kidney disease, vision loss, heart attack, stroke and hypertension.

- **Control inflammation.** Blood glucose spikes can cause inflammation in general but also in the lining of the blood vessels, because the spikes produce free radicals that damage healthy cells.

A flattened curve will help prevent the overproduction of insulin and stress hormones such as cortisol, which increase blood pressure.

When our blood glucose curve is flattened, we have more energy, focus and a better mood; reduce our sugar cravings; and can better manage our weight. We also lower our risk of diabetes

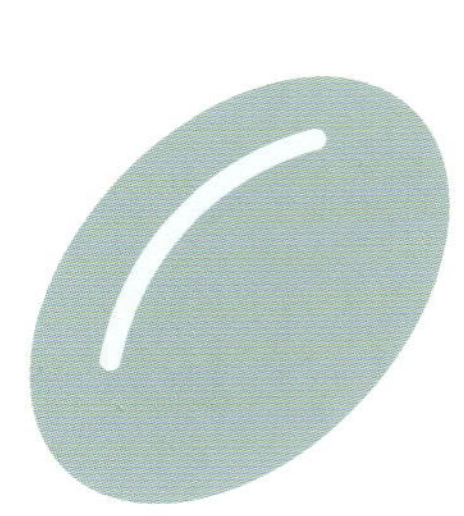

complications, including microvascular and macrovascular complications that affect the eyes, kidneys, heart and nerves.

A flattened curve is so important for our overall health and wellbeing. It is really an underrated hack for better energy, fewer cravings, better focus and concentration plus productivity and mood.

You don't need to give up carbohydrates, but make them a part of a complete meal.

It's such a huge win for long-term health.

HOW DO YOU FLATTEN THE GLUCOSE CURVE?

The best way to flatten the glucose curve naturally is to combine both diet and lifestyle changes:

- **Exercise regularly.** This increases insulin sensitivity and helps the muscles use glucose for energy, lowering blood glucose. Muscles use glucose, so your body doesn't need to store as much. Resistance training, swimming, cycling, brisk walking, running, dancing and hiking are all good options. Aim for at least 150 minutes per week.

- **Reduce or avoid refined carbs and added sugar.** This includes sweets, treats, white bread and pasta, white rice, and soft drinks. Avoid sugar spikes by choosing low-GI whole grains, fruit, vegetables and legumes.

- **Get enough fibre in your diet.** This is so important! Recent research shows that 83% of Australians aren't getting enough fibre in their diet. Fibre slows down the absorption of carbohydrates, which means a more consistent blood glucose level. Oats, legumes, nuts, seeds and non-starchy vegetables are all good sources of fibre.

- **Eat probiotic-rich foods.** Options include sauerkraut, kimchi, miso, tempeh, tofu, kombucha and yoghurt. Also take a good-quality probiotic daily.

- **Get on top of stress.** Cortisol is a stress hormone that can raise blood glucose levels. Try stress-less techniques such as

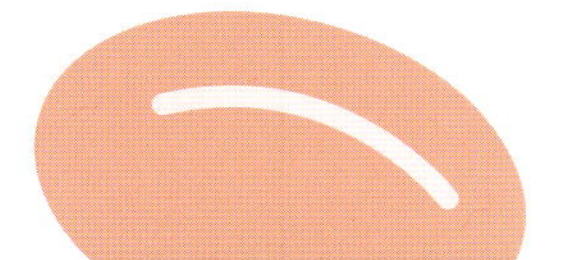

deep breathing, mindfulness, resting, going for walks and meditation. Always seek help from a healthcare professional if the stress is too much.

- **Sleep well.** Poor sleep increases cortisol, which raises blood glucose and hunger hormones.

- **Drink enough water.** Being dehydrated can cause your body to release more sugar and reduce the kidneys' ability to remove excess glucose. My tip is to drink enough water so your urine is a light yellow colour. Of course, avoid cordial, sugary drinks and sugary fruit juices!

- **Don't skip meals.** Skipping meals or eating large portions can really dysregulate blood glucose. Make sure meals are healthy and balanced, including all your macronutrients: fats, proteins and complex carbohydrates.

- **Get to and maintain a healthy weight.** This is a given for treating all chronic disease, because it lowers inflammation and improves blood glucose control. My 10:10 Plan is excellent for weight loss.

- **Monitor your blood glucose,** especially if you already have diabetes. You'll see the effect of these changes!

MUSCLES AND BLOOD GLUCOSE

Muscle is a core foundation for good health and longevity. We all start gradually losing muscle around age 40, a process called sarcopenia. I am so aware of the importance of muscle. I train 6 days a week, roughly 10 hours per week. My training involves a mix of reformer Pilates (which I love), weights, running, using a cross-trainer and HIIT training. I tell my children I'm taking care of their future by exercising because I won't be a burden on them when I'm older, I don't want them to spend their lives being my carers. My goal is to age with strength, independence, stability and mobility. Exercise should be a non-negotiable for everyone, like brushing your teeth. Just find what you love and do it.

Muscle plays a central role in nearly every aspect of your health!

- Muscle helps regulate metabolism, controlling how your body burns calories and manages blood glucose.

- Muscle is essential for preventing type 2 diabetes and maintaining a healthy weight.

- Strong muscles support your joints, bones and overall mobility, which are key for independence, especially as you age.

- Maintaining muscle can lower your risk of chronic diseases such as heart disease; protect you from falls and injuries; and boost your mental health, immune system and longevity.

- Muscle is linked to healthy aging, better quality of life and overall health and wellness.

MUSCLES – A GLUCOSE SINK

Skeletal muscle is the largest tissue in the body that absorbs glucose from the blood. When you eat and your blood glucose rises, insulin instructs your muscle cells to absorb glucose, converting it into energy or storing it as glycogen for later use.

Muscle cells are extremely responsive to insulin.

In healthy people, skeletal muscle removes around 60% to 80% of glucose from the blood after a carbohydrate-rich meal.

Insulin binds to receptors on the muscle cell surfaces, allowing glucose to enter. In type 2 diabetes, the muscle cells become less sensitive to insulin. This insulin resistance means glucose struggles to be taken up by muscle after meals, causing blood glucose to remain high.

Muscle insulin resistance is often the earliest defect in prediabetes and type 2 diabetes.

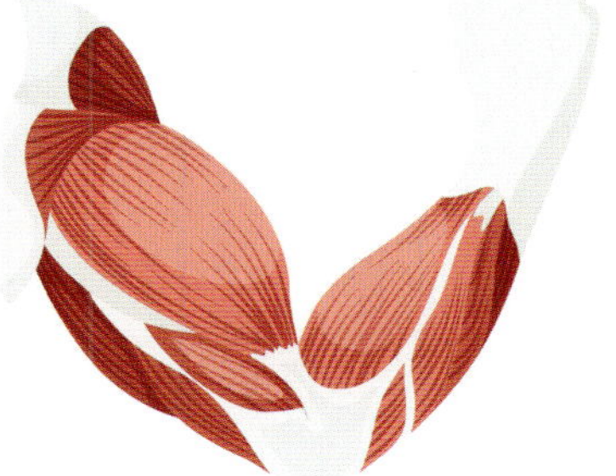

MUSCLES, EXERCISE AND GLUCOSE

Physical activity lets muscle cells absorb glucose without needing insulin. When we do activities such as walking, lifting or cycling, glucose is transported to the muscle cells even if insulin signalling is impaired. This is why exercise is so effective at lowering blood glucose – even for people with insulin resistance or diabetes.

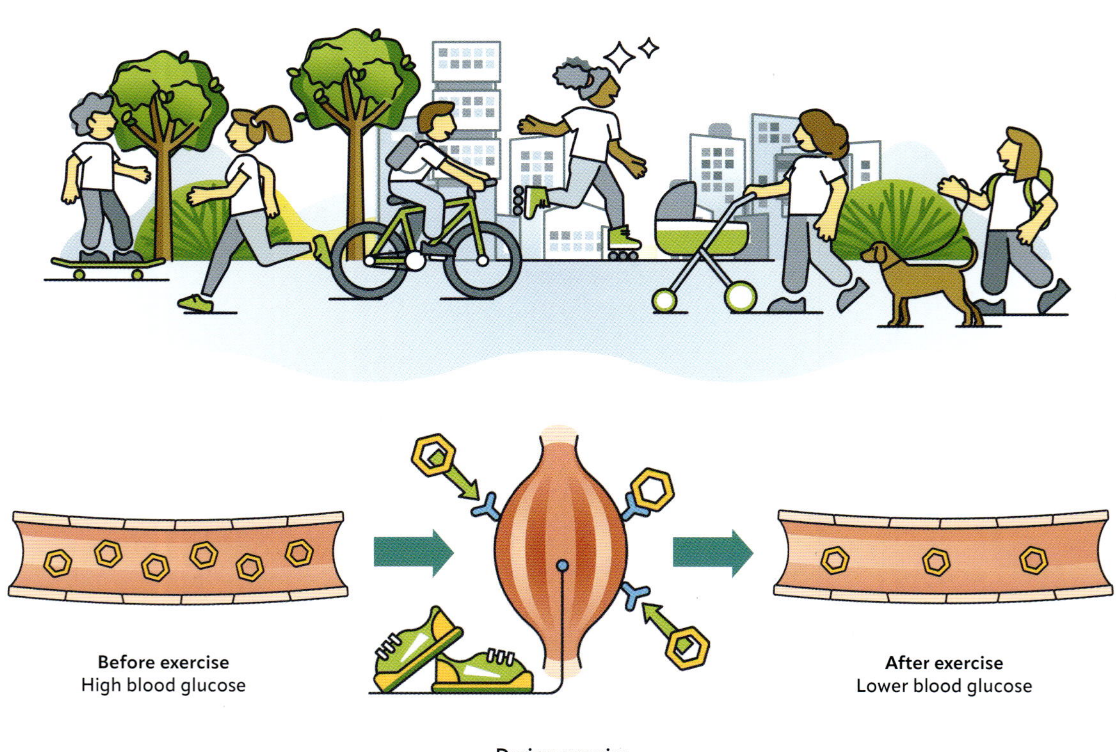

Muscles store some incoming glucose as glycogen. When the body needs energy, the muscles can break down glycogen, which in turn helps maintain blood glucose levels. Greater muscle mass means more tissue for disposing of glucose. This contributes to improved insulin sensitivity, lower fasting blood glucose and healthier HbA1c levels.

Strength training, in particular, builds muscle while also improving insulin's action in the body. When you are next walking or exercising, think of what is happening inside your body.

One of my primary focuses when helping clients lose weight
is to ensure I'm preserving their muscle. Losing muscle due to
aging, incorrect weight loss, inactivity or illness makes it harder
to clear glucose, making blood glucose harder to control. This is
an especially big concern for people with diabetes. Lower muscle
mass means higher blood glucose, more medications and greater
risk for complications.

But exercise doesn't just give short-term improvements.
Regular activity increases the capability and number of glucose
transporters, and it enhances our ability to generate energy
(mitochondrial function) and our insulin sensitivity.

So what are you waiting for?

If you don't already exercise, think of what kind of movement you
love. It could be swimming, running, dancing, Pilates, cycling,
power walking, rowing or hiking. Find what you love, make
it a regular part of your routine and think about why you are
exercising and how you are regulating your blood glucose – that's
what I do!

WHAT DOES A GLUCOSE SPIKE AND DROP FEEL LIKE?

People are often surprised when they find out what a glucose spike
feels like. The assumption is that it's a boost in mood, laughing, all
high on sugar but it's actually far from this. A glucose spike doesn't
feel good at all.

A blood glucose spike can feel like:

- increased thirst (dry mouth)
- frequent urination
- fatigue or feeling unusually tired
- blurred vision
- headaches
- difficulty concentrating or feeling foggy
- irritability, anxiety or restlessness.

TYPE OF DROP	SYMPTOMS
MODERATE DROP	• Feeling shaky, trembling or weak • Sweating, chills or clamminess • Hunger or nausea • Rapid or irregular heartbeat ('thumping' heart) • Dizziness, light-headedness or feeling faint • Headache • Tingling or numb lips, tongue or cheeks • Anxiety, irritability, impatience or nervousness • Moodiness • Difficulty concentrating, confusion • Blurred or double vision • Fatigue, drowsiness or lack of energy
SEVERE DROP	• Loss of coordination or slurred speech • Behaviour changes, confusion or acting strangely • Seizures or convulsions • Loss of consciousness (passing out)
NOCTURNAL (NIGHT-TIME) DROP	• Nightmares, sweating, or waking up confused or tired

HYPOGLYCAEMIA

A 'hypo' (short for hypoglycaemia) is when your blood glucose drops too low, falling below what your brain and cells need for energy. Hypos can be very serious. They are dangerous because our brain depends on a constant supply of glucose to function well. If your blood glucose dips too much, you can feel confused, dizzy or weak. You could lose consciousness or, in the worst case, have a seizure or even die. If left untreated, they can be increasingly difficult to notice, increase the risk of accidents and be dangerous to health.

Managing hypos is extremely important when you're starting a weight-loss program. Many of my patients with type 2 diabetes wear a continuous blood glucose monitor when they start the program to track their blood glucose levels.

LOSING WEIGHT AND HYPOS

To lose weight, you need to reduce your carbohydrate and calorie intake. If you are on antidiabetic medications or insulin, the body may be expecting your earlier elevated blood glucose, so without the carbohydrate intake, the medications can lower the blood glucose too far.

When people start exercising along with dieting, it can further lower blood glucose, increasing the risk of a hypo. As you lose weight, you should adjust your medication accordingly. The original dose may be too high for your new weight and food intake, making the blood glucose drop more rapidly.

- **Early symptoms.** Sweating, shakiness, hunger, blurred vision, feeling irritable, fast heartbeat and anxiety.

- **Severe symptoms.** Confusion, inability to concentrate, clumsiness, weakness, slurred speech, seizures and even unconsciousness.

MANAGING HYPOS

This is your top priority, especially if you are diagnosed with diabetes. First, you need to learn to recognise when a hypo is starting.

- My go-to for a hypo for my patients is fruit or honey. The guideline is to have 15 grams of carbohydrate – this will reverse hypoglycaemia quickly.

- Fruit provides fast-acting carbohydrates that are quickly absorbed into your bloodstream.

- Options include grapes, raisins, bananas, apples and oranges.

- Other options are orange or apple juice, glucose tablets or jelly beans, if fruit isn't available.

- Once the hypo has settled and resolved, have a small snack to prevent another drop, such as wholemeal bread or crackers.

Preventative steps:

- Wear a continuous blood glucose monitor or make sure you are monitoring your blood glucose well.

- Plan your meals.

- Keep on top of your diabetic medications, because you may need to adjust them on your weight-loss journey.

Learn to be aware of the symptoms and how to act quickly. Also stay in touch with your healthcare provider.

BLOOD GLUCOSE AND KETOSIS

Ketosis is a metabolic state in which our body burns fat for fuel instead of glucose. This can happen with dieting and fasting, but also with insulin resistance, because the body's cells are less responsive to insulin. This means there is a build-up of glucose in the blood, rather than it getting into the body's cells, and the body switches over to breaking down fat for energy.

Over time, insulin resistance can lead to lower insulin levels and the body can stay in ketosis, lowering the blood pH to an acidic level, known as ketoacidosis. This is seen in T1D. In T2D, insulin levels do decrease over time, but not to a level that causes the blood to become acidic.

Ketoacidosis is one of the big complications we see with diabetes – it can be life threatening.

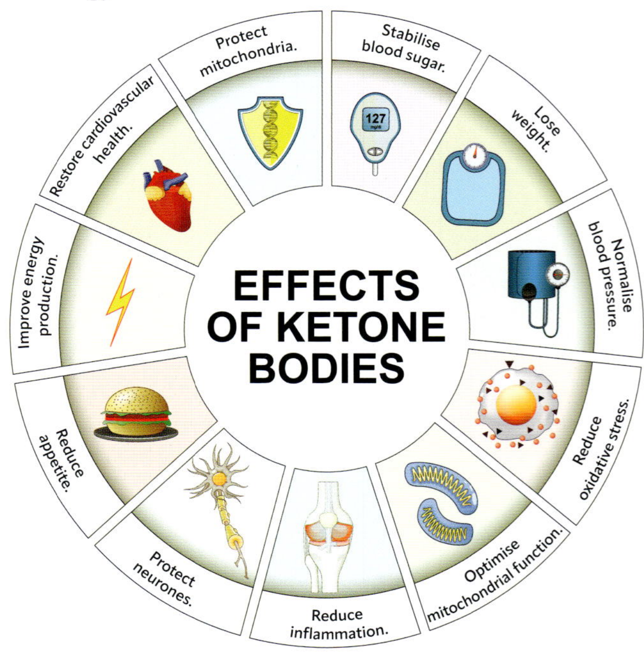

HARNESSING KETOSIS

As a practitioner, my favourite method for weight loss is to put the body into ketosis. I do this not with the traditional keto diet, but with The 10:10 Plan, which is a high-protein, low carbohydrate diet. There is something amazing about the feeling of being in true ketosis. You are getting a constant supply of energy, and you can feel so clear-headed, energised, motivated and positive. I love it!

How ketosis works in a few steps:

1. For whatever reason (insulin resistance, dieting or fasting), the body goes into ketosis.

2. Fat cells (triglycerides) are converted to ketones in the liver. The fat cells are first broken down into fatty acids and glycerol in a process called lipolysis.

3. The fatty acids are taken to the liver and undergo a process called beta-oxidation, where they are broken down into smaller units called acetyl-CoA. The acetyl-CoA is then converted into ketone bodies.

4. Ketones are released into the bloodstream and used as a form of energy. All body tissues and our brain can use ketones for energy.

WHAT ABOUT THE KETO DIET AND DIABETES?

People with T2D need to be careful following the traditional keto diet to avoid the risk of ketoacidosis. With my T2D patients, I do need them to have carbohydrates in their daily diet. I usually add half a banana or another carb of their choice.

The pancreas and diabetes

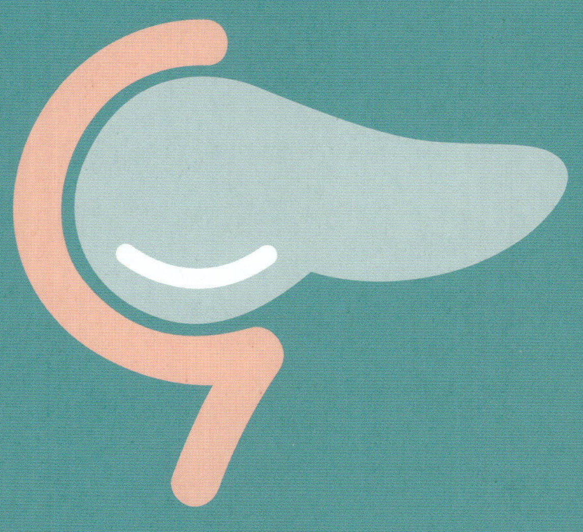

To really understand diabetes, you need to know about the pancreas, the organ at the core of diabetes. Our amazing pancreas is part of our digestive system. Its main roles are digestion and blood sugar regulation.

ANATOMY OF THE PANCREAS

The pancreas is a large organ located in the upper abdomen behind the stomach. It is surrounded by the gall bladder, liver, spleen, small intestine and stomach. Because it's deep in your belly, pancreatic disease is hard to diagnose; people often don't find out until it's too late.

The pancreas looks like a sweet potato in size and shape. I love how we can compare organs to fruit and vegetables. It has a somewhat bulbous head and neck, and a narrow body with a point at the end. Imagine it lying on its side – it's around 15 cm long, about the length of your hand. The outer layer of the pancreas has the texture of a corn cob, and it weighs about 92 grams – about the same as a small tin of tuna.

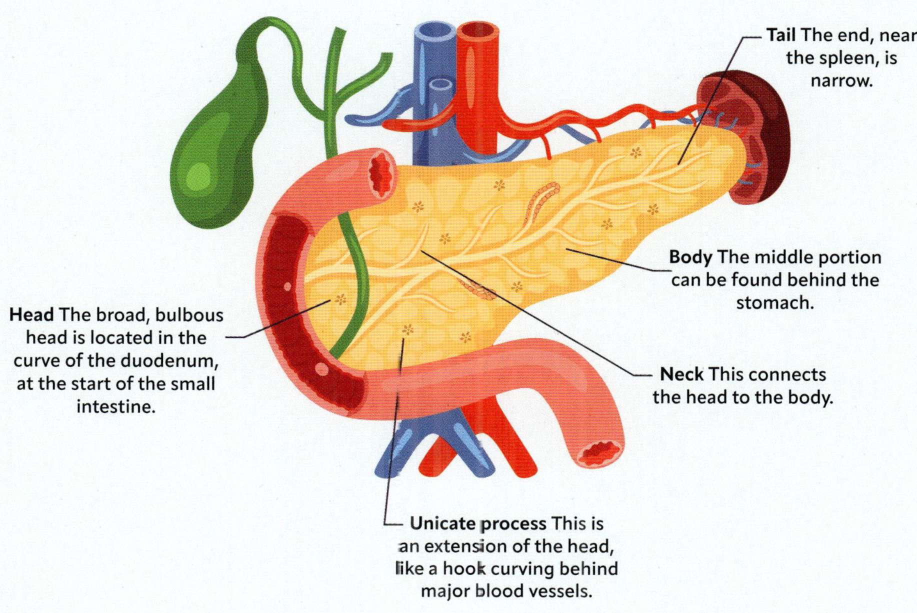

The pancreas has two duct systems:

1. **Main pancreatic duct** (duct of Wirsung): This runs through the pancreas, joining the common bile duct to drain digestive enzymes into the duodenum via the ampulla of Vater.

2. **Accessory pancreatic duct** (duct of Santorini): This is smaller and drains into the duodenum separately.

Main functions of the pancreas:

- **Digestion.** Making enzymes to break down food

- **Blood glucose regulation.** Producing hormones to regulate blood glucose – insulin and glucagon

- **Appetite.** Producing hormones that regulate appetite

- **Stomach acid stimulation.** Making hormones to stimulate stomach acids

- **Emptying the stomach.** Producing hormones to tell the stomach when to empty.

Think of the pancreas as a factory with two production lines: exocrine, making digestive enzymes such as lipase, proteases and amylase that break down the food in the small intestine; and endocrine, making hormones such as insulin to control sugar in your bloodstream, glucagon to help raise blood glucose, and somatostatin to help regulate digestion.

When our blood glucose is too high, the pancreas makes insulin to lower it, and when it's too low, the pancreas makes glucagon to increase it. The balancing of sugar is so important for our overall health but also to support other organs such as the brain, kidneys, liver and our heart.

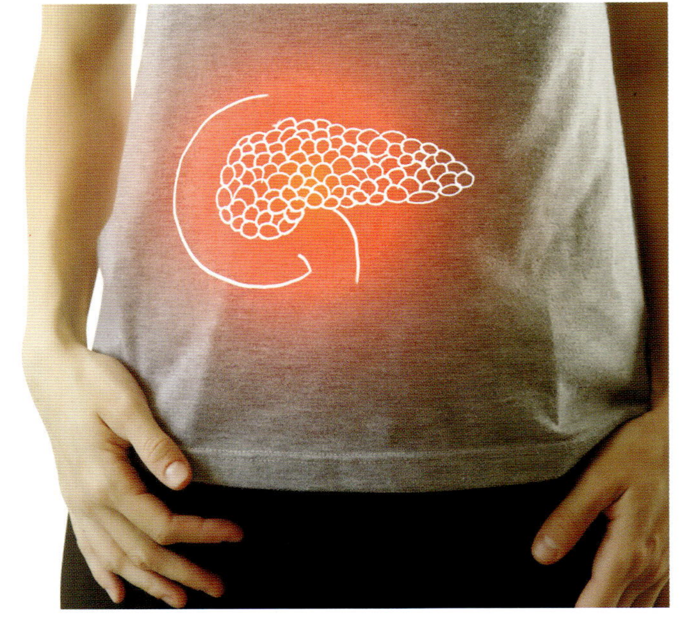

A SUPPORT FOR DIGESTION

Our pancreas makes 2–4 litres of enzyme-rich fluids daily – a lot of liquid when you really think about it. The amount depends on how much food you eat daily. Here is a snapshot of how food is broken down, so you can better understand the pancreas.

When food enters your stomach, the pancreas releases liquid into small tubes (or ducts) that flow into your main pancreatic duct. This connects with your bile duct, which moves bile (which is made in the liver and helps to break down fats) from the liver to your gallbladder. From the gallbladder, the liquid travels to the small intestine (duodenum). Then together, the bile and pancreatic liquids arrive in the duodenum to break down the food.

CONDITIONS AND DISORDERS THAT CAN AFFECT THE PANCREAS

- **Type 1 diabetes.** When your pancreas does not make enough insulin.

- **Type 2 diabetes.** When your body still makes insulin but it is not utilised correctly.

- **Hyperglycaemia.** This is when your body produces excess glucagon, resulting in high blood glucose.

- **Hypoglycaemia.** This is when there is too much insulin, causing blood glucose levels to drop.

- **Pancreatitis.** This is inflammation of the pancreas; it can be chronic or acute. Digestive enzymes become activated within the pancreas and cause tissue damage. Common causes are heavy alcohol use, gallstones, medications or genetic factors.

- **Pancreatic cancer.** Cancerous cells in the pancreas can be very difficult to detect and treat. The pancreas is called the 'silent' organ, because it doesn't show symptoms when something goes wrong and people don't usually find out until it is too late.

SYMPTOMS OF AN UNHAPPY PANCREAS

Here are some general symptoms of an unhappy pancreas:

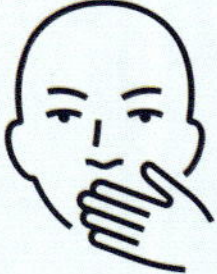 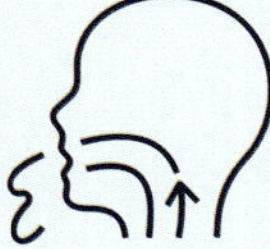

Unexplained nausea or vomiting

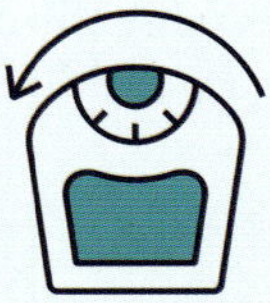

Unexplained weight loss

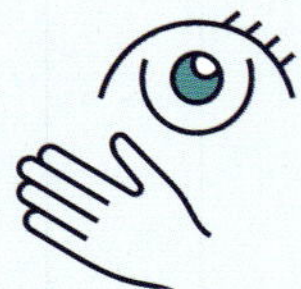

Jaundice (yellow eyeballs and skin)

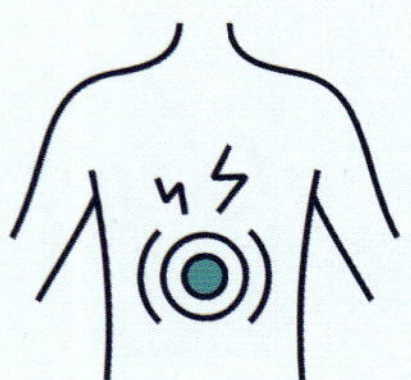

Back pain

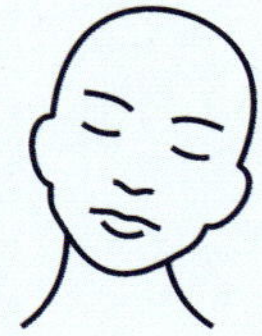

Fatigue

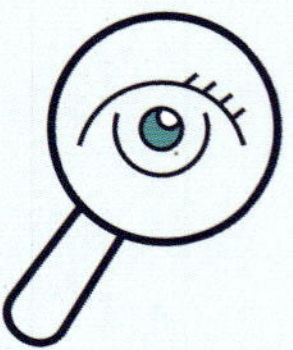

Blurry vision

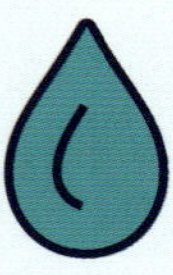

Thirst

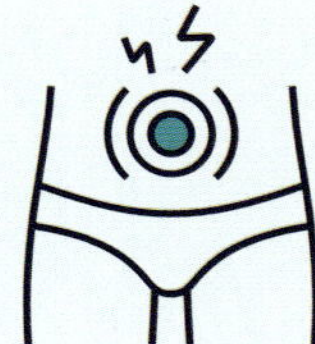

Abdominal pain

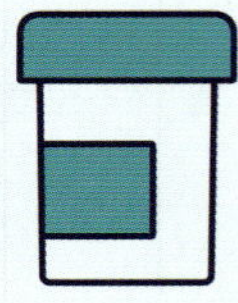

Dark urine

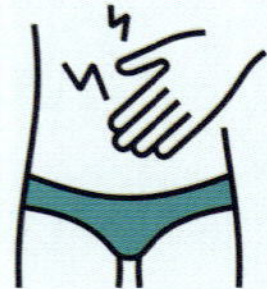

Frequent trips to the bathroom

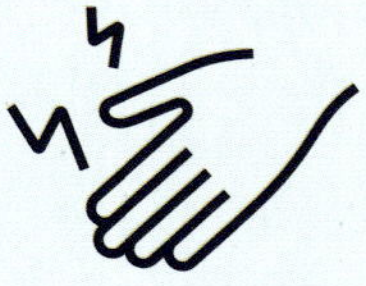

Tingles in the hands and feet

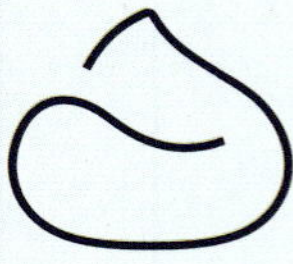

Light-coloured greasy stools (not your classic brown)

TESTING FOR PANCREAS HEALTH

Given the pancreas is deep in the abdomen, testing can be difficult. The options are:

- abdominal ultrasound
- blood tests
- endoscopic ultrasound
- angiography
- MRI (magnetic resonance imaging)
- CT (computed tomography) scan
- faecal elastase test (to determine if your pancreas is making digestive enzymes).

Some of the most common treatments for treating the pancreas include dietary changes; insulin replacement; medications; cancer treatments such as radiation, surgery and chemotherapy; and surgery. The first thing I tell my patients with pancreas issues is to stop drinking alcohol and change their diet.

Like our amazing liver, parts of the pancreas can be removed, and some people can even get a pancreatic transplant. Unlike the liver, however, the pancreas cannot regenerate. Removing a pancreas is extremely rare and would only ever happen if you had a massive injury, really severe pancreatitis or pancreatic cancer. If your pancreas was removed, you'd need to control your blood sugar for the rest of your life.

Other ways you can support your pancreas:

- **Get to and maintain a healthy weight for your height.** This will reduce your risk of type 2 diabetes and gallstones that cause pancreatitis.

- **Manage any medications.** Only take what you need and always get regular check-ups.

- **Reduce or ideally avoid alcohol.** Drinking alcohol increases your risk of pancreatitis and pancreatic cancer.

- **Stop smoking.** Smoking increases your risk of pancreatitis and pancreatic cancer.

- **Stay hydrated.** Aim to drink 30 ml per kilogram of your own body weight daily.

- **Eat smaller and more frequent meals.** Don't overload the pancreas.

- **Eat and live well.** Enjoy real wholefoods, do regular exercise, stress less and make sure you do regular annual check-ups.

BEST AND WORST FOODS FOR OUR PANCREAS

BEST FOODS	LIMIT SEVERELY (A COUPLE OF TIMES PER MONTH) OR IDEALLY AVOID
Lean protein – chicken, eggs, beans, lentils, tofu, turkey, fish and dairy. Make sure you have protein with every meal. A good guide is the size of your palm is your protein portion per meal.	**Fatty meats** – pork belly, beef brisket, duck.
Good fats – avocado, nuts, healthy nut butters, seeds, walnuts, fatty fish. Include fats daily. An easy way is to snack on nuts every day or add avocado to breakfasts or lunches.	**Fried foods** (the body struggles to digest these) – chips, fries, doughnuts, fried chicken.
Fruit and vegetables – think of the rainbow, lots of different types. Seasonal is best and aim for 3 cups leafy greens daily.	**Sugary, refined processed foods** – simple sugars such as pastries, cakes and biscuits, ice cream.
Whole grains – choose wholegrain products such as brown rice and oats.	Refined grains and white carbs – white bread, regular pasta, white rice and other low-fibre, highly processed grain products.
Fibre (something we don't get enough of) – fruit, vegetables, whole grains.	**Margarine**, mayonnaise and oily sauces.
Antioxidants – berries daily is amazing, plus the leafy greens.	**Alcohol.**

NUTRIENTS THE PANCREAS LOVES

Certain vitamins and minerals support the pancreas, helping it perform its digestive and hormonal functions effectively. The pancreas does not like processed foods, junk foods, soft drinks and excess alcohol. Supplements can help along the way for that extra boost, but healthy food is best. Aim for a balanced diet rich in lean proteins, complex carbohydrates, good fats, wholefoods, fruit and vegetables to give your pancreas the love it needs.

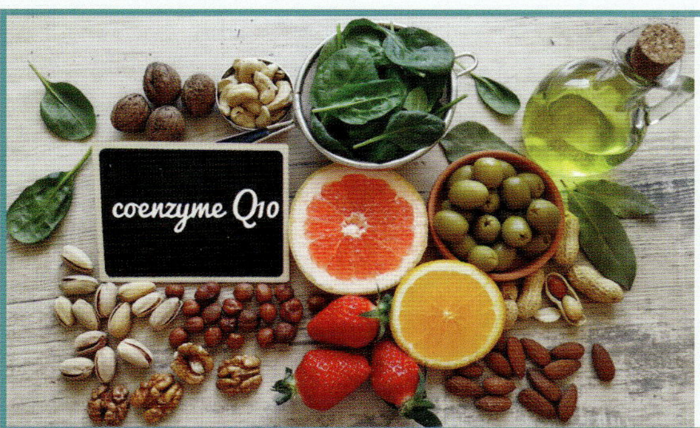

COENZYME Q10

This antioxidant helps protect the pancreas from oxidative damage. CoQ10 can also help with energy production. Research shows that it may help improve insulin sensitivity.

Sources: Greens such as spinach and broccoli, fatty fish, whole grains, organ meats such as liver

CHROMIUM

Chromium is a trace mineral that plays a role in insulin action, and carbohydrate, fat and protein metabolism. In people with poor insulin sensitivity or low chromium status, supplements may modestly improve insulin action and some blood-sugar-related markers, but it is not a primary treatment for diabetes, heart disease or weight management.

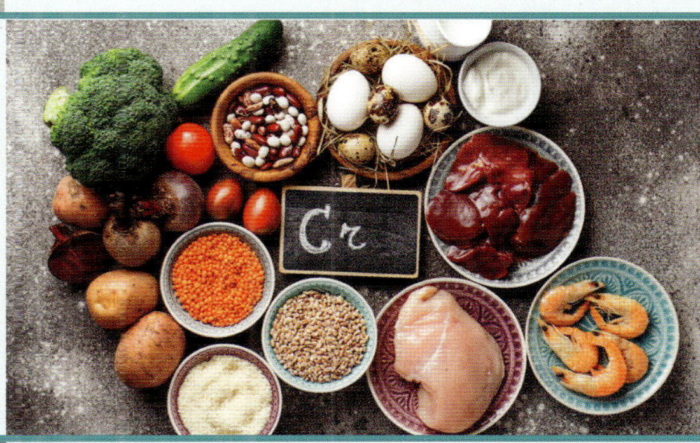

MAGNESIUM

Did you know that about 60% of Australians are magnesium-deficient? Magnesium is so important for enzymes in the pancreas to function properly, as well as blood glucose regulation. Magnesium deficiency can be linked to insulin resistance and type 2 diabetes.

Sources: Dark leafy greens, almonds, pepitas, cashews, legumes, whole grains

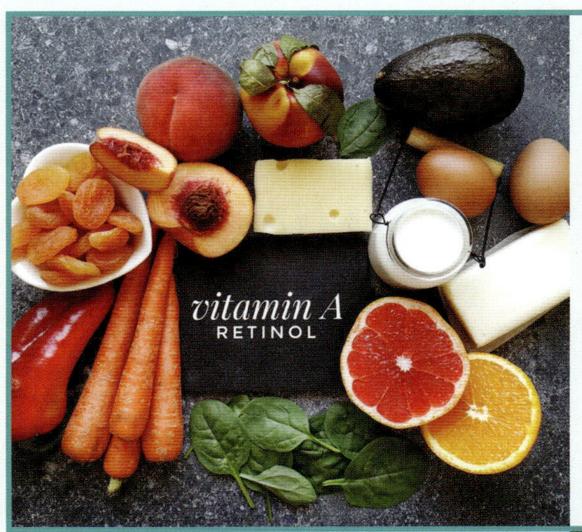

VITAMIN A

This vitamin supports immunity, which in turn protects the pancreas. Vitamin A is important for healthy cell function.

Sources: Carrots, sweet potato, kale, pumpkin, mango, rockmelon, spinach

VITAMIN B (B1, B3, B6, B12)

B vitamins are so important for energy. They support metabolic function; brain health; red blood cell formation; skin, hair and nails; heart health; immunity; and the nervous system. B1 helps with glucose metabolism, B3 supports insulin functioning, and B6 and B12 regulate blood glucose and can help reduce inflammation.

Sources: Meat, chicken, dairy, eggs, whole grains, organ meats, milk, bananas, potatoes, nuts, fish

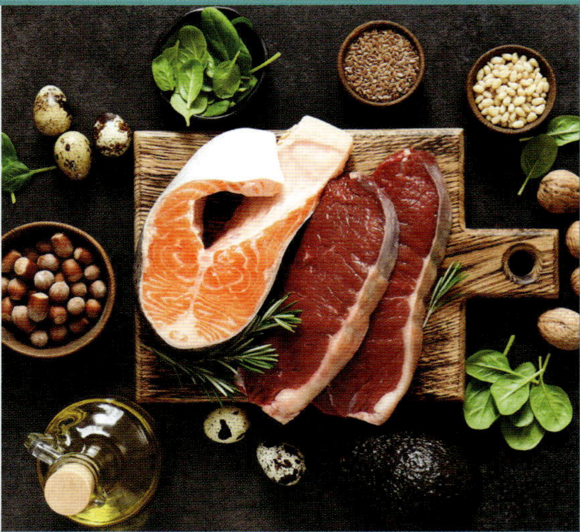

VITAMIN C

Not only is vitamin C amazing for our immune system, which most of us are aware of, it is also important for iron absorption and collagen uptake. Did you know that vitamin C is a powerful antioxidant that can protect the pancreas from oxidative stress? Oxidative stress damages cells, including the cells that produce insulin. Being involved in synthesising collagen and repairing tissues means vitamin C is excellent for the health of our pancreas.

Sources: Strawberries, guava, broccoli, capsicum, kiwifruit, lemons, oranges

VITAMIN D

This vitamin helps regulate insulin secretion and improve your sensitivity to insulin. Low vitamin D is linked to type 2 diabetes and a dysfunctional pancreas.

Sources: Egg yolks, sundried mushrooms, fortified dairy products, fatty fish such as mackerel and salmon

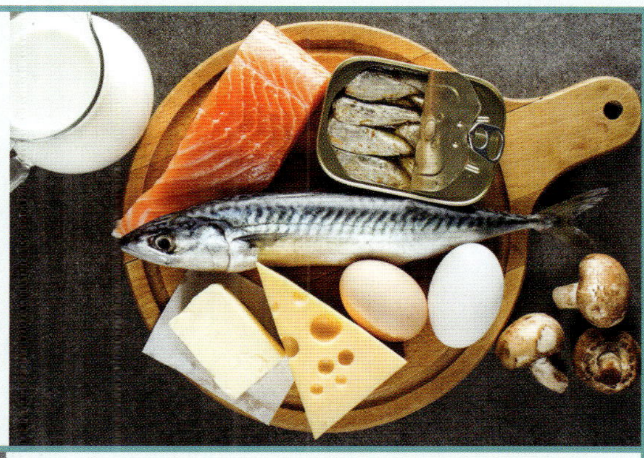

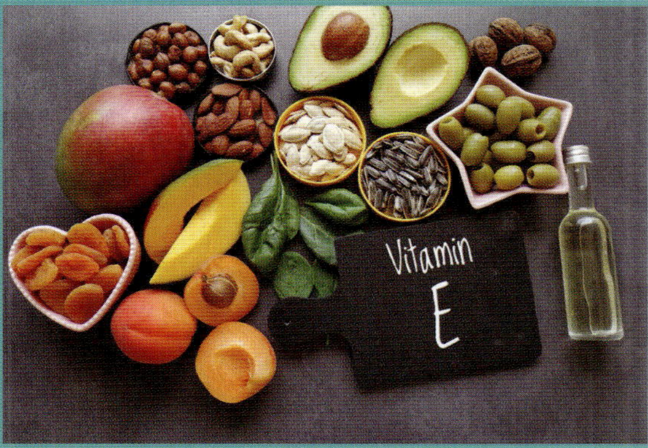

VITAMIN E

This antioxidant can help protect the pancreas from oxidative damage and can lower the risk of pancreatitis and pancreatic cancer.

Sources: Spinach, nuts, seeds, vegetable oils

ZINC

Zinc is so good for our immune system but also plays a role in the storage, synthesis and release of insulin in the pancreas. It can also lower inflammation and plays a role in pancreatic cell regeneration.

Sources: Meat such as pork and lamb, chicken (legs and thighs), oysters, beans, nuts, seeds, whole grains

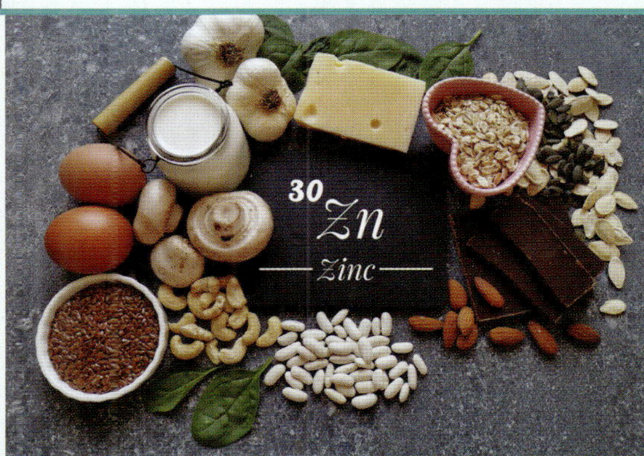

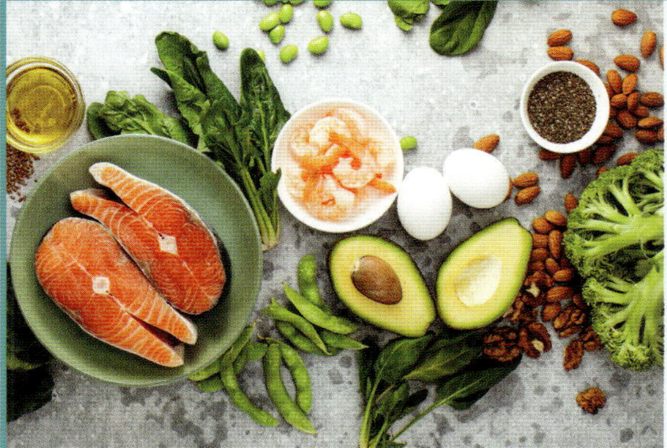

OMEGA-3 FATTY ACIDS

These fatty acids are anti-inflammatory, so lower inflammation in the pancreas.

Sources: Linseeds (flaxseeds), walnuts, chia seeds, fatty fish, cod liver oil

OXIDATIVE DAMAGE AND ANTIOXIDANTS

I use the words oxidative damage, free radicals and antioxidants a lot when writing. Here is what these terms mean.

OXIDATIVE DAMAGE

This occurs when the body's DNA, lipids, proteins and cells are damaged by free radicals.

Free radicals are highly reactive compounds that can damage the body's tissues and organs if left unchecked. These unstable molecules have unpaired electrons so they need to steal electrons from healthy cells to become stable. They are like scavengers destroying healthy cells in our body. This damages healthy cell membranes, proteins, lipids and the genetic material inside the cell. When free radicals exceed the body's ability to counteract them, oxidative stress and damage occur.

Sources of free radicals and oxidative damage include pollution, UV radiation, smoking, fatty and sugary diets, alcohol and stress as well as inflammatory diseases and chronic infections.

Oxidative damage in the pancreas can impair the function of the beta cells (insulin-producing cells), disrupt enzyme production, and increase inflammation. The health consequences can be diabetes, with the damage contributing to insulin resistance, as well as pancreatitis, cancer and organ aging, increasing the risk of chronic disease.

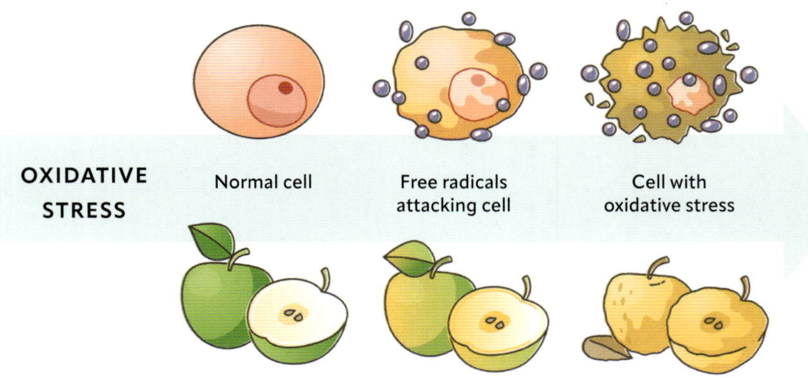

ANTIOXIDANTS

Our body naturally produces free radicals when cells are using oxygen to generate energy, but environmental factors also increase their production. Antioxidants are compounds that can neutralise free radicals by donating an electron to stabilise them. In this way, they reduce oxidative stress and protect the body from cellular damage.

Different types of antioxidants include vitamins A, C and E; minerals such as selenium and zinc; and phytonutrients (plant-based antioxidants) including flavonoids, polyphenols and lycopene. Enzymes such as glutathione, catalase and superoxide dismutase also have antioxidant properties.

Antioxidants have many health benefits: supporting immunity, delaying aging, preventing inflammation, and reducing the risk of chronic disease and skin disorders. Sources of antioxidants are berries, leafy greens, nuts and seeds, whole grains, herbal and green tea, dark chocolate, tomatoes, sweet potatoes, carrots, legumes and citrus.

HOW TO NEUTRALISE FREE RADICALS

Along with eating healthy foods, you can beat oxidative stress through exercising regularly, reducing exposure to toxins such as alcohol and smoking, sleeping well, and managing stress. Therefore, you're reducing your risk of chronic diseases such as diabetes, heart disease and cancer.

I love to get people thinking about their health from the inside, not just the outside.

With good nutrition, exercise, stressing less, sleeping well and living a healthy lifestyle, you improve the chances of your pancreas keeping up and supporting your journey to long-term good health and wellness.

FAT IN THE PANCREAS

Just like fat in our liver, fat build-up in our pancreas is harmful. It increases our risk of disease. Fat builds up because of insulin resistance and obesity. When the body consumes more energy than it can store in subcutaneous fat tissue under the skin, the excess dietary fat begins to accumulate in organs such as the liver, heart, skeletal muscle and pancreas. This is known as 'ectopic' fat deposition.

Called pancreatic steatosis, fat in the pancreas impacts the functioning and health of beta cells, which produce insulin and are essential for blood sugar regulation.

NAMING CONVENTIONS

Pancreatic steatosis is also known as 'non-alcoholic fatty pancreas disease', mainly due to its links to obesity, excess caloric intake and insulin resistance.

While non-alcoholic fatty liver disease (NAFLD) was renamed metabolic dysfunction–associated steatotic liver disease (MASLD) to remove stigma, sadly the same has not happened for non-alcoholic fatty pancreatic disease, which really needs to change. So I prefer to use terms like 'pancreatic steatosis' and 'fatty pancreas'.

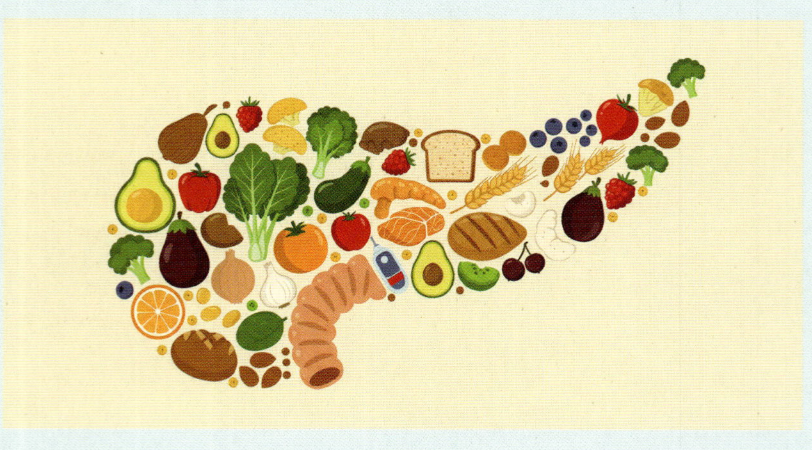

What a fatty pancreas does:

- **Lipid toxicity.** Too much fat in the pancreas can lead to lipid toxicity. Fatty acids damage beta cells, causing cell stress, inflammation and even the death of cells. This further reduces insulin cell production and speeds up diabetes progression.

- **Beta cell damage.** Beta cells are responsible for producing and releasing the hormone insulin, which regulates blood glucose levels. Pancreatic fat around beta cells can interfere with their ability to determine blood glucose levels and properly release insulin, leading to insulin resistance.

- **Inflammation.** Pancreatic fat also increases inflammation within the organ, further increasing insulin resistance and tissue scarring.

- **Poor blood glucose control.** High levels of pancreatic fat are linked to poor blood glucose control, loss of beta cell functioning and an increased risk of complications.

- **Exocrine and endocrine malfunction.** Fat in the pancreas impacts both its exocrine (enzyme) and endocrine (hormone) functioning. Fat accumulation in the islets of Langerhans (where beta cells produce insulin) contributes to cellular dysfunction, reduces insulin secretion and promotes beta cell death (apoptosis).

- **Adipokines.** Also called adipocytokines, these are bioactive signalling proteins secreted mainly by fat tissue that regulate metabolism, inflammation, appetite, insulin sensitivity and cardiovascular function by communicating with organs such as the liver, skeletal muscle, immune system and brain. In visceral obesity, adipose tissue becomes dysfunctional, with an altered adipokine profile that promotes insulin resistance and increase production of pro-inflammatory mediators, thereby contributing to metabolic and cardiovascular disease.

Other factors that cause fat to build up in the pancreas include genetics, cortisol, sex hormones, age and of course diet. Note that beta cell mass decreases with age.

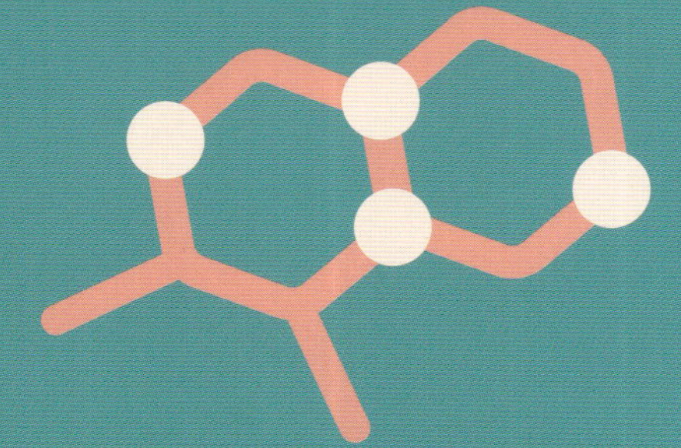

CHAPTER 6

Insulin and insulin resistance

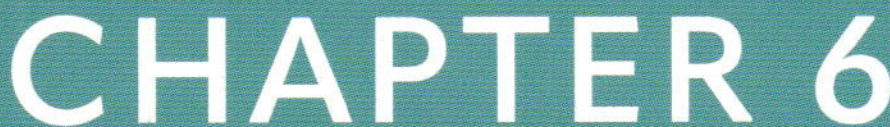

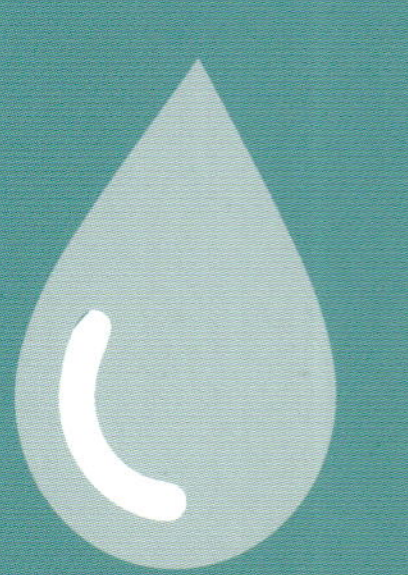

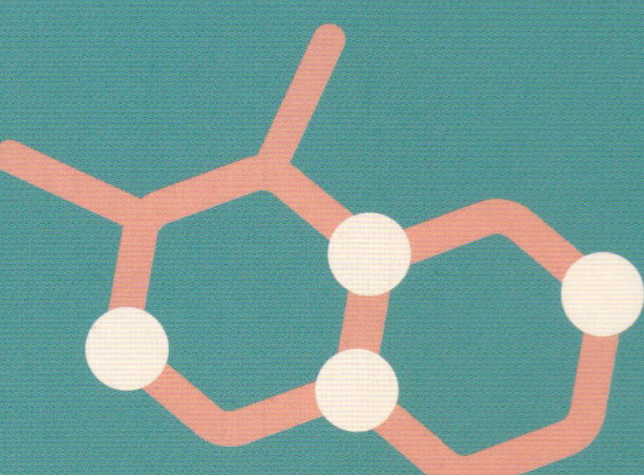

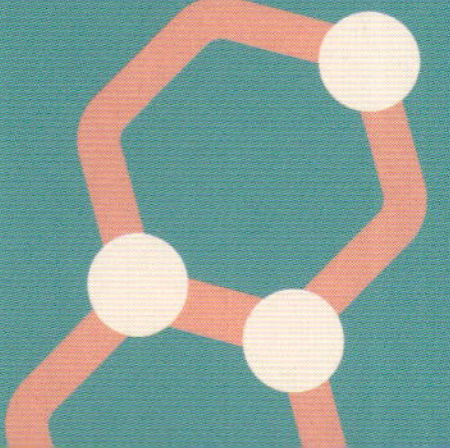

I've really been looking forward to writing this chapter. I want to share everything insulin and insulin resistance – the start of disease. If you can recognise the signs and symptoms of insulin resistance early, you can get on top of disease progression. Preventative medicine is the key.

Insulin is a real buzz word now in the health space. So many influencers and health experts throw the word around like they do protein! Insulin can have both a good and a bad reputation: good for managing our blood sugar, and bad for being the master fat-locking hormone. But like all hormones in our incredible human body, it has a very important role.

WHAT IS INSULIN?

Many people think of insulin as a medication used to treat diabetes but it's so much more than that. Insulin is a hormone produced by beta cells in the pancreas that controls blood glucose levels. Its main function is to transport glucose from the bloodstream into the body's cells, where it can be used for energy or stored for when needed. Think of insulin as a chaperone for glucose.

When we eat, our blood glucose rises, which triggers our pancreas to release insulin into our bloodstream. Insulin then signals the cells of our muscles, liver and fat to start absorbing glucose. When insulin binds to a liver cell, the liver cell makes fat, and when it binds to a muscle cell, the muscle makes protein. As the glucose is absorbed, our blood glucose returns to normal.

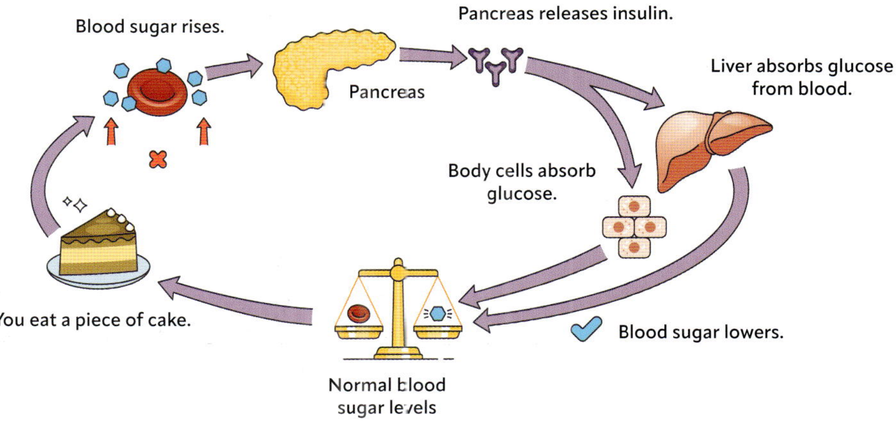

Our whole body needs insulin. Our brain needs glucose for energy and neuron growth, our ears use glucose to hear, our heart needs energy and blood pressure managed, and our muscles need to produce protein and energy. Our ovaries and testicles also need glucose for healthy hormone production, our bones use it for energy and growth, and our nerves need glucose for growth, repair and energy.

It makes you think about how important insulin is to our overall health.

Insulin is vital for maintaining our blood glucose levels and metabolising energy. The liver stores excess glucose as glycogen or fat in adipose tissues. In normal healthy functioning, this pathway stops the body from breaking down fat and protein. But when the body can't produce enough insulin, or our cells become resistant to it, our blood glucose stays elevated, causing type 2 diabetes.

THE ANABOLIC (BUILDING) HORMONE

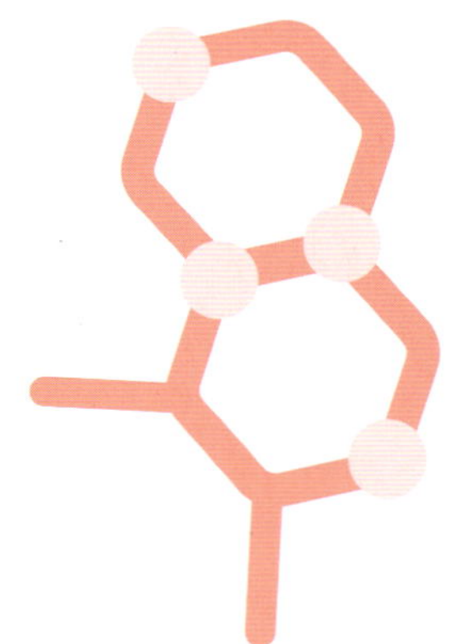

Insulin's major role is to ensure energy from food is efficiently used and stored, which makes it essential for growth, tissue maintenance and metabolic balance. It's often referred to as our main anabolic hormone because it supports the body's processes of building and storing energy, promoting the synthesis of large molecules from smaller ones. Specifically, insulin stimulates the uptake and storage of glucose, amino acids (protein) and fat (triglycerides) in adipose tissue while inhibiting their breakdown – hence the building hormone!

This means insulin also has a role in repair and growth because of its capacity to drive all the anabolic (building) processes – it does so much more than people think.

Insulin strongly influences tissue repair, growth and muscle building.

When our insulin is low, our body transitions to breaking down your stored fat and (if protein intake or energy availability is inadequate) muscle for energy. This contributes to weight loss. You need healthy levels of insulin for moving glucose and other nutrients into cells, supporting glycogen replenishment, and enabling muscle growth and repair. Insulin is a key building (or anabolic) hormone in human physiology.

With type 2 diabetes, this finely tuned process is disrupted. Cells become resistant to insulin's signal, so the body often will produce more insulin, yet it still struggles to store and use nutrients effectively.

INSULIN'S KEY ACTIONS

- **Insulin helps to build and store complex molecules in the body.** This helps cells grow, repair and store energy.

- **It helps muscle and fat cells to absorb glucose from the blood.** Glucose is stored as glycogen (in muscle and liver) or converted into fat (in adipose tissue).

- **Insulin increases the uptake of amino acids by cells.** It activates pathways that build proteins, supporting muscle growth and repair. It also influences protein metabolism throughout the body, supporting cell growth and survival.

- **It's the master fat-locking hormone. Insulin helps create fats from glucose (lipogenesis) and suppresses fat breakdown (lipolysis).** This encourages the body to store fat rather than release it for energy.

- **Insulin helps your body to use fat as energy.** Insulin is an anabolic hormone that helps your body manage energy. It regulates carbohydrate, lipid and protein metabolism and also influences immune function and brain function. In adipose tissue, insulin increases uptake and storage of fat and suppresses fat breakdown (lipolysis).

- **You need insulin for immune system and brain health.** Insulin regulates energy use and glucose uptake in some immune cells, and may play a role in learning and memory.

- **It helps your body regulate sodium and kidney function.** Research shows insulin sensitivity and resistance in immune, kidney and bone cells, making it a complex hormone.

HOW DO YOU MEASURE INSULIN?

You can have high insulin levels without having type 2 diabetes. Called hyperinsulinemia, the condition is most commonly associated with insulin resistance. Insulin resistance is where the body's cells don't respond well to insulin, so the pancreas produces more of it to keep blood glucose within a normal range.

With insulin resistance, the symptoms are really subtle at first: sugar cravings, struggling to focus, weight gain or fatigue. You can have insulin resistance for years before your blood glucose becomes abnormal, especially if you are overweight or obese, have other metabolic conditions, or have a rare genetic condition.

You can measure insulin through a fasting blood test and an oral glucose tolerance test. This is a good test to add to your annual check-ups; it's the earliest warning sign of future metabolic disease and a hallmark of prediabetes and insulin resistance.

HIGH INSULIN LEVELS DESTROY THE METABOLISM

Hyperinsulinaemia, or high blood insulin, damages our metabolism in so many ways and yet we never really think about this. High insulin really does set the stage for obesity, T2D, metabolic syndrome and just drives chronic disease.

Chronically high insulin signals the body to store more fat, particularly around the organs, instead of burning it, leading to central obesity (belly fat) and fatty liver. It also prevents the release of stored fat for use as energy and makes weight loss harder. This drives insulin resistance.

High insulin lowers blood sugar after meals, triggering hunger, sugar cravings and overeating, which compounds fat gain and metabolic dysfunction. It also raises blood pressure, which is dangerous for our heart health, and increases low-density lipoprotein (LDL) cholesterol, leading to fatty liver, cancer and autoimmune problems. The cells also become metabolically inflexible, leading to persistent low energy and feeling tired. This is because they lose the ability to switch between using glucose and fat as fuel.

Over time, elevated insulin impairs blood sugar regulation. The pancreas can't keep up production, so blood sugar elevates and the result is prediabetes.

High insulin levels sabotage the metabolism by driving fat storage, blocking fat-burning, raising sugar cravings, increasing blood pressure, skewing cholesterol, promoting inflammation, and setting the stage for diabetes and heart disease.

If you have diabetes, you already have coronary artery disease and the damage probably started in your 30s.

UNDERSTANDING INSULIN RESISTANCE

In 2025, about 1.5 million Australians have type 2 diabetes, which is driven by insulin resistance. The thing about insulin resistance, however, is that it begins around 10–15 years before you see a diabetes diagnosis. Slowly and silently, it causes metabolic and vascular damage. Cases of type 2 diabetes in Australia have tripled in the past 20 years. The exact prevalence for insulin resistance is unknown. With many cases going undiagnosed, up to 2 million Australians could have diabetes.

Globally, insulin resistance affects a substantial portion of adults. It's commonly estimated to affect from 20% to over 50% of the population, depending on age, region and risk factors. It is especially prevalent in older adults and those with obesity or prediabetes.

Up to 88% of people in the USA could have insulin resistance, with more than half not even knowing they have it.

WHAT IS INSULIN RESISTANCE?

There are several different kinds of insulin resistance. Most people get insulin resistance from poor diet and lifestyle choices, but some rare types are linked to immunity or genetics. The most common type is manageable, reversible and preventable.

- **Common type.** Most people with insulin resistance have it because they are overweight, don't exercise enough or have too much belly fat. It is linked to the progression to type 2 diabetes.

- **Genetic types.** Some people have rare, inherited problems in their bodies' insulin system, which make insulin work poorly.

- **Autoimmune type.** In rare cases, the body makes antibodies that block insulin from working properly.

Insulin resistance is the first step on the road to diabetes. Your body's muscle, fat and liver cells stop responding effectively to insulin. The cells fail to take up glucose and, in turn, the pancreas compensates by releasing more insulin. This leads to hyperinsulinemia, or high circulating insulin levels.

Over time, if insulin resistance is untreated and the pancreas can't keep up, the result is high blood sugar (hyperglycaemia) then prediabetes and type 2 diabetes.

Chronically high glucose levels can be deadly.

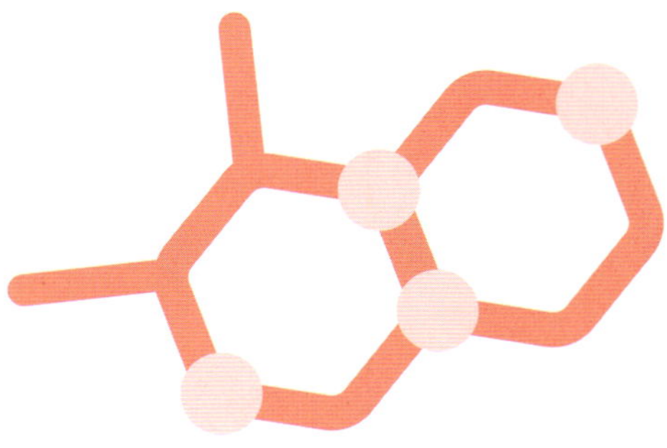

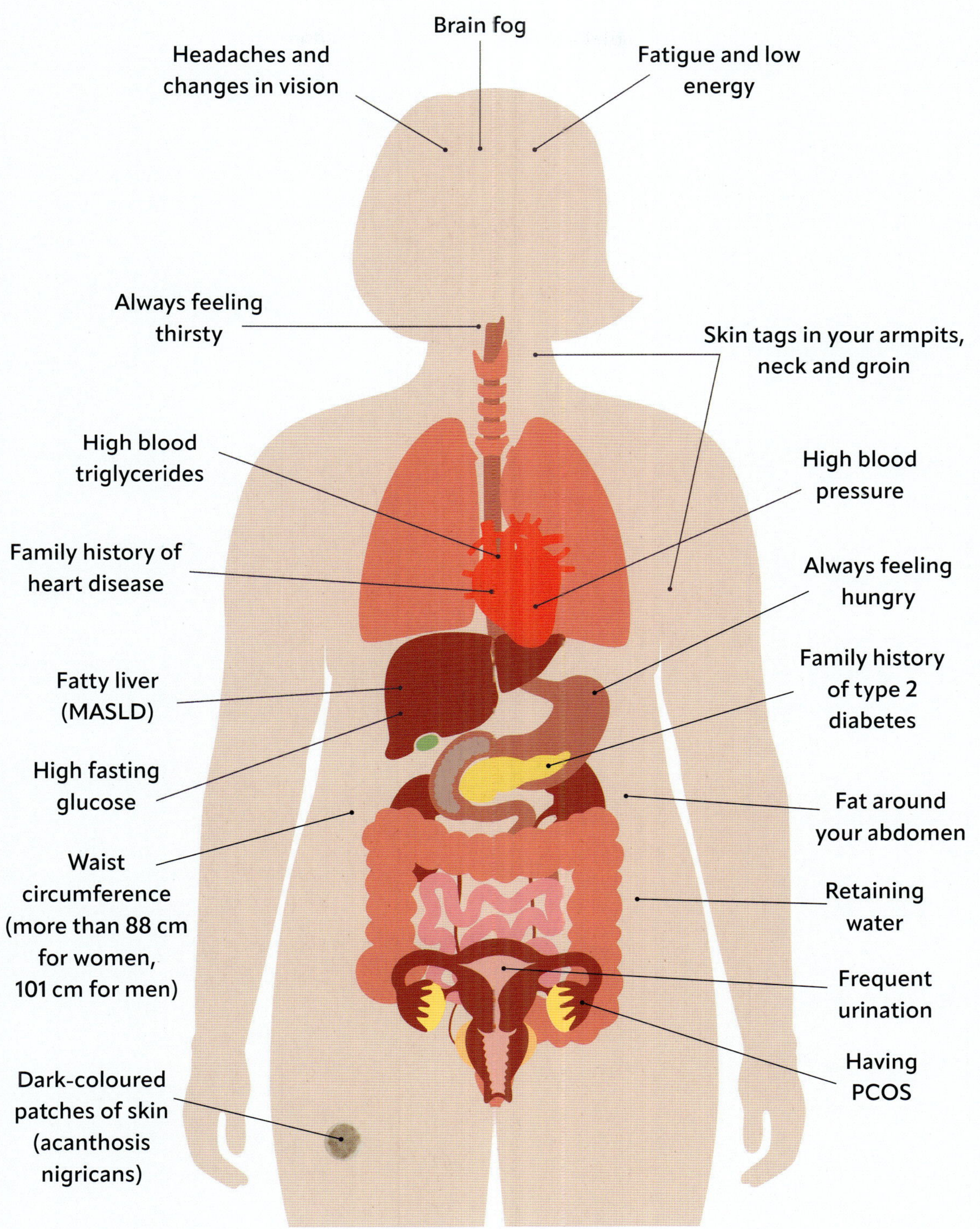

SIGNS YOU COULD BE INSULIN RESISTANT
Brain fog
Headaches and changes in vision
Fatigue and low energy
Always feeling thirsty
Skin tags in your armpits, neck and groin
High blood triglycerides
High blood pressure
Family history of heart disease
Always feeling hungry
Fatty liver (MASLD)
Family history of type 2 diabetes
High fasting glucose
Fat around your abdomen
Waist circumference (more than 88 cm for women, 101 cm for men)
Retaining water
Frequent urination
Having PCOS
Dark-coloured patches of skin (acanthosis nigricans)

WHAT HAPPENS WHEN YOU HAVE INSULIN RESISTANCE

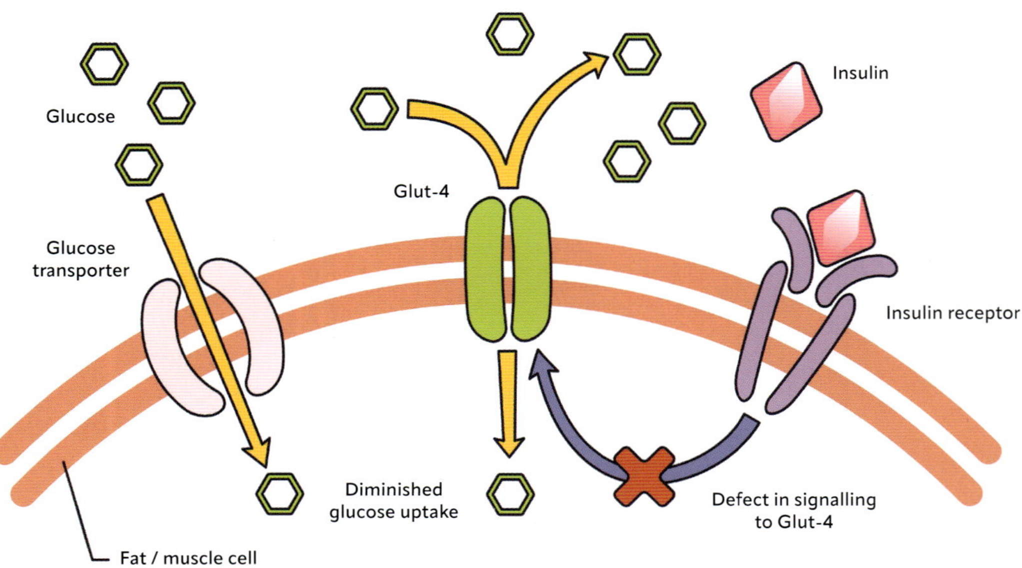

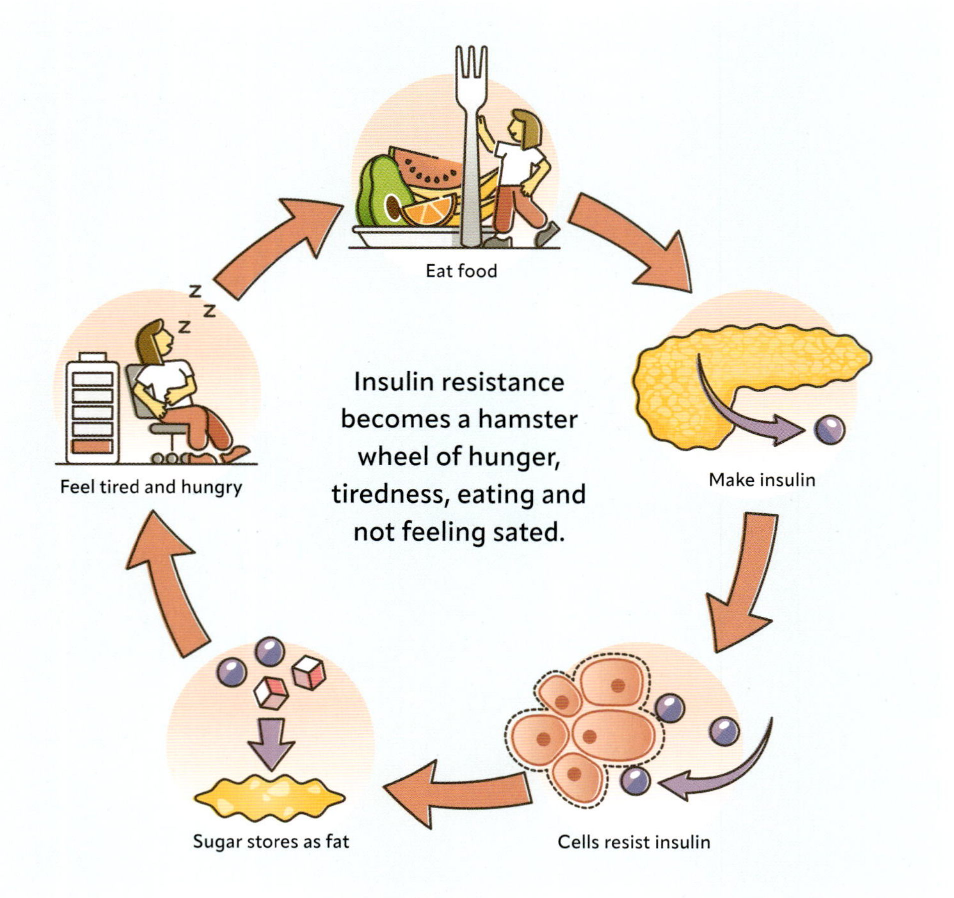

METABOLIC SYNDROME

Insulin resistance is a feature of metabolic syndrome, the name for a cluster of conditions that increase your risk of chronic kidney disease, stroke, type 2 diabetes and heart disease. Risk factors include:

- high triglycerides
- low HDL levels
- high LDL levels
- central obesity (abdominal fat)
- high blood pressure
- elevated fasting blood glucose.

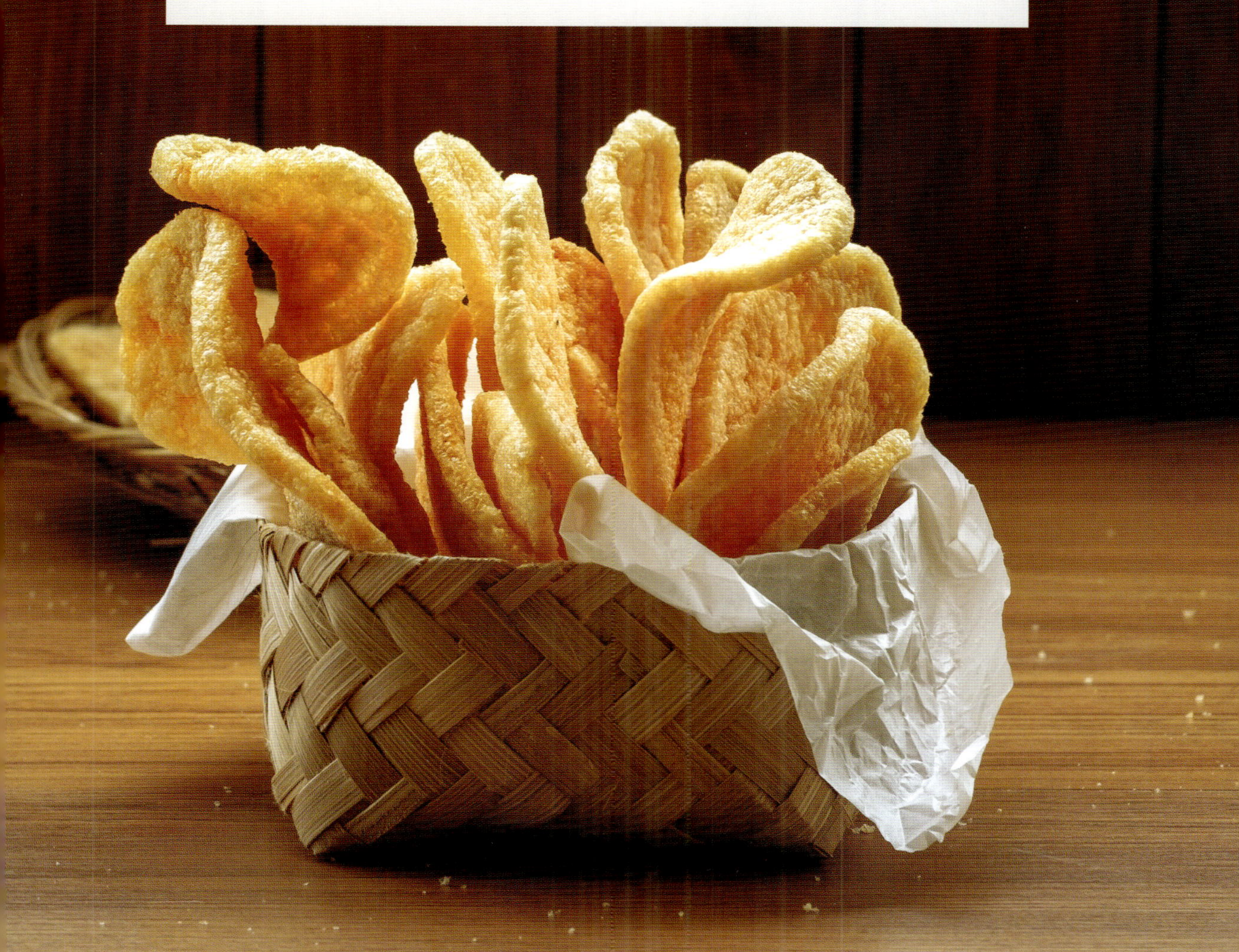

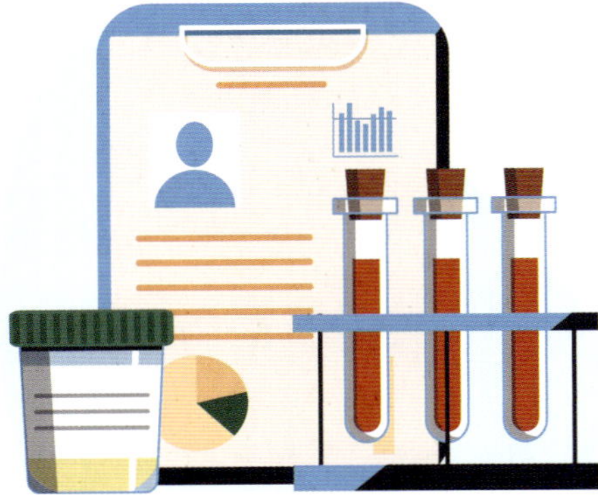

DIAGNOSIS

There is no single test to diagnose insulin resistance. Your doctor will check your:

- fasting glucose levels

- body's response to sugar via a glucose tolerance test

- haemoglobin A1c

- lipid profile (cholesterol and triglycerides).

You may need to wear a continuous glucose monitor.

Get a full check-up by your doctor, who will ask about your family and medical history, look at physical signs such as skin changes (like acanthosis nigricans), and perform blood tests. Your doctor will consider all the risk factors.

You cannot let insulin resistance go untreated.

The first step is to get to a healthy weight, exercise and change your diet to improve insulin sensitivity.

I have treated so many people with insulin resistance. It's hard in the beginning, you feel like you're pushing mud uphill, but perseverance is key. But once your body is healthy again, you can almost see it and it is amazing. In my clinic, I normally see a big change when the person has lost about 10 kg of fat.

INSULIN RESISTANCE AND DISEASE

Insulin resistance is linked to a range of diseases, such as metabolic, cardiovascular, endocrine, hepatic (liver) and neurological diseases. Causes can include metabolic syndrome, sedentary lifestyle, inflammation, family history, abdominal fat and genetics.

TYPE 2 DIABETES

Insulin resistance is the first step on the path towards T2D. The associated complications of insulin resistance and T2D are retinopathy (damage to the eyes that eventually destroys vision), nephropathy (kidney disease), neuropathy (damage to the nerves) and cardiovascular disease.

METABOLIC SYNDROME

This is a cluster of heart disease risks (high cholesterol, high blood pressure, low HDL, high LDL, abdominal fat, elevated fasting blood glucose), which are all underpinned by insulin resistance.

CARDIOVASCULAR (HEART) DISEASE

Insulin resistance is a risk factor for heart disease, including stroke, heart attack and coronary artery disease. Insulin resistance drives chronic inflammation, high cholesterol and high blood pressure. It also causes atherosclerosis (the narrowing and hardening of the arteries), which leads to stroke, heart attack and artery disease. Even without diabetes, insulin resistance is a strong driver for cardiovascular disease.

MASLD (FATTY LIVER DISEASE)

MASLD is linked to insulin resistance, especially in those who are overweight or obese. Insulin resistance increases the circulation of free fatty acids. Over time, these deposit in the liver, starting the progression of liver disease.

PCOS

This condition is the most common cause of infertility in women. It is characterised by irregular periods, excess male hormones, hirsuteness, thickening of the waist and polycystic ovaries.

Most women with PCOS will be resistant to insulin. When elevated, insulin will stimulate the production of too much ovarian androgen, affecting the reproductive system and increasing the risk of heart disease, T2D and being overweight.

HIGH BLOOD PRESSURE (HYPERTENSION)

Insulin resistance and high blood pressure go hand in hand. Insulin resistance leads to stiff arteries, causes the kidneys to retain sodium and creates endothelial dysfunction (where the inner lining of the blood vessels does not function properly). All this causes hypertension.

DYSLIPIDAEMIA (ABNORMAL FAT LEVELS IN THE BLOOD)

Insulin resistance changes the metabolism of lipids (fats), leading to high triglycerides, increased LDL and lower HDL. This is a driver for heart disease, in particular atherosclerosis.

EXCESS WEIGHT (OBESITY)

Excessive weight gain, especially around the abdomen, is worsened by insulin resistance. This, in turn, drives fat storage. Insulin resistance is closely related to the hormones ghrelin and leptin, which regulate our hunger, metabolism and energy. Fat distribution matters more than total fat mass too: visceral fat is metabolically active in ways that promote insulin resistance.

CHRONIC KIDNEY DISEASE

Insulin resistance is now recognised as a risk factor for kidney disease. Both are included in metabolic syndrome. Insulin resistance contributes to kidney disease by causing inflammation and high blood pressure – you can really see the cycle.

ALZHEIMER'S DISEASE (TYPE 3 DIABETES)

A lot of research suggests that insulin resistance can drive Alzheimer's disease. The chronic inflammation underpinning insulin resistance drives the decline in cognition and neurodegeneration.

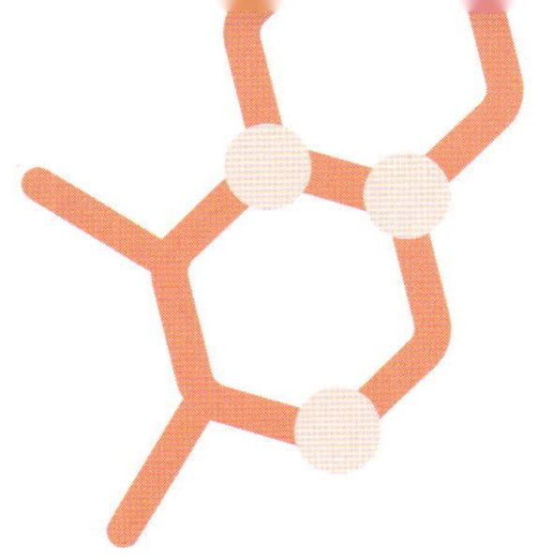

HORMONES AND INSULIN RESISTANCE

Hormones can influence how effectively our body responds to insulin.

- **Oestrogen.** This hormone is important for our insulin sensitivity. Oestrogen improves our sensitivity to insulin by helping our cells better respond to it.

- **Progesterone.** While the role of progesterone is nowhere as significant as oestrogen in its impact on insulin resistance, it's important because it balances with oestrogen.

- **Testosterone.** Insulin resistance is linked to lower testosterone secretion, which implies that testosterone supports insulin function and glucose metabolism. Women have testosterone in much smaller amounts than men, but it still contributes to our metabolic regulation.

- **Cortisol.** Hormones such as cortisol can worsen or even cause insulin resistance by increasing blood sugar, and can interfere with insulin signalling.

Our hormone–insulin interactions shed a light on why hormonal changes during different life stages can impact our metabolic health.

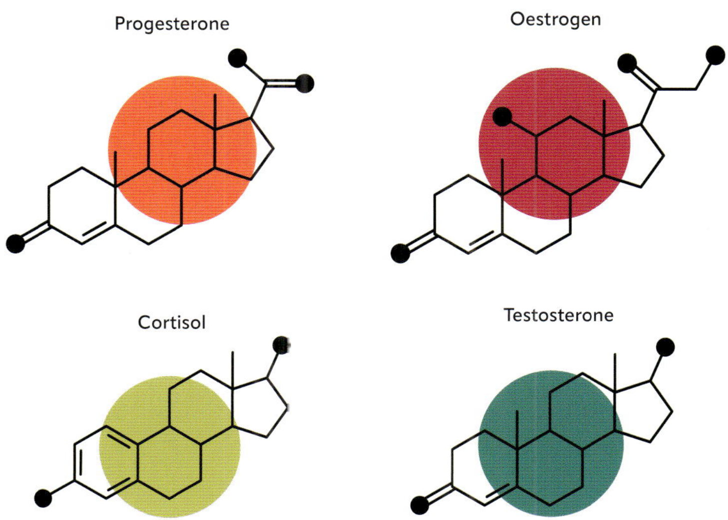

HORMONES AND THE MENSTRUAL CYCLE

Insulin, oestrogen and progesterone are closely interconnected in how they affect metabolism and insulin sensitivity throughout the menstrual cycle, during menopause, or when undertaking hormone therapy.

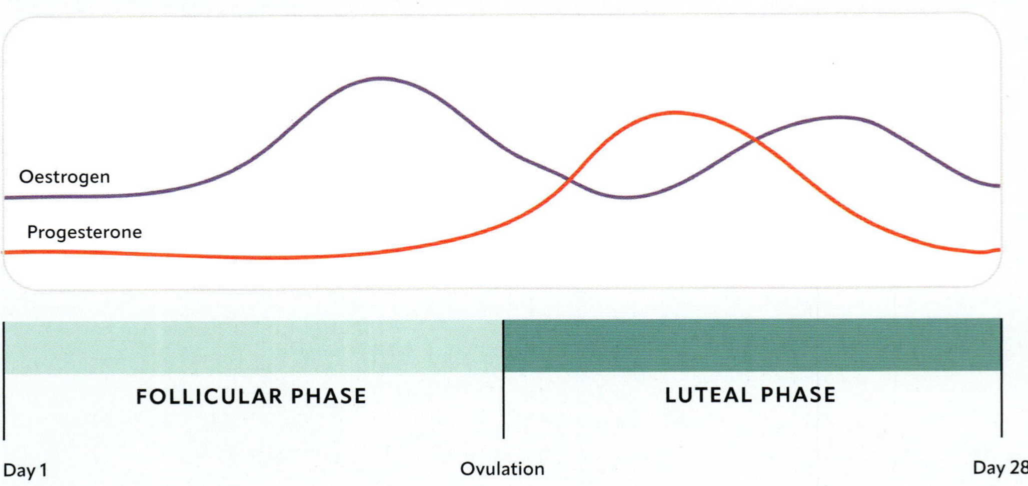

OESTROGEN	PROGESTERONE
Oestrogen helps the body use insulin more efficiently. Higher oestrogen levels, such as during the follicular phase of the menstrual cycle, are associated with better glucose metabolism and lower insulin resistance. Low oestrogen levels (such as after menopause) can lead to decreased insulin sensitivity and a higher risk of developing insulin resistance and metabolic issues. This is one of the many reasons why postmenopausal women struggle with their weight.	Progesterone tends to increase insulin resistance, especially during the luteal phase of the menstrual cycle, when its levels are high. This hormone can hinder insulin's action on tissues such as fat and muscle, which may cause higher post-meal blood glucose and less efficient glucose uptake. High progesterone often makes blood glucose control more difficult, which can be observed in both natural menstrual cycles and with some hormone therapies.

Now you can see why female weight can fluctuate over the course of the menstrual cycle. Higher estrogen in the follicular phase improves insulin sensitivity, while higher progesterone in the luteal phase reduces it, making blood sugar harder to control at that time.

MENOPAUSE AND INSULIN RESISTANCE

Oestrogen levels decline during menopause; this is linked to insulin resistance. The decreasing oestrogen makes the body less responsive to insulin, thus increasing the risk of insulin resistance as well as type 2 diabetes, heart disease and other chronic non-communicable diseases.

The decline of oestrogen in menopause reduces our sensitivity to insulin, leading to a higher blood glucose and insulin resistance. Menopause is also linked to having more visceral and abdominal fat. This is partly due to lower levels of adiponectin, a protein that helps improve our sensitivity to insulin.

Hormone replacement therapy (HRT) can help reduce insulin resistance and improve metabolic health, but my biggest bit of advice is when going through menopause is to manage your diet and lifestyle choices. Make sure you're exercising regularly and eating well to help manage insulin resistance. This is what I am doing with huge success.

INFLAMMATION AND INSULIN RESISTANCE

Insulin resistance is closely related to chronic inflammation, which has a big impact on the progression and development of insulin resistance, especially if you have type 2 diabetes. Chronic inflammation, especially in fat tissue, produces too many chemical messengers called pro-inflammatory cytokines. These chemicals mess with the way insulin works by blocking the signals that tell cells to take in glucose from the blood. This disruption happens in places like fat tissue, the liver and muscle cells, making them more resistant to insulin.

- **Fat (adipose) tissue is a huge contributor to inflammation.** Within the adipose tissue, fat cells and immune cells such as macrophages release inflammatory cytokines in response to excess nutrient intake and obesity. This creates a vicious cycle of inflammation and an impaired insulin response.

- **Stress switches on inflammation.** When certain immune sensors in the body (such as Toll-like receptors) detect stress or damage, they can switch on inflammation. This produces harmful molecules that can block insulin from working properly.

- **Oxidative stress makes inflammation worse.** High blood glucose and fat levels in the blood add to this problem by creating oxidative stress, which damages cells and results in even more inflammation. This combination not only makes the body resistant to insulin, but can also harm the beta cells in the pancreas that make insulin, so they produce less of it.

- **It becomes a vicious cycle.** Inflammation causes insulin resistance, and insulin resistance causes more inflammation, a cycle that progressively damages your blood glucose control.

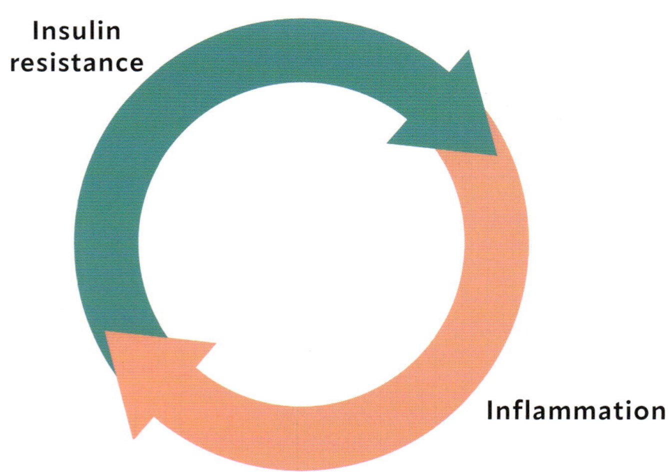

Inflammation causes insulin resistance mainly through pro-inflammatory cytokines and activated immune pathways that disrupt insulin signalling and beta cell function. This inflammation–insulin resistance cycle is central to the development of type 2 diabetes and other metabolic diseases.

Certain lifestyle factors will increase insulin resistance:

- **Having a poor diet.** If you eat a lot of highly processed foods, sugary drinks, refined carbohydrates and bad fats, you'll get continuous spikes in blood sugar, impacting insulin production and function. It's so important for your diet to be rich in healthy wholefoods, whole grains, vegetables and lean proteins.

- **Not exercising regularly.** Lack of physical activity reduces the muscles' uptake of glucose, making the muscle cells less responsive to insulin. Exercise improves the function of insulin.

- **Having too much body fat.** Visceral (abdominal) fat has a strong link to insulin resistance because it releases inflammatory substances that interfere with the insulin signalling.

- **Smoking.** Tobacco use is linked with an increased risk of insulin resistance.

POOR SLEEP AND INSULIN

Sleep is so important! When we don't sleep enough, our body produces more inflammatory markers such as C-reactive protein, which interfere with the insulin's ability to work effectively.

I always tell my patients to test C-reactive protein levels annually to watch for any trends.

Sleep deprivation disrupts the hormones cortisol and catecholamines, which regulate metabolism and insulin sensitivity. Lack of sleep causes higher blood glucose and fat levels in the blood, creating oxidative stress (which is the body's natural defence system not being able to keep up). This damages the cells responsible for insulin production and action. This will then decrease the sensitivity to insulin in the muscles and liver, which means glucose is not taken up efficiently.

The loss of sleep can also impair beta cells in the pancreas, which will secrete less insulin and – you probably guessed it – worsen blood glucose control. A vicious cycle takes place where insulin resistance triggers more inflammation and inflammation disrupts the function of insulin.

Chronic poor sleep or sleep deprivation triggers inflammation, hormone imbalances, oxidative stress and metabolic disturbances that make insulin less effective, increasing the risk of insulin resistance and type 2 diabetes. Sleep is so important for healthy insulin functioning and glucose metabolism.

How much sleep do you need?

7–9 hours a night – this is how much sleep an adult needs.

CHRONIC STRESS AND INSULIN RESISTANCE

Stress increases our resistance to insulin primarily through inflammation and oxidative stress. The hormone cortisol is raised when you have ongoing (chronic) psychological stress. Too much cortisol can increase inflammation and oxidative stress, which are linked to insulin resistance. Oxidative stress damages insulin-producing beta cells in our pancreas, reducing insulin production and making us more resistant to insulin.

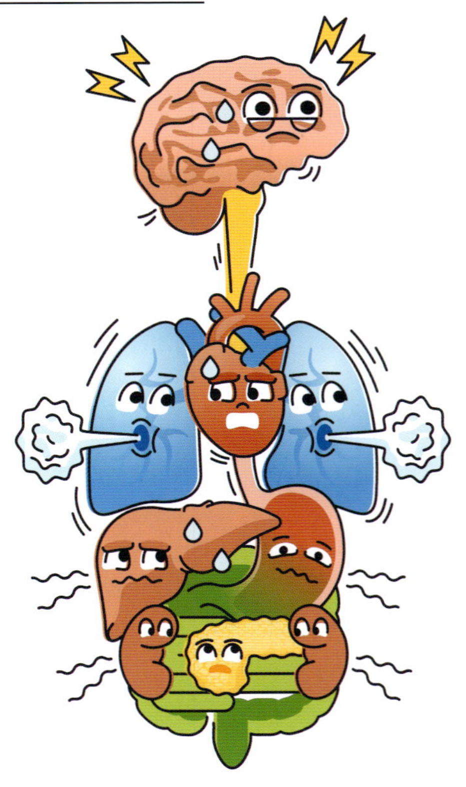

MEDICATIONS AND INSULIN RESISTANCE

Some medications such as corticosteroids and beta blockers can worsen insulin action:

- **Corticosteroids** (such as prednisone) can make it harder for insulin to work. They block the signals insulin uses to move glucose into cells, making your body store more fat around the belly. They can also raise blood sugar levels and, if used for a long time, may cause diabetes in some people.

- **Beta blockers** (used for heart problems and high blood pressure) can sometimes make insulin less effective. They may slow the flow of blood to muscles, so those muscles take in less glucose, and they may also reduce the amount of insulin your body releases. Some newer beta blockers don't have this problem.

A lot of people take unnecessary medications, and I also work with patients to reduce their medications. Taking something you don't need can be dangerous to your health.

Make sure you're only taking the medications you need.

Many of my patients and people on my programs find they can reduce or remove some medications as they reach their health goals and a healthy weight. So please always check with your healthcare provider whether you need medications and always review them.

INSULIN AS A MEDICATION

People need to take insulin as a medication when their body either cannot make enough insulin or cannot use insulin to control blood glucose levels. This happens mainly in the following types of diabetes:

- **Type 1 diabetes.** The pancreas stops making insulin because the body's immune system attacks the insulin-producing cells, so people must take insulin to survive and manage their blood glucose levels.

- **Type 2 diabetes.** The body becomes resistant to insulin or doesn't make enough insulin over time. When lifestyle changes and other medications aren't enough to control blood glucose, people may need insulin injections to help bring blood glucose into a healthy range.

Taking insulin as medicine helps move glucose from the blood into the body's cells for energy, preventing high blood glucose and serious complications such as heart problems, kidney damage and nerve issues.

EXERCISE AND INSULIN RESISTANCE

I love this! Exercise is absolutely medicine. In all my treatment plans, exercise is essential. It's the key to quality of life, mental health, longevity and, yes, reducing insulin resistance.

Exercising helps your body use insulin better, especially in the muscles. When you exercise, your muscles take in more glucose from your blood, even without insulin. After exercising, your insulin sensitivity stays higher for many hours, meaning insulin works more effectively to control your blood glucose.

Here's how muscle regulates your blood glucose. Muscle takes in glucose from the blood through the action of the glucose transporter protein GLUT4, which moves to the muscle cell surface in response to insulin or muscle contractions, allowing glucose to enter muscle cells for energy or storage.

Exercise also helps reduce visceral fat (which releases substances that drive insulin resistance). Losing this fat by being active makes your cells respond better to insulin. Both aerobic exercises (such as walking, cycling) and resistance exercises (such as weightlifting) can improve insulin sensitivity by different mechanisms.

Even a single session of moderate exercise can increase your muscles' glucose uptake by about 40%, and regular exercise improves your insulin sensitivity over time. This makes exercise an effective way to prevent or manage type 2 diabetes and related health problems.

So think about what exercise you could do. I tell my patients to find something they love – it could be hiking, bushwalking or dance classes – and to just move and get their heart rate up. Aim for at least 30 minutes per day of cardiovascular exercise and do resistance training around three times a week.

30 minutes a day – your target for cardio exercise.

BENEFITS OF EXERCISE

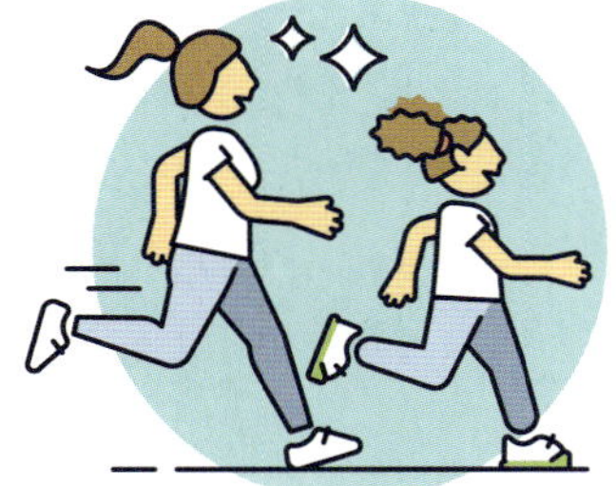

Improved functional mobility

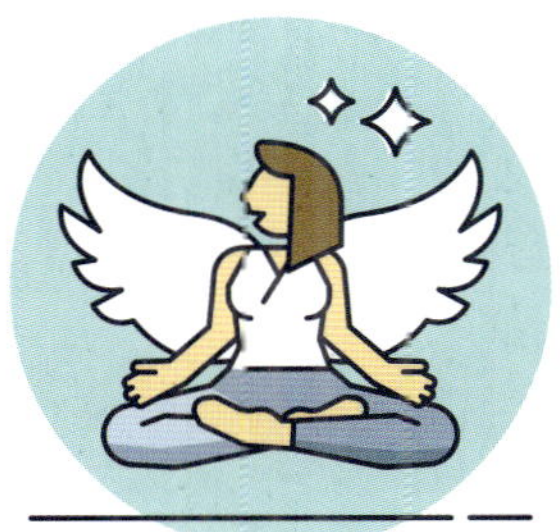

Stress and anxiety relief

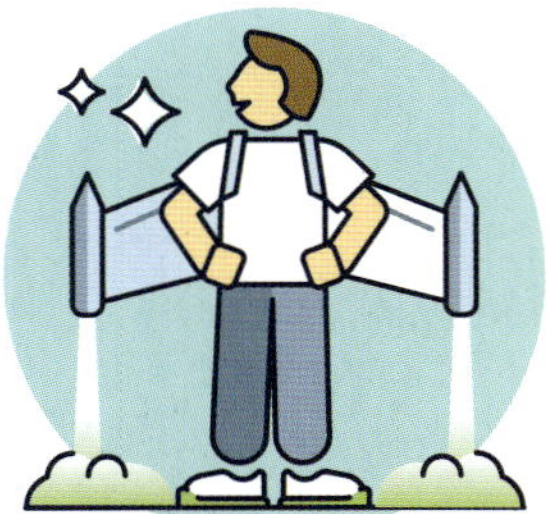

Increased energy levels

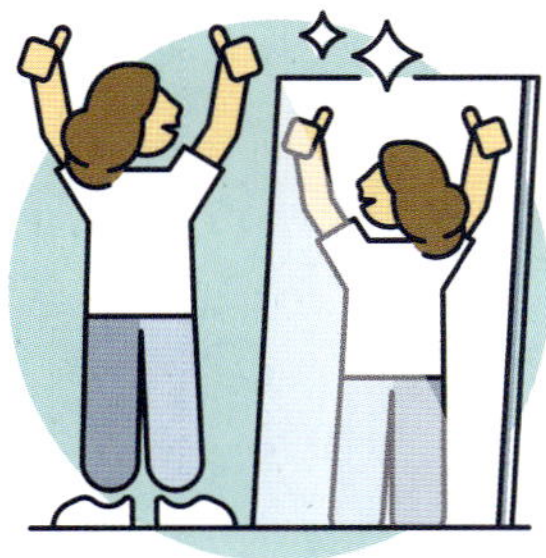

Higher self-esteem

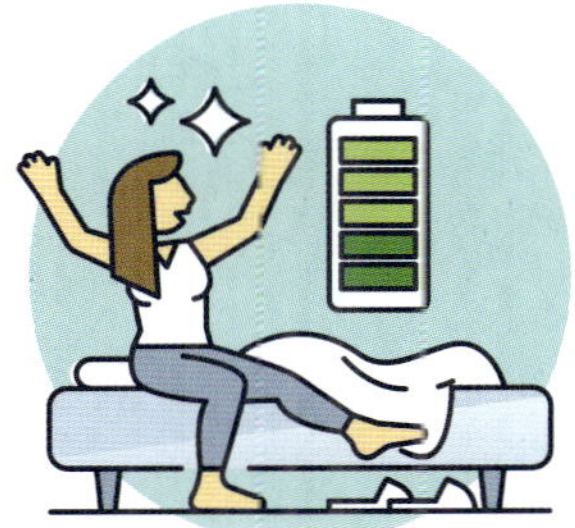

Better sleep

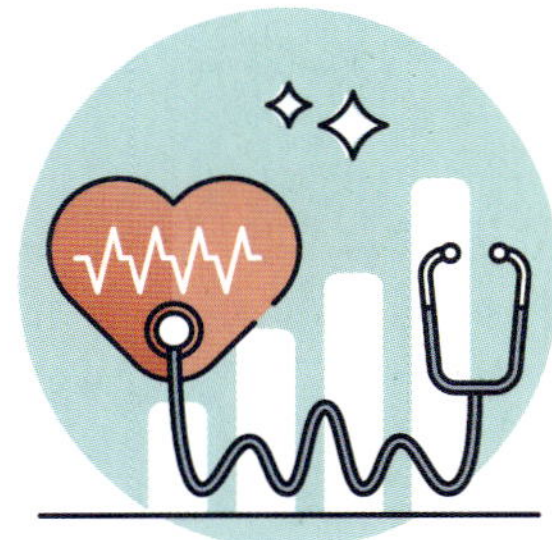

Improved overall health

Muscle is so important for regulating blood sugar! Muscle is active tissue so needs regular movement. Exercising is one of the best ways to keep insulin working well and prevent diabetes. I swear by exercise! I run four or five times per week and do about three or four reformer Pilates classes per week. Twice a week, I do resistance training.

FATTY PANCREAS AND INSULIN RESISTANCE

Fat builds up in the pancreas when people are overweight, don't eat healthy food, get older or drink too much alcohol. Some medicines and health problems can also contribute to fatty pancreas. Too much fat in the pancreas can damage the beta cells that make insulin. This means your body doesn't make enough insulin, making it harder to control blood glucose.

People who already have a higher risk for diabetes are affected more by this problem. In short, fat in the pancreas makes it harder for your body to handle glucose, especially if you're at risk for diabetes. The solution – get to a healthy weight and learn how to stay there.

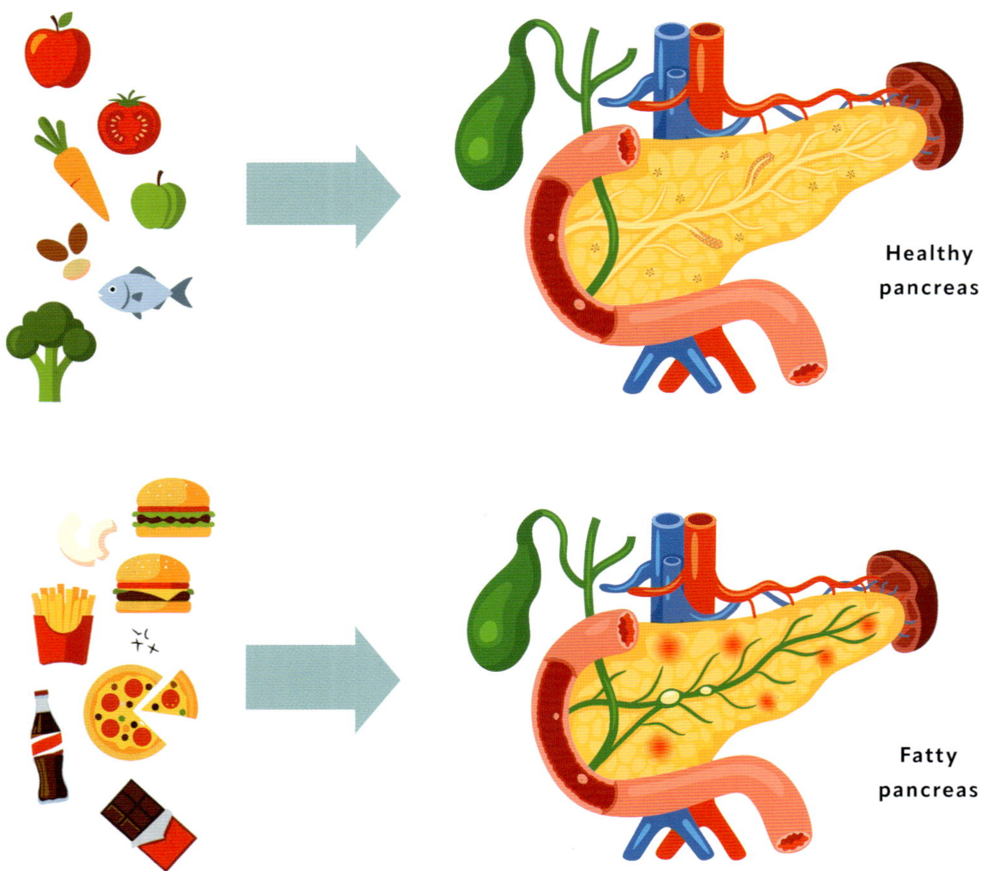

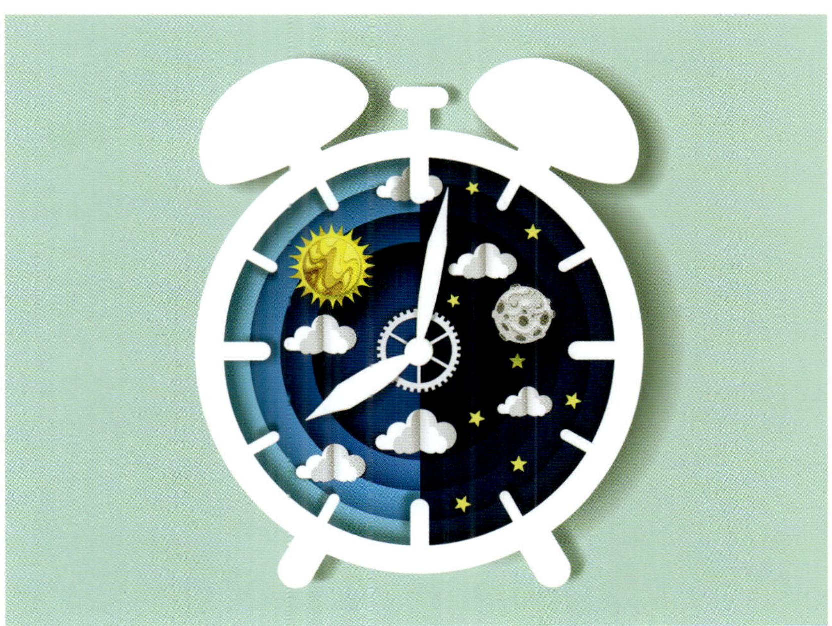

INSULIN AND OUR CIRCADIAN RHYTHMS

Circadian rhythms impact our body in so many ways. The release of hormones aligns with our circadian rhythms, so what we eat at different times of day will affect how our body processes food.

First, I want to explain what our circadian rhythms are. They are natural cycles of mental, physical and behavioural changes that happen over a day or 24 hours. They are regulated by our brain's internal master clock. The rhythms align with the day–night cycle and many body processes such as the sleep–wake cycle, hormone release, body temperature and metabolism.

The suprachiasmatic nucleus, or our master clock, is located in the hypothalamus and is light-sensitive – light is the signal that aligns our circadian rhythms with the external environment. Circadian rhythms are also regulated by the timing of our meals and physical activity. When our circadian rhythms are disrupted, such as in shift work, exposure to artificial light, and even poor and irregular sleep, it can have a negative effect on our health, leading to sleep disorders, weight gain, inflammation and moodiness.

Our sensitivity to insulin, or how effectively our bodies respond to insulin, fluctuates across the day. This is how it looks.

Now I know what you're thinking, and it's what I've been telling my patients for my whole career as a clinical nutritionist: eat your largest meal and carbohydrates during the day and have dinners carb-free for your long-term health and wellness. This leverages your body's natural insulin sensitivity for much better glucose control.

WAKING UP AND EARLY MORNING	EVENING AND NIGHT-TIME
We are most sensitive to insulin in the morning after waking up and in the first part of the day. Our insulin sensitivity peaks in the morning. This means our body utilises glucose from food way more efficiently at breakfast than at dinner. Our tolerance to glucose is high during the day and slowly declines as the day goes on. **Insulin sensitivity is highest – this is what we want.**	Our insulin sensitivity drops in the evening and night-time. A gradual drop happens from the afternoon and its lowest point is in the late evening and overnight. Our body is less efficient at processing glucose from the food we eat late in the day and at night. **Insulin sensitivity is lowest – we need to be mindful.**

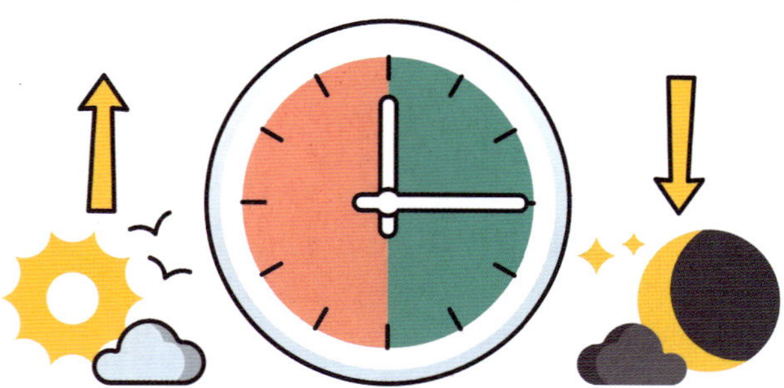

I have lived by this for all my adult life and it's what I recommend when maintaining a goal weight – to enjoy your carbs at breakfast and lunch but avoid them at dinner. The key here is working in with our circadian rhythms and hormones to optimise our metabolism as well as lower our risk of diabetes.

You need to think of insulin resistance as the quiet driver behind all those serious chronic diseases. The best treatment is with lifestyle and dietary changes, and early detection is best to avoid progression of disease.

TIPS FOR INSULIN SENSITIVITY

Following these simple steps can help your body keep insulin working well, lowering the risk of insulin resistance and type 2 diabetes.

- **Eat a balanced diet.** Choose wholefoods such as vegetables, fruits, whole grains, lean proteins and healthy fats. Avoid too much sugar, processed foods and refined carbs, which can make insulin work less well.

- **Stay active.** Regular exercise helps your muscles use sugar better and makes insulin more effective. Aim for activities such as walking, cycling or any movement you enjoy.

- **Maintain a healthy weight.** Carrying less visceral (belly) fat improves how your body responds to insulin.

- **Get enough good sleep.** Poor or not enough sleep can make insulin work less effectively, so try to rest well every night.

- **Manage stress.** Chronic stress can hurt insulin sensitivity, so find ways to relax, such as meditation, hobbies or spending time with loved ones.

- **Don't smoke.** Smoking increases insulin resistance and has associated health risks.

- **Limit alcohol.** Drinking too much alcohol can interfere with insulin function.

- **Stay hydrated.** Drinking enough water supports your overall metabolism.

Small lifestyle changes over time make a big difference. Be consistent and make these tips your way of life.

NATURAL WAYS TO REDUCE INSULIN RESISTANCE

Lowering insulin resistance needs a holistic approach. These lifestyle modifications each contribute by lowering insulin demand, improving insulin signalling pathways, reducing systemic inflammation and enhancing the body's ability to regulate blood sugar effectively. Combining these strategies yields the best results for reversing insulin resistance. Aim to make them a way of life rather than a short-term fix.

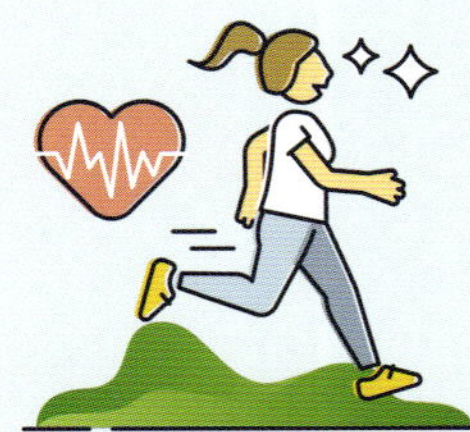

WALKING AFTER A MEAL

I love this one. Walking soon after eating helps to lower postprandial (after-meal) blood glucose levels by increasing the muscles' glucose uptake and improving insulin sensitivity.

Studies show that even short walks (10–30 minutes) after meals reduces blood glucose spikes more effectively than a single exercise session at another time of day. And it's just so easy to turn into a routine. Make it a time to think and be mindful – even go for a walk with a loved one. I think it's something everyone should do.

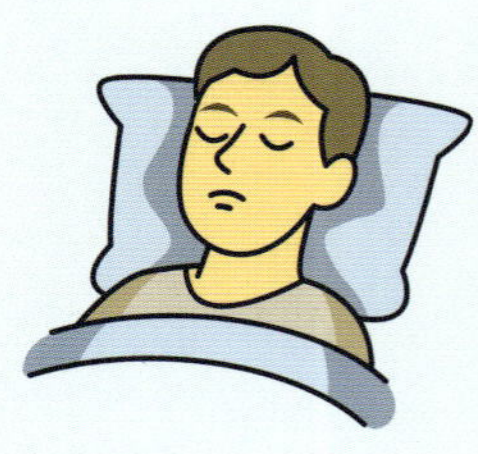

GOOD SLEEP IS WHERE THE MAGIC HAPPENS!

Getting enough high-quality sleep supports insulin sensitivity by regulating the hormones involved in glucose metabolism. These include insulin, cortisol and growth hormone.

Poor sleep increases inflammatory markers and stress hormones, promoting insulin resistance. Restoring proper sleep patterns improves blood glucose control and lowers insulin resistance by helping to reduce systemic inflammation and optimising metabolic hormone balance.

AVOID SNACKING AND GRAZING THROUGHOUT THE DAY

Reducing frequent snacking, picking and grazing throughout the day, or unnecessary caloric intake between meals, prevents your blood glucose and insulin levels from being constantly elevated. This lowers insulin demand and helps break the cycle of hyperinsulinemia (excess insulin), which drives insulin resistance.

Limiting snacking supports periods of lower insulin secretion, allowing your body's cells to regain insulin sensitivity over time and improving metabolic flexibility.

SKIPPING DINNER

Intermittent fasting approaches such as skipping dinner reduce the daily insulin load and extend fasting periods, promoting lower insulin levels and enhancing insulin sensitivity. Periods without food intake help the body to better regulate glucose homeostasis, decrease insulin secretion, and activate pathways related to cellular repair and fat metabolism. Collectively, these reduce insulin resistance.

AVOID LATE-NIGHT EATING

Not eating food late at night aligns your eating patterns with the body's natural circadian rhythms, when insulin sensitivity is higher earlier in the day and lower at night. Late-night eating is linked to impaired glucose tolerance and increased insulin resistance. By restricting food to daytime hours, your insulin sensitivity improves, and your night-time insulin and glucose levels are lower.

LIMITING GRAINS

Eating fewer refined grains and high-GI carbs lowers glucose and insulin spikes, which contribute to chronic insulin resistance. Choosing fibre-rich whole grains instead improves glucose metabolism and moderates insulin response. Some people – especially those with insulin resistance – may benefit from limiting their total grain intake to reduce their glycaemic load and improve insulin sensitivity.

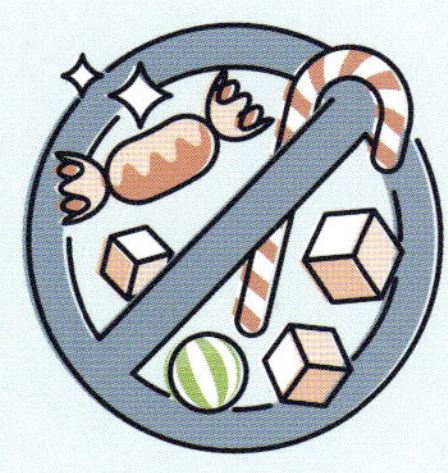

QUITTING SUGAR

Minimise added sugars to avoid rapid blood glucose surges and subsequent high insulin release, helping to reduce these driving factors for insulin resistance. High sugar intake promotes fat accumulation (especially visceral fat), inflammation and metabolic dysfunction, worsening insulin sensitivity. By cutting out sugary foods and beverages, you'll have more stable blood glucose, less chronic insulin elevation and better metabolic health.

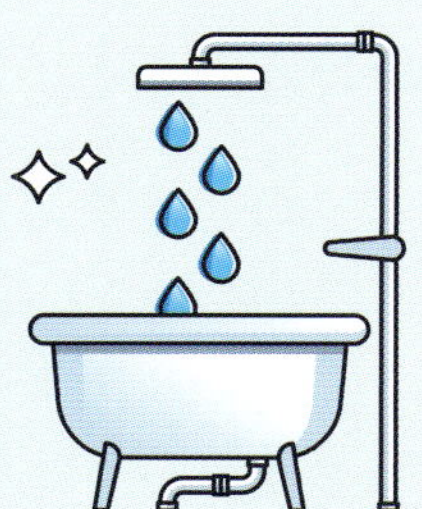

COLD SHOWERS

Cold exposure – such as cold showers and ice baths – activates brown adipose tissue, which increases glucose uptake for heat production and improves whole-body insulin sensitivity. Clinical studies show cold therapy can boost insulin sensitivity by significant margins in insulin-resistant individuals. Cold showers may also reduce inflammation and stimulate metabolic rate, improving glucose metabolism, though they should be an adjunct rather than a standalone therapy.

INSULIN RESISTANCE BY THE NUMBERS

Insulin resistance can last for many years, even up to 10 years or more before you see any symptoms or progression to prediabetes. Over time, the body gradually becomes less responsive to insulin, but the pancreas compensates by making more insulin to keep blood glucose normal.

10–15 years: how long you can have insulin resistance without knowing it.

Many people have insulin resistance without knowing it, because there are often no symptoms for a long period. If you don't address insulin resistance with lifestyle changes, it can eventually worsen, leading to higher blood glucose, prediabetes or diabetes.

5–10 years: how long you can have prediabetes before it progresses.

You can have prediabetes for many years before it progresses to type 2 diabetes if you don't make any lifestyle changes. Some people with prediabetes never develop diabetes, especially if they start exercising more, eating healthier and losing weight, which can prevent or even reverse prediabetes. Most people don't notice any symptoms during this time, so get regular check-ups to detect it early.

6–10 years: reduced life expectancy if you don't manage type 2 diabetes.

Type 2 diabetes is for life – it's a chronic condition that doesn't go away, though you can put it into remission with major lifestyle changes or weight loss. Type 2 diabetes can reduce your life expectancy, especially if it's diagnosed at a younger age or you don't manage your blood glucose.

3–10 years: increased life expectancy if you manage type 2 diabetes well.

With good treatment and healthy habits, however, people can live many years with type 2 diabetes and may even extend their life expectancy by 3–10 years, compared to poorly controlled cases. Remember, you can reverse type 2 diabetes and bring it into remission, especially early after diagnosis, if you make substantial weight loss and lifestyle changes.

46% of patients who lose weight go into remission after 1 year.

Major clinical trials show that up to 46% patients who lose about 10% to 15% of their body weight are in T2D remission one year later, with about 36% remaining in remission after two years. Over longer periods, remission rates drop, with 13% of patients still in remission after five years. This is why diet and lifestyle changes need to be a way of life, not just for a short period of time. You can't go back to your old ways.

Remission is much more likely in people with a recent diagnosis (within 6 years) and lower initial blood sugar levels. This is why I always tell my patients to get regular check-ups, stay on top of your health, and don't ignore signs or symptoms.

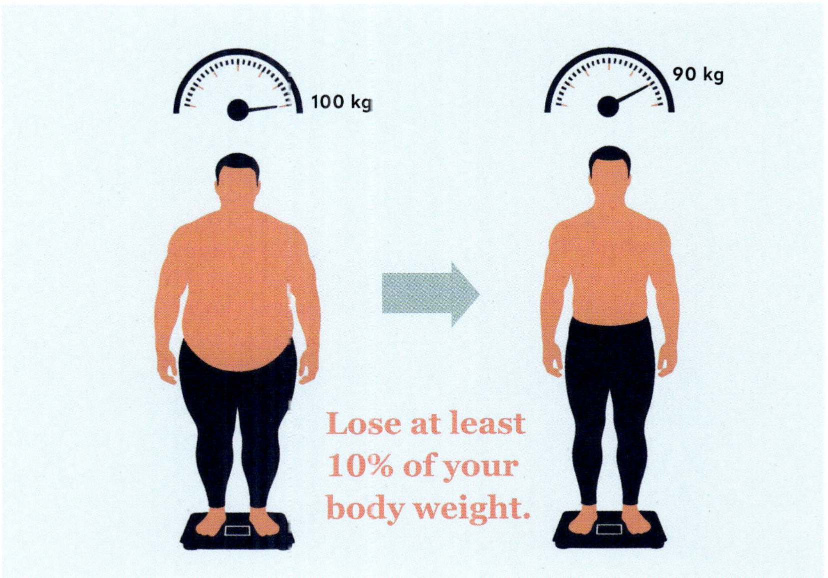

CHAPTER 7

Type 2 diabetes and complications

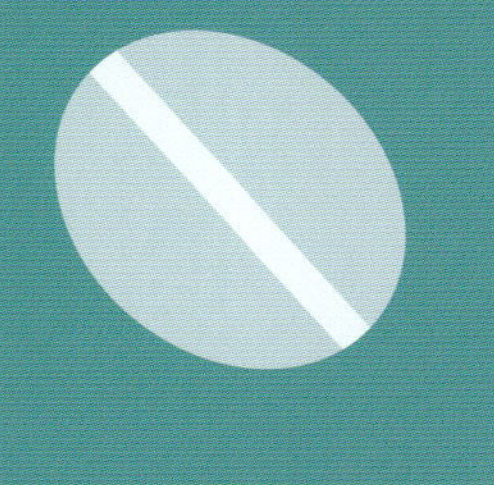

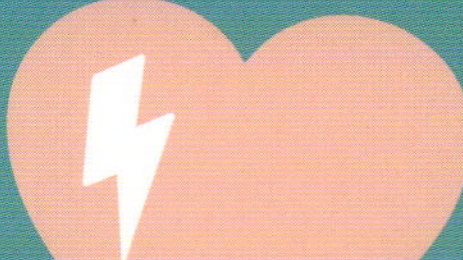

THE PROGRESSION TO TYPE 2 DIABETES

For many of my patients who have shared their type 2 diabetes journey with me, it all starts with obvious symptoms and signs. The most common symptoms are feeling thirsty all the time, going to the bathroom to wee a lot, and feeling hungry all the time even though you're eating regular meals and snacks. You complain of feeling tired or low energy all the time, and you could have lost weight without trying in some cases.

People may notice their vision being blurry; tingling, numbness or pain in the hands or feet; and poorly healing cuts, wounds or sores. Some see lots of infections, urinary tract infections or even thrush. Another complaint is skin changes: dark areas around the neck or armpits.

These symptoms don't just start overnight – they develop gradually and can be unnoticed for years. If you have a family history of diabetes, are overweight and don't exercise, you are at a much higher risk.

SYMPTOMS OF TYPE 2 DIABETES

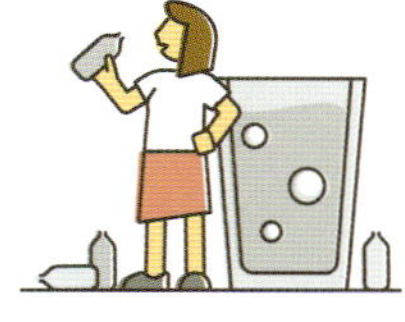

Always thirsty

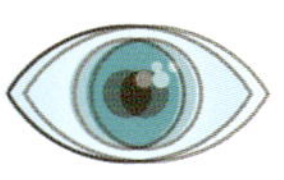

Blurry vision

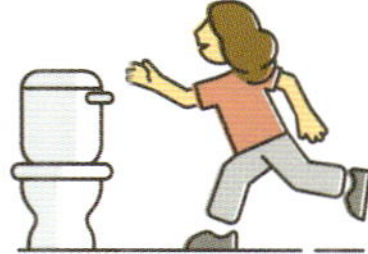

Needing to urinate often

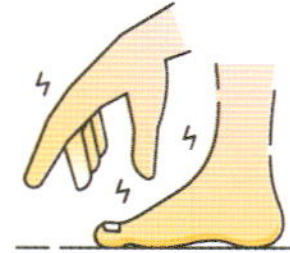

Pain in the hands and feet

HOW DOES THIS HAPPEN?

The progression to type 2 diabetes comes through worsening insulin resistance and declining pancreatic beta cell function. Insulin resistance and beta cell dysfunction start many years before a diabetes diagnosis – up to 10 years. The beta cells initially increase insulin output then decline before diabetes can develop.

STAGE	DESCRIPTION	INSULIN RESISTANCE	BETA CELL FUNCTION	BLOOD GLUCOSE
1. Normal metabolism	Body cells respond normally to insulin. Insulin easily moves glucose into cells.	Normal	Fully functional	Normal (3.5–5.5 mmol/L fasting)
2. Early insulin resistance	Cells start to respond less effectively to insulin (due to genetics, diet, inactivity or fat accumulation).	Mildly increased	Producing more insulin to compensate (hyperinsulinemia)	Normal
3. Compensated prediabetes	Insulin resistance worsens. The pancreas increases insulin output to maintain near-normal glucose. Beta cells start showing signs of stress.	Moderate–high	Working harder; pancreas is enlarged and overstressed	Slightly elevated (5.6–6.9 mmol/L fasting)
4. Beta cell fatigue and failure	Beta cells begin to fail. Insulin secretion can't keep up with rising resistance. Chronic inflammation in the pancreas and liver dysfunction worsens.	High	Declining; function begins to drop	Rising (glucose above normal range)
5. Transition to type 2 diabetes	Beta cell failure reaches a critical threshold; insulin levels fall while glucose rises sharply.	Very high	Significantly reduced, many beta cells damaged or lost	High (≥7.0 mmol/L fasting or ≥11.1 mmol/L post-meal)
6. Established type 2 diabetes	Persistent hyperglycaemia because insulin output is inadequate. Chronic inflammation continues, damaging pancreatic and liver tissue.	Severe	Poor insulin production capacity	Chronically elevated

THE MENTAL AND EMOTIONAL JOURNEY

In my experience, people go through a range of emotions when they find out they have type 2 diabetes. I've warned some patients they're on their way to a diagnosis who have not believed it could happen to them. Finding out you have type 2 diabetes can trigger a complex mental and emotional journey.

- **Shock and disbelief.** The diagnosis can be unexpected, especially if you had no clear symptoms before. You may feel confusion and anxiety about what the diagnosis means for your health and lifestyle.

- **Denial and downplaying.** You may refuse to accept the diagnosis or downplay its seriousness, especially if you feel fine physically. This can delay important lifestyle changes or treatment.

- **Shock and fear.** The worry about potential complications such as heart disease, vision loss, or kidney problems can feel overwhelming.

- **Anger and frustration.** Maybe you'll feel angry and frustrated. You could feel upset or resentful, wondering why this happened to you or blaming yourself for lifestyle factors.

- **Guilt and self-blame.** It's hard not to feel guilt over your past habits or choices. I find this one challenging as a practitioner. You may feel sadness or depression as you realise diabetes is a lifelong condition that needs to be managed. Life is so different now.

- **Overwhelm.** All the changes you are faced with can feel overwhelming. Change starts with understanding the disease; managing your blood sugar, diet, exercise, doctors' appointments and medication; and seeing someone like me to help change your diet.

I find that time is one of the world's greatest healers. Many move towards acceptance as they learn more about diabetes and gain confidence in managing it.

The diabetes journey is unique to each person. You just need to go through the process, starting with denial and fear; then, when you're ready, comes understanding and acceptance. The best part is to get proactive with managing your condition, doing lots of research and getting a plan in place. Many people I work with really understand their health and its importance, and are inspired for a positive health outcome. I'll always encourage my patients to aim for reversal and show them it can be done.

Here is the journey, starting at the day you are diagnosed.

TIMELINE OF YOUR DIAGNOSIS JOURNEY

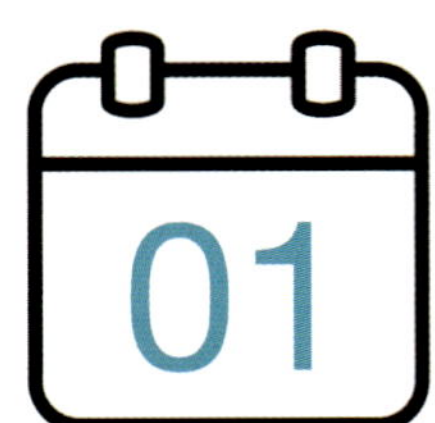

DAY 1

When you're diagnosed, chances are you're sitting with your doctor. Usually, you will be given a comprehensive approach that will combine medication if needed and lifestyle changes.

The initial approach will emphasise a healthy diet, regular physical activity, weight control, quitting smoking or vaping (if you do), and limiting or ideally avoiding alcohol. These changes help control your blood glucose and reduce complications. Even losing 5% to 10% of your body weight can improve blood glucose control and potentially induce remission in early diabetes. The doctor will recommend weight loss in most cases.

Your doctor will recommend changes to your diet to help manage your blood glucose levels and weight. Eating a well-balanced diet is just so important. Everyone is different, there is no one-size-fits-all, but the general guidelines include:

- eating a wide variety of nutrient-rich foods, such as whole grains, vegetables, fruits, lean proteins and healthy fats

- evenly spacing your meals throughout the day

- not skipping meals if you're on medications that can cause blood sugar to go too low

- practising portion control.

They will encourage you to exercise more. As we've seen, exercise helps you manage your blood glucose levels, lose weight and lower your risk of complications from type 2 diabetes. After all, as I always say, exercise is medicine. The exercise recommendations are:

- getting at least 150 minutes of moderate to vigorous intensity aerobic exercise per week, spread over multiple days

- completing two to three sessions of resistance exercise or strength training per week, spread over non-consecutive days

- limiting the amount of time you spend engaging in sedentary behaviours

- not going more than 2 days in a row without physical activity.

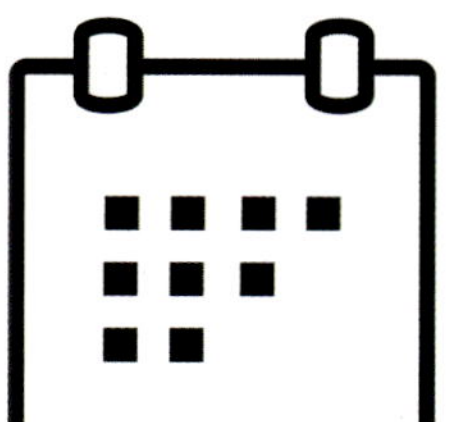

FIRST 1–2 WEEKS

Depending on the case, you may be prescribed medication. If you don't have contraindications, the first-line medication is metformin. Metformin helps lower blood glucose by improving insulin sensitivity and reducing the liver's glucose production. If you don't achieve your blood glucose targets with lifestyle changes and metformin, you may need other medications, such as sulfonylureas, DPP-4 inhibitors, SGLT-2 inhibitors or insulin.

- **Learn how to monitor your blood glucose.** The main goal in treating diabetes is to keep your blood glucose levels within the target range. You will have regular blood tests such as HbA1c, and your doctor may suggest an at-home blood glucose monitoring kit to check how the treatment is going and manage the risk of glucose highs and lows. This part is really important – many of my patients wear a continuous glucose monitor on the back of their arm that is linked to their phone, which I highly recommend.

- **Get the education and support you need.** There is so much to learn in the early stages. From the very start, you need to be fully educated on everything from medication and complications to nutrition, exercise and self-care. Type 2 diabetes is a serious condition. Healthcare professionals such as diabetes educators, clinical nutritionists and dieticians can help you manage the disease and ideally improve your outcomes.

Type 2 diabetes is a disease of the diet – treat it by changing your diet and lifestyle!

FIRST THREE MONTHS, AND ONGOING

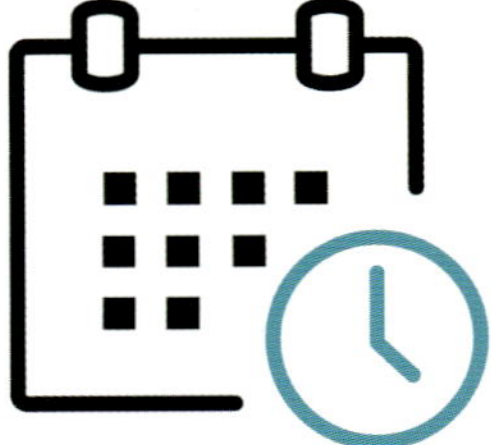

When starting on your journey to manage type 2 diabetes, the doctor may encourage you to make ongoing changes to your diet, exercise routine or other lifestyle habits. They might prescribe one or more medications. They will also schedule regular check-ups and blood tests.

Let your doctor know if you notice changes in your symptoms or blood glucose levels. Type 2 diabetes can change over time, and your doctor may adjust your treatment plan to meet your evolving needs.

Many people simply stay on the medication, visit the doctor and live with diabetes. But others really want to make the change – to reverse the disease and live a long and healthy life. This is where I come in – once someone is ready to learn how to reverse T2D with diet and healthy lifestyle changes. I love these motivated patients who come in ready to change!

It's so rewarding to see these patients get their health back, feeling confident, positive and in control.

The thing about T2D is that you can put it into remission for the rest of your life by changing your diet.

TYPE 2 DIABETES AND DIARRHOEA

This can be a huge embarrassment to many, but people with type 2 diabetes need to be aware of it. Diarrhoea can be extremely distressing for the patient. Here are the causes:

- **Autonomic neuropathy.** This is the most common cause, resulting from damage to the nerves that control involuntary body functions, including movement in the digestive tract. In people with long-standing or poorly controlled diabetes, high blood sugar can gradually harm these nerves, leading to erratic signalling. As a result, the intestines may move food too quickly (causing diarrhea), too slowly (causing constipation) or alternate between the two. It often shows up as frequent, watery diarrhea, especially overnight.

- **Metformin.** Some diabetes medications, most commonly metformin, can cause gastrointestinal side effects, with diarrhoea being one of the most frequent.

- **GLP-1 receptor agonists.** Other medications such as GLP-1 receptor agonists (e.g. Wegovy, Ozempic), can sometimes cause changes in bowel habits, from chronic constipation to diarrhoea. These medications slow stomach emptying, speed up movement through the intestines, disrupt gut signalling and can alter the gut microbiome, resulting in diarrhoea.

- **Exocrine pancreatic insufficiency.** This is when the pancreas is not making digestive enzymes. Diarrhoea or loose stools are the result.

- **Other factors.** These include small intestinal bacteria overgrowth (SIBO) and food intolerances such as lactose intolerance, non-celiac sensitivity and celiac disease. Nerve damage can affect how the body reabsorbs bile, which aids digestion. Poor reabsorption is linked to triggering diarrhoea.

If you're suffering from constant diarrhoea, remember to hydrate.

And always have regular check-ups with your healthcare provider.

COMPLICATIONS OF TYPE 2 DIABETES

In most cases, type 2 diabetes comes with complications. Chronic high blood glucose levels damage your nerves, organs and blood vessels over the years, which started back with insulin resistance then prediabetes and now type 2 diabetes. Chronic high blood glucose increases inflammation and oxidative stress, harming the body's tissues. Remember, diabetes is caused by the body's inability to produce or utilise insulin, leaving blood sugar levels high.

TIMELINE OF COMPLICATIONS

The complications of type 2 may develop not long after you have been diagnosed. Whether you develop complications depends on your age, overall health, blood glucose control, diet, lifestyle and any other conditions.

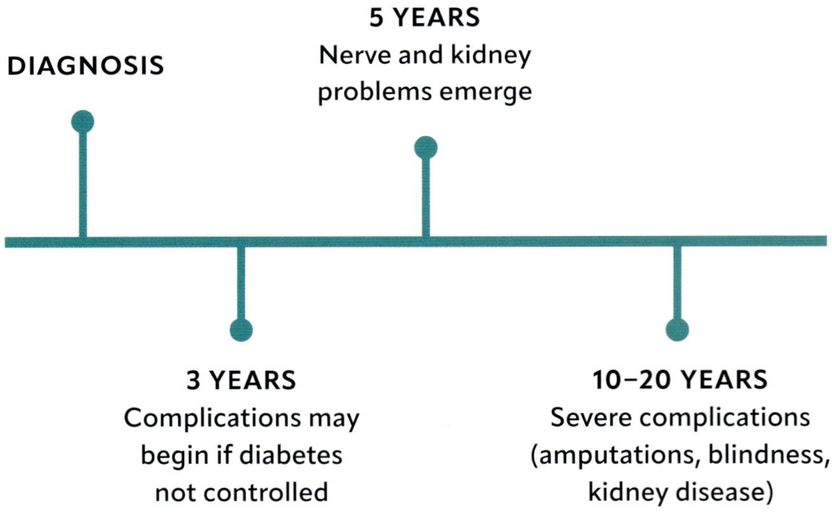

If you are young when diagnosed, you'll see the complications earlier as well. There is no one-size-fits-all regarding when these complications will present – certain factors can influence them. If you don't manage your blood glucose well, have high blood pressure and cholesterol, eat an unhealthy diet, make poor lifestyle choices and smoke, these factors will speed up complications. But if you choose to manage your heart health, blood pressure, cholesterol and blood glucose properly, you can delay the severity, onset and general presentation of these complications.

This is why having your regular annual health check-ups, getting a diagnosis early, then making the changes to a healthy diet and lifestyle are just so important to reverse these complications.

ACUTE (SHORT-TERM) COMPLICATIONS

CONDITION	WHAT IT IS	SYMPTOMS
DIABETIC KETOACIDOSIS (DKA)	When the body breaks down fat too quickly because it lacks insulin. The body is producing ketones that make the blood become acidic.	• Frequent urination • Nausea • Vomiting • Abdominal pain • Rapid breathing • Extremely thirsty • Feeling confused • Coma (worst-case scenario, more common in T1D but can occur with T2D)
HYPOGLYCAEMIA (LOW BLOOD GLUCOSE)	When blood glucose levels become dangerously low. It can be caused by missing meals, excessive exercise and some medications.	• Blurred vision • Feeling dizzy • Loss of consciousness • Seizures • Irritable • Sweaty and shaky
HYPERGLYCAEMIA (HIGH BLOOD GLUCOSE)	When blood glucose levels are way too high.	• Frequent urination • Thirsty • Blurred vision • Feeling tired

CHRONIC (LONG-TERM) COMPLICATIONS

PART OF BODY	WHAT IT IS	BEST FOODS	LIFESTYLE CHOICES
BLOOD VESSELS	High blood glucose damages the lining of blood vessels, which leads to microvascular damage. This will hinder nutrient and oxygen supply to tissues, causing damage to nerves, kidneys and eyes.	• Leafy greens (spinach, kale) • Beetroot • Cruciferous vegetables • All berries • Citrus • Fatty fish (mackerel, sardines, salmon) • Nuts and seeds • Extra-virgin olive oil • Avocado oil • Whole grains (oats, quinoa, lentils, chickpeas, legumes) • Fibre	• Regular aerobic exercise • Strength training • Stop smoking • Blood pressure management • Cholesterol management • Weight management • Blood glucose management • Sleep well (7–9 hours a night) • Stress less
HEART	Diabetes increases the risk of heart attacks, strokes, high blood pressure and peripheral artery disease because of poor blood flow to the limbs. Atherosclerosis (hardened arteries) increases the risk of stroke and heart disease. People with diabetes are often obese and have high cholesterol.	• Whole grains • Fatty fish rich in omega-3 (salmon, mackerel) • Nuts (walnuts, almonds) • Olive oil • Leafy greens • Berries • Legumes and high-fibre foods	• Regular aerobic exercise (walking, cycling) • Weight management • Quitting smoking or vaping • Blood pressure and cholesterol control • Stress management
THE KIDNEYS	Nephropathy is damage to the kidneys' filtering units, which means protein can leak out (microalbuminuria). If untreated, it will progress to kidney failure. When fully advanced, the patient will need a kidney transplant or dialysis.	• Low-sodium diet • Moderate protein intake from plant-based sources (beans, lentils) • Fresh fruits and vegetables • No processed foods high in phosphorus and potassium	• Blood glucose management • Blood pressure management • Hydration
EYES	Blindness caused by injury to the blood vessels in the retina (also known as diabetic retinopathy) will increase the risk of glaucoma and cataracts. Early stages are asymptomatic but without proper treatment, blindness will occur.	• Foods high in antioxidants and vitamins A, C, E and zinc (carrots, kale, spinach, citrus fruits, nuts, seeds)	• Good blood glucose control • Blood pressure management • Regular eye check-ups • Not smoking

PART OF BODY	WHAT IT IS	BEST FOODS	LIFESTYLE CHOICES
FEET	Reduced blood flow means a loss of sensation in the feet, and also causes infections and ulcers. In some cases, sadly, amputation is needed.	• Nutrient-rich diet to support wound healing • Vitamin C (citrus, capsicum, strawberries, kiw fruit) • Zinc (nuts, seeds) • Protein (lean meats or plant sources)	• Proper foot hygiene • Comfortable shoes • Blood glucose control • Regular foot inspections • Not walking barefoot
NERVES	High glucose causes nerve damage (neuropathy): tingling, loss of sensation, pain and numbness in the hands and feet. If autonomic nerves are affected, it can mean problems with bladder control, bladder dysfunction, digestion (gastroparesis), sexual function, and abnormal heart rate or blood pressure issues.	• Foods that support nerves and reduce inflammation • B vitamins (leafy greens) • Omega-3s and vitamin D (fatty fish). • Vitamin E (nuts and seeds) • Magnesium and B vitamins (whole grains) • Vitamin B12 (eggs and lean meats) • Antioxidants (colourful fruits and veggies) • Fibre and folate (legumes)	• Regular exercise • Maintaining a healthy weight • Not drinking alcohol • Not smoking • Blood glucose control • Protecting your feet with good shoes • Getting enough sleep • Stress management
IMMUNE SYSTEM	High glucose impairs the immune response. This means healing is slow and there is a greater frequency of infections and they can be severe. Infections can impact the gums, urinary tract and skin.	• Vitamin C (citrus fruits, berries, red capsicum) • Vitamins A, C (leafy greens) • Probiotics (yoghurt, kefir, kimchi) • Anti-inflammatory, antiviral foods (garlic, ginger, turmeric) • Vitamin E, omega-3s (nuts, seeds, fatty fish)	• Eating a variety of wholefoods • Limiting processed foods and sugar • Exercising regularly (150+ min/week) • Getting enough sleep • Managing stress with relaxation techniques • Not smoking • Moderate alcohol consumption • Maintaining social connections • Getting regular check-ups

OTHER CONDITIONS

Type 2 diabetes increases your risk for conditions such as elevated cholesterol, high blood pressure, fatty liver, dementia, hearing loss, sleep apnoea, skin conditions such as bacterial and fungal infections, osteoporosis, and mental health issues such as depression and anxiety.

These complications are caused by long-term damage from high blood glucose levels that harm organs, nerves and blood vessels.

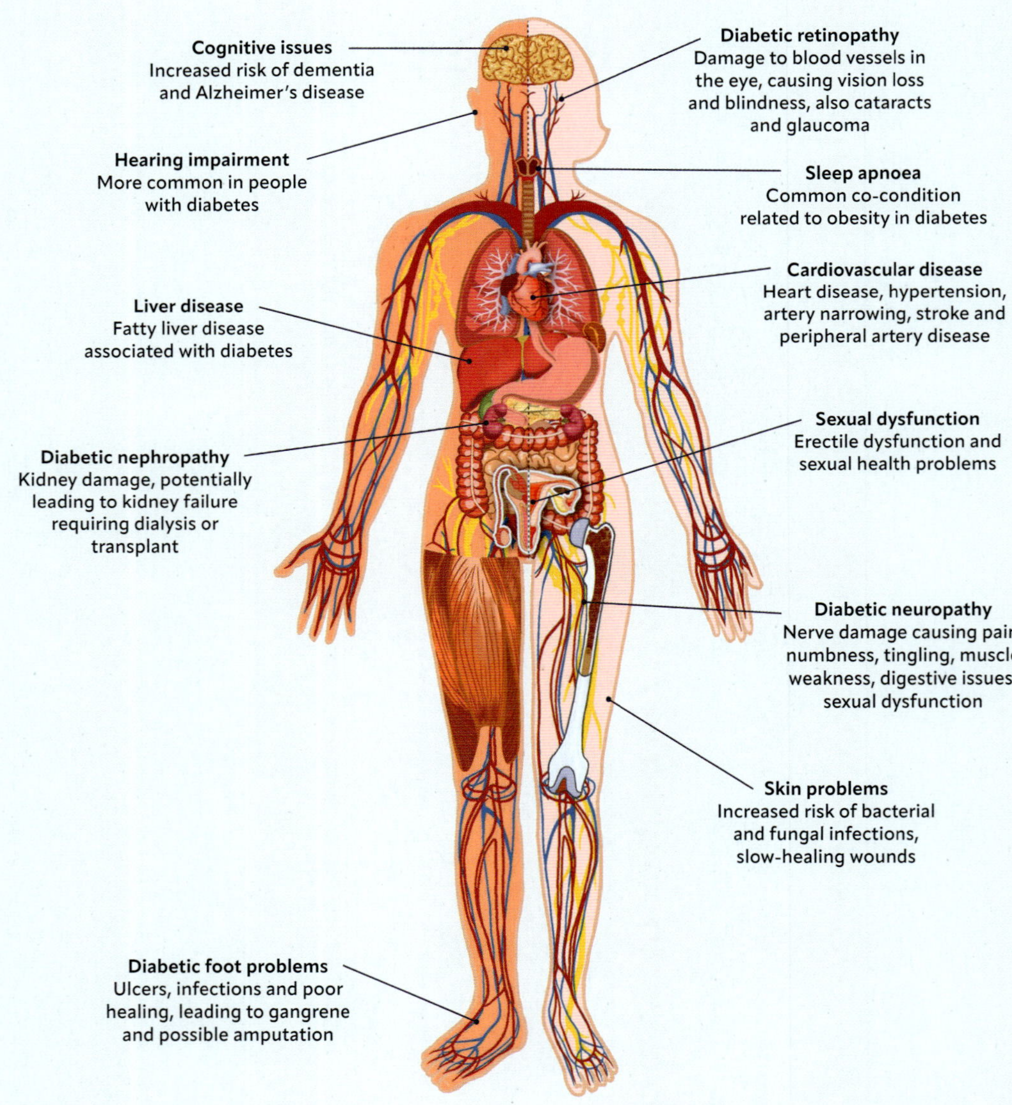

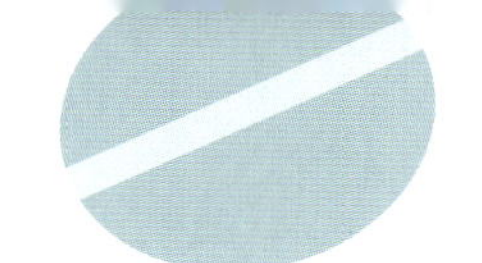
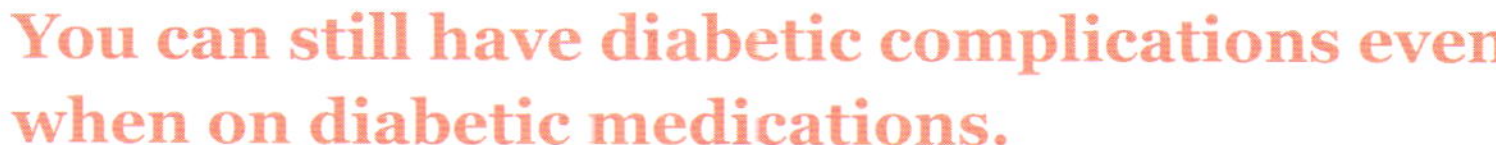

You can still have diabetic complications even when on diabetic medications.

The reasons for this include:

- **The progressive nature of diabetes.** Over time, it can be harder to control blood glucose with medications, and your treatment needs recalibrating. In some cases, even with medication, blood sugar levels aren't in the normal range. Years of small, repeated elevations in blood glucose can still damage the organs, eyes and blood vessels, leading to complications.

- **Not taking medications.** People can sometimes forget to take their medication. Cost may be an issue. People may not stick to the regime or even not understand the instructions.

- **Comorbidities.** If you have other health conditions such as elevated blood pressure and cholesterol, and continue with poor diet and lifestyle choices (smoking, lack of exercise, stress, poor sleep), this can lead to complications. People's genetics are another factor.

The longer you have diabetes, the higher your risk for developing complications, regardless of medication. Most likely, you had the complications before you were prescribed the medication. So you can't just go to a doctor get a script and your T2D will be managed or treated – you can still have complications.

As I always say, the progression of disease is individual; it's the same with medication response. Some people don't respond as well to medication and so their diabetes is harder to control.

Medications can reduce but will not eliminate complications.

Diabetes management needs to start with making diet and lifestyle changes; regularly monitoring your blood pressure, blood glucose, cholesterol; and taking a comprehensive approach.

IMMUNE SYSTEM ISSUES

Having type 2 diabetes changes your immunity in many ways. For starters, the chronic high blood glucose impairs the ability of your white blood cells to fight infections and respond rapidly. This makes it harder for your body to handle bacteria, viruses and fungi, and increases the length of infections.

Type 2 diabetes also causes chronic inflammation throughout the entire body, triggered by high blood glucose and inflammation from fat cells (yes, these cells can do that). The inflammation damages organs, reduces your immunity, and feeds diabetic complications such as heart disease and neuropathy. Your immune cells, such as neutrophils, lymphocytes and macrophages, don't function as well and the body's ability to make antibodies is also lessened.

This poor immunity means people with diabetes are way more prone to infections, such as infections in the respiratory system and urinary tract. And because the blood flow is poor and immunity is impaired, cuts or injuries take a long time to heal, leading to increased infections.

Our immune system matters in type 2 diabetes because:

1. **High blood glucose suppresses the functioning of immune cells.** High blood glucose impairs the activity of neutrophils, macrophages and T cells, which are crucial for identifying and destroying pathogens. This makes infections (such as urinary tract or skin infections) more frequent and harder to control. This is a real telltale sign of type 2 diabetes.

2. **Chronic inflammation and oxidative stress.** Constant high blood glucose causes oxidative stress, an overproduction of reactive oxygen species (ROS). This damages immune cells and disrupts insulin signalling. This creates a vicious cycle of inflammation, insulin resistance and just exhausting the immune system.

3. **Reduced circulation and healing.** Poor vascular function in diabetes limits oxygen and nutrient delivery to tissues. We address circulation in week 4 of The 9-week program. This delays wound healing and reduces local immune responses. When I say 'local', I mean local to the wounds.

- **Gut microbiome imbalance.** High-sugar or highly processed diets damage the gut microbiota, increasing gut permeability, more commonly known as 'leaky gut', and inflammation. A balanced gut is essential for a strong immune system as around 70% of immune tissue lies in the gut wall. To learn more about gut health you can get a copy of my book *The Gut Repair Plan.*

- **Higher susceptibility to infections.** People with type 2 diabetes are more prone to respiratory and viral infections because of the immune dysregulation caused by insulin resistance and chronic inflammation.

BREAST CANCER AND TYPE 2 DIABETES

Looking at all the research, I felt this was worth highlighting. A woman with type 2 diabetes has an increased risk of developing breast cancer. Large-scale reviews and multiple recent studies consistently show a 10% to 30% increased risk of breast cancer for women with T2D, even after adjusting for shared risk factors such as age and body mass index.

Several meta-analyses found women with T2D have between 15% to 27% higher risk of developing breast cancer, especially after menopause. The risk is more for certain types of breast cancer such as ER-negative (oestrogen receptor negative).

Chronically high insulin levels can stimulate cell cancer growth. And chronic high blood sugar fuels cancer cells because they need glucose for energy. Diabetes increases systemic inflammation that can alter sex hormones, plus obesity, poor diet, lack of exercise and older age increase the risk of both type 2 diabetes and breast cancer.

Controlling your diabetes, maintaining weight, getting regular screening and making lifestyle modifications can lower the risk. Make sure you're on top of your breast cancer screening, keep your blood glucose stable, do regular exercise, eat healthy and be proactive with your health.

OTHER CONSIDERATIONS

Metabolic (bariatric) surgery can produce high rates of diabetes remission, particularly in people with obesity.

New medications (GLP-1 agonists, such as Mounjaro, and SGLT-2 inhibitors) improve blood glucose and often help with weight loss, but they typically manage diabetes rather than induce sustained remission. Interestingly, in my clinical experience most of my patients with T2D have not had success with taking weight-loss injections (such as Ozempic). Many have been on the medication for about 2 years and have had waves of being on and off the medication.

These patients have had way more success with my weight-loss plan than with the weight-loss injections. The surprise I see on my patients' faces when I work with them and get results in weeks versus the years they've spent on medications – they feel frustrated that they've lost years to the disease. Now I'm not telling people to not take medication – that's not my objective here. Education is so important when it comes to understanding diabetes; my aim is to teach people how to eat to stay in remission for life.

JENNY'S STORY

When I started treating Jenny, she'd had T2D for about 5 years. Two years ago, she did Ozempic for 12 months and her weight never changed. She stopped, then tried it again. Again, her weight was unchanged; she was still more than 100 kg. Jenny came to see me for help with losing weight, and with my program started losing 1 kg per week. We are still working together to reach her health goal, but it brings me back to the need to treat the disease by treating the cause – change the diet!

Many of my patients with insulin resistance and T2D have poor gut health: altered gut microbiome, leaky gut and inflammation. Think about the challenges of poor gut health when getting to a health goal. For more on gut health, see my book *The Gut Repair Plan*.

Important limitations:

- **Remission is not the same as cure.** The underlying tendency for diabetes remains and can return if you don't maintain lifestyle changes.

- **Remission is most achievable soon after diagnosis.** It's less likely in long-standing diabetes or without substantial weight loss.

In many cases, you can reverse insulin resistance and T2D by losing substantial weight and changing your lifestyle, especially if you start early. New therapies may expand these possibilities, but sustained remission depends on keeping the weight off and maintaining healthy habits – this is the only true way and the key to success!

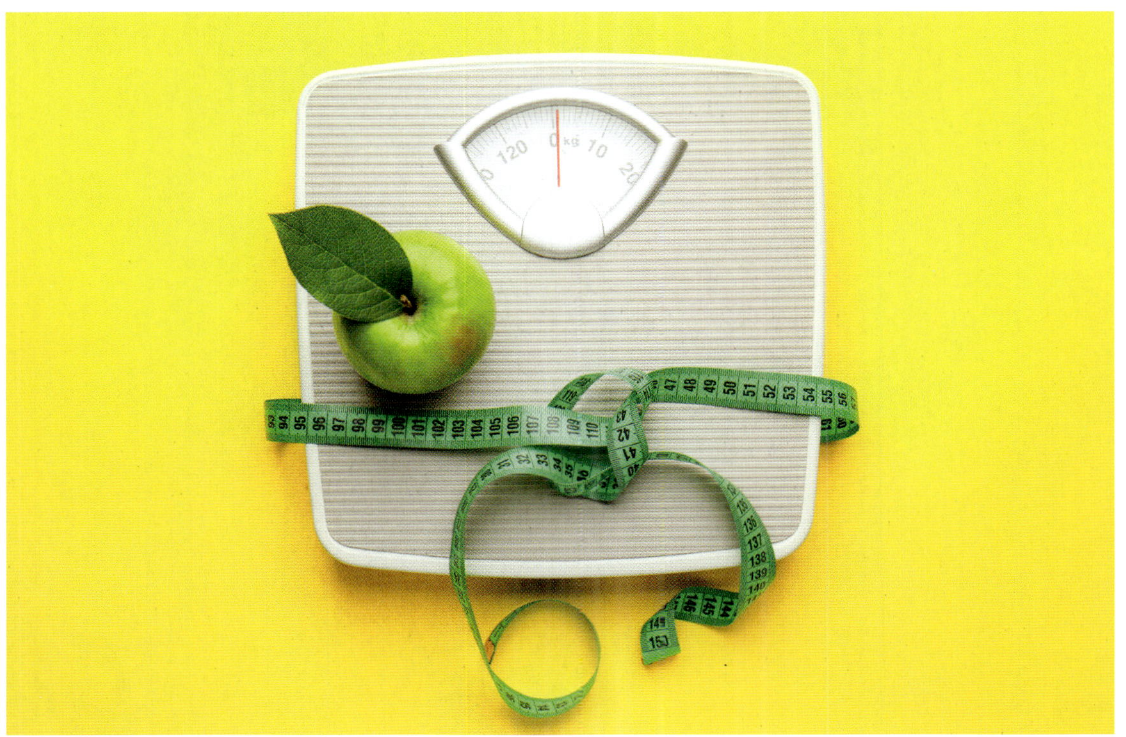

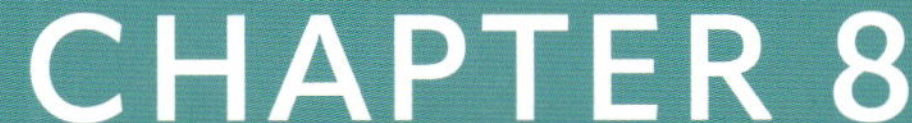

CHAPTER 8

Comorbidities and type 2 diabetes

A comorbidity is a medical condition that exists alongside a diagnosis. Comorbidities occur for lots of reasons, such as shared risk factors such as poor diet, smoking, genetics, lack of exercise, inactivity and environmental factors. Many people who have diabetes, for instance, are likely to be overweight or have high blood pressure.

In general, comorbidities are more common in people as they age, and in those who don't exercise, have a poor diet and live an unhealthy lifestyle.

Some diseases with similar biological mechanisms can arise from the same pathway, such as inflammation, hormonal imbalance, poor immune system function or blood vessel damage. A disease can also lead to a new problem, such as diabetes causing nerve and eye damage. There can be genetic conditions or chronic infections, and sometimes coincidence, especially as people age. Mental health and lifestyle factors may play a part, such as an illness causing depression.

Comorbidities can be:

- chronic conditions – hypertension, heart disease or arthritis
- physical or mental conditions – anxiety and depression
- related or even unrelated to the primary disease.

Comorbidities can affect your overall health, and impact the treatment plan. Most people I treat for weight loss in my clinic have one or more of the following:

- depression
- high blood cholesterol
- PCOS
- insulin resistance
- prediabetes
- diabetes
- anxiety
- poor gut health
- high blood pressure
- arthritis
- fatty liver disease.

I still need to treat these diseases while helping them lose weight.

When you have two or more chronic conditions, this is referred to as a 'multimorbidity'. This is very common in my experience. When multiple medical conditions are present in a person at the same time, they affect each other and the person's overall health.

WHAT CAUSES COMORBIDITIES IN PEOPLE WITH T2D?

Type 2 diabetes shares risk factors with conditions such as heart disease, high blood pressure, dyslipidaemia (high fat in the blood) and obesity: being sedentary (not exercising), smoking, poor diet, unhealthy lifestyle and genetics.

- **Chronic inflammation.** Conditions such as hypertension, kidney disease and heart disease stem from chronic inflammation, insulin resistance and damage to blood vessels. These are all central to diabetes.

- **High blood glucose.** The continual high blood glucose in diabetes directly damages nerves and blood vessels, increasing complications such as eye, nerve and kidney disease.

- **Ongoing metabolic stress.** As diabetes progresses over time, you're more likely to develop other chronic conditions due the ongoing metabolic stress.

- **Aging.** You're at higher risk of chronic diseases as you age. Much depends on the support older people have with managing their health.

- **Mental health problems.** Depression, anxiety and other mental health problems are more prominent in people with diabetes, because of the emotional burden of living with a chronic disease as well the inflammation and hormonal changes that take place.

At diagnosis:

77% of people have 1+ comorbidities
44% of people have 2+ comorbidities
30% of people have 3+ comorbidities

After 10 years:

60% of people have 3+ comorbidities

Among older people:

95% of people have comorbidities

This really highlights the fact that most people who live with T2D have multiple health conditions that require treatment along with diabetes.

MEDICATIONS AND COMORBIDITIES

Someone with T2D who has three comorbidities will likely be prescribed multiple daily medications, typically between four and seven separate medicines per day, sometimes more. They can include:

- at least one or two diabetes medications (these may be combined or separate)

- several cardioprotective medicines (commonly for blood pressure and cholesterol)

- additional medications for comorbidities such as neuropathy, depression or gastric symptoms.

Five years after diagnosis, people take on average six medications (often including one diabetes medicine, four for cardiovascular protection, and one for another condition). In some cases, and especially with older adults or those with more complex conditions, patients may take up to nine different medications daily.

This level of 'polypharmacy' increases the complexity of your regimen and the risk of medication interactions. So you and your healthcare provider must regularly review medicines for their safety and effectiveness, and simplify whenever possible.

POLYPHARMACY AND THE LIVER

Taking multiple medications daily with type 2 diabetes and three comorbidities impacts your liver health:

- **Metabolic dysfunction steatotic liver disease (MASLD).** Your risk of significant liver damage increases with obesity, metabolic syndrome and polypharmacy. Both the underlying diseases and medications can contribute to liver injury, including steatosis (fatty liver), fibrosis or even cirrhosis.

- **Drug–drug and drug–food interactions.** These can overwhelm the liver's ability to process toxins and medications safely. Adverse effects include impaired drug metabolism, or even drug-induced liver injury, especially if you are older or have a pre-existing liver condition.

- **Medications may influence liver health.** Some diabetes medications such as GLP-1 therapies and possibly Metformin may help reduce liver fat, and slow and improve MASH (metabolic dysfunction-associated steatohepatitis). Certain states and specific blood-pressure medications appear to slow the fibrosis progression in people with fatty liver disease. Poorly controlled diabetes clearly worsens outcomes for your liver, so insulin and other glucose-lowering medications can protect the liver when they help achieve good control rather than being harmful.

Be aware that daily use of several medications in people with T2D and three comorbidities increases the risk of liver-related problems, which always need ongoing care, monitoring and proper management. I tell my patients their doctor should routinely assess liver health, look for signs of adverse effects and adjust medication regimens. Don't get complacent with your treatment.

While the liver is incredible and takes a lot of assault, it does have a breaking point. For more on the liver, see my bestselling book *The Liver Repair Plan*.

COMMON COMORBIDITIES WITH TYPE 2 DIABETES

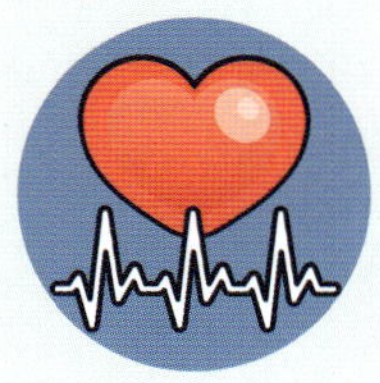

CARDIOVASCULAR DISEASES

Because of hypertension and dyslipidaemia, people with T2D have a higher risk of cardiovascular diseases such as coronary heart disease, heart failure and stroke. Cardiovascular disease is the main cause of death among people with diabetes. Diabetes makes arteries stiff and prone to blockages, raising the risk of heart attacks and contributing to poor circulation, particularly in the legs and feet.

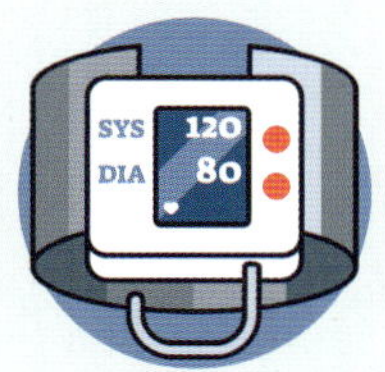

HYPERTENSION (HIGH BLOOD PRESSURE)

Two-thirds of people with diabetes have or will develop hypertension. This is because elevated blood glucose damages blood vessels, making them less elastic, so the heart works harder to pump blood. This greatly raises the risk of heart attacks, strokes, kidney damage and vision problems.

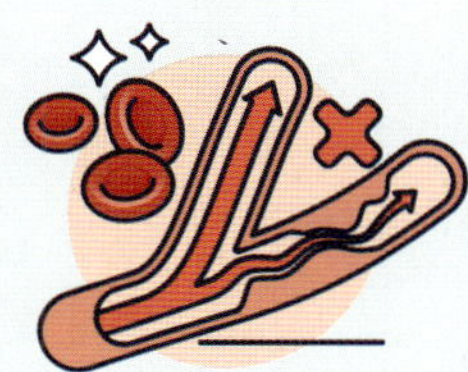

DYSLIPIDAEMIA (ABNORMAL CHOLESTEROL)

Dyslipidaemia is characterised by high triglycerides, low HDL ('good' cholesterol), and high LDL ('bad' cholesterol) to the point where the doctor will recommend a statin in your medication regime. Dyslipidaemia increases the risk of atherosclerosis, heart attacks and strokes. Almost one-third of people with diabetes have high cholesterol, and most have some kind of lipid abnormality.

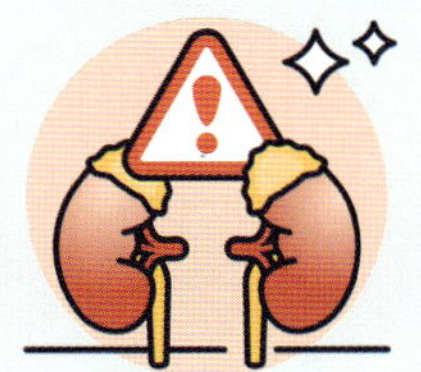

CHRONIC KIDNEY DISEASE

Persistently high blood glucose and blood pressure damage the small blood vessels in the kidneys, affecting their ability to filter blood. Over time, this can lead to chronic kidney disease and eventually kidney failure. In the worst-case scenario, you'll need dialysis or transplantation. Diabetes is the leading cause of chronic kidney disease worldwide.

OBESITY

Obesity shares causal pathways with T2D (especially central abdominal obesity). Up to 90% of adults with type 2 diabetes are obese. Obesity increases insulin resistance and the risk of cardiovascular disease, sleep apnoea, joint problems and some cancers. Managing your weight is crucial to improving both diabetes and its comorbidities.

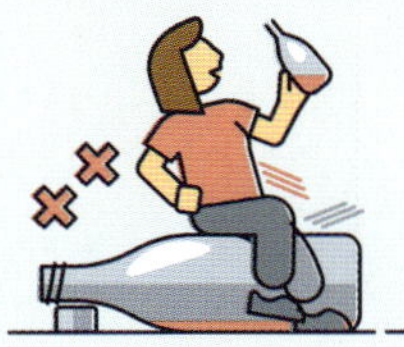

LIVER DISEASE (MASLD)

Obesity and insulin resistance in people with T2D often contribute to fat accumulation in the liver, leading to metabolic dysfunction associated with steatotic liver disease (fatty liver). This can progress to inflammation (hepatitis), scarring (cirrhosis) and even liver cancer.

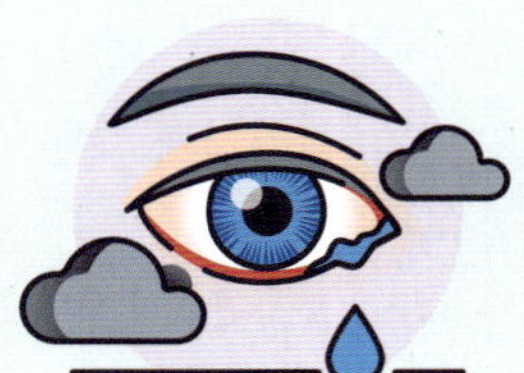

MICROVASCULAR COMPLICATIONS (RETINOPATHY, NEPHROPATHY, NEUROPATHY)

Microvascular complications develop gradually, so be aware and address small signs and symptoms, because they really are life-changing.

- **Retinopathy:** Damage to the eye's blood vessels can lead to vision loss and eventual blindness.
- **Nephropathy:** Kidney damage results in protein in the urine and kidney failure.
- **Neuropathy:** Nerve damage, especially in the feet, causes numbness, tingling and pain, and raises the risk of foot

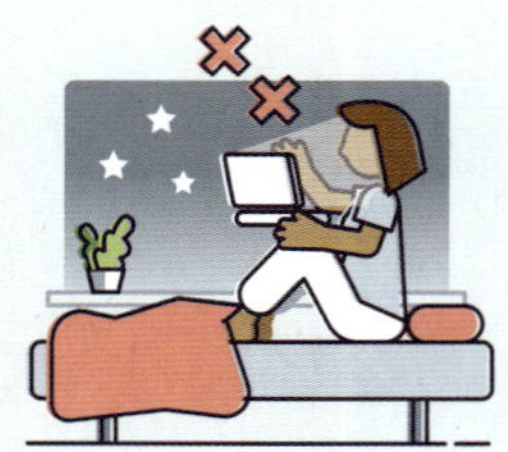

MENTAL HEALTH DISORDERS (DEPRESSION, ANXIETY)

People with T2D are twice as likely to have depression or anxiety. Effects can be from coming to terms with the disease and managing the disease. Many people with T2D have poor gut health, which also increases the risk of anxiety and depression.

Mental health conditions really do need treatment because they can make self-management harder and can worsen glycaemic control, leading to poorer health outcomes, progressing the disease faster than it otherwise would.

Stay connected with your healthcare provider because they may pick up issues and get an action plan in place. People with depression are not motivated and many won't even realise they could be developing depression in the early stages.

SLEEP DISORDERS

Diabetes makes sleep disturbances more frequent. Conditions such as sleep apnoea, restless leg syndrome and insomnia are more common in people with diabetes, interfering with daily functioning and potentially worsening blood glucose control.

Sleep is king when it comes to overhauling your health. It's so important for your hormonal health, program compliance, mental health, motivation, mood and quality of life.

CANCERS

Type 2 diabetes is associated with a higher risk of certain cancers, including liver, pancreatic, endometrial and colorectal cancer. Contributing factors may include chronic inflammation, insulin resistance and obesity.

Make sure you're checking your C-reactive protein and erythrocyte sedimentation rate in every blood test you do, to keep track of trends or trajectories. Get routine colonoscopies.

Of course, getting to a healthy goal weight is essential. For more, please see my weight-loss program The 10:10 Plan.

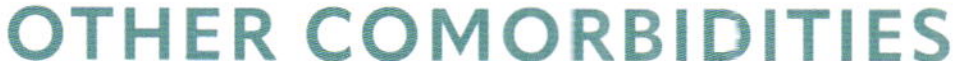

OTHER COMORBIDITIES

Most people with T2D will experience multiple comorbidities as they age, making the disease much more complex than impaired glucose metabolism. Frequently reported conditions include:

- osteoarthritis (due to excess weight and joint stress)

- asthma and other lung conditions (possibly related to inflammation)

- autoimmune and connective tissue diseases.

Managing diabetes effectively means paying attention not only to your blood sugar levels but also to your heart, kidney, nerve, mental and overall metabolic health. Early intervention, ongoing treatment and a holistic approach are absolutely essential to reduce your risk of comorbidities and complications, and improve your quality of life.

GUT HEALTH AND DIABETES

I want to touch on the relationship between our gut health and type 2 diabetes. Taking care of our gut is essential for a holistic approach when treating disease.

Research shows that people with T2D have a less diverse gut microbiome and an imbalance between healthy and unhealthy bacteria. Chronic high blood glucose makes the gut less hospitable for beneficial bacteria. Many people with T2D also have diets low in fibre and high in processed carbohydrates and fats, are less physically active, and have high stress, all of which decrease beneficial bacteria.

Chronic inflammation and leaky gut syndrome make the gut lining more permeable, leading to less diverse gut microbiota. Medications such as antibiotics can cause gut dysbiosis. And some diabetics have genetic predispositions and live in environments that can influence the strains of bacteria.

HOW DO GUT MICROBES INFLUENCE DIABETES?

Gut bacteria help to break down complex carbohydrates and produce short-chain fatty acids that improve insulin sensitivity. A disrupted microbiome may produce fewer short-chain fatty acids, leading to poorer insulin regulation and higher blood glucose.

Leaky gut syndrome, where microscopic gaps in the intestinal lining allow bacterial fragments to enter the bloodstream, is caused by an unhealthy gut. This triggers inflammation throughout the body, which is a major contributor to insulin resistance and type 2 diabetes progression.

Gut microbes can also affect how our body absorbs nutrients and metabolises medications, such as metformin. Some interesting research suggests that metformin's effect on lowering blood glucose partly relies on its impact on gut bacteria. See how amazing our gut is!

Certain bacteria can influence the production of hormones in the gut (such as GLP-1), which impact hunger, satiety and insulin release.

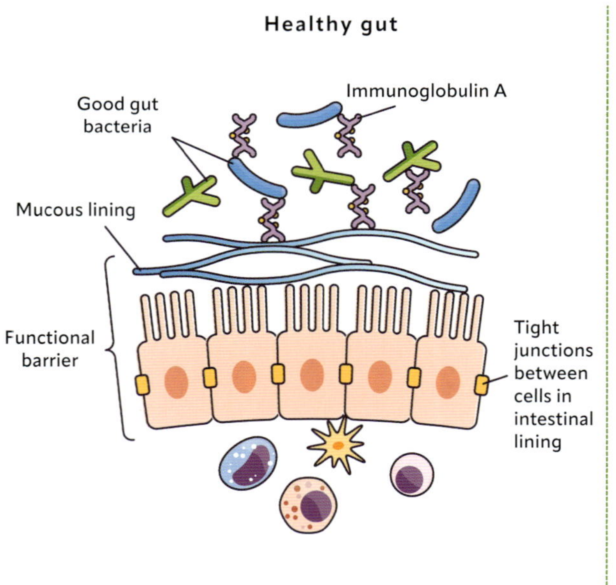

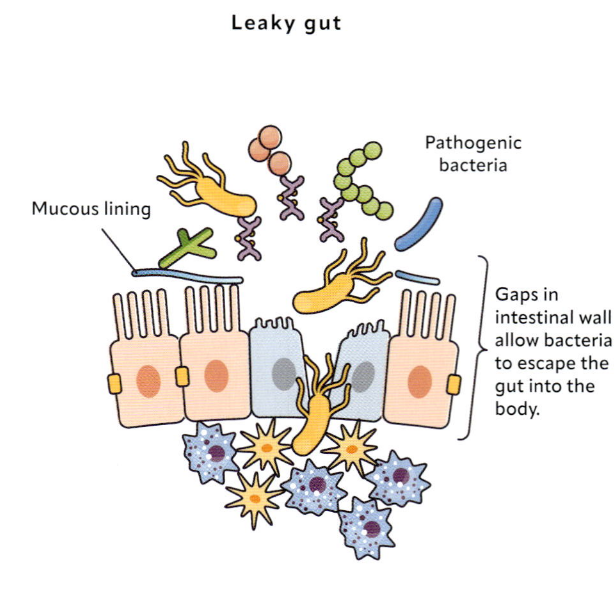

What we eat impacts the health of our liver. Our gut bacteria can either help prevent or promote fatty liver disease. Bacterial by-products and gut inflammation impact liver function. So taking care of our gut when treating T2D is really important. I suggest eating lots of probiotic-rich foods, but also you can take a probiotic daily to support your gut. I certainly do.

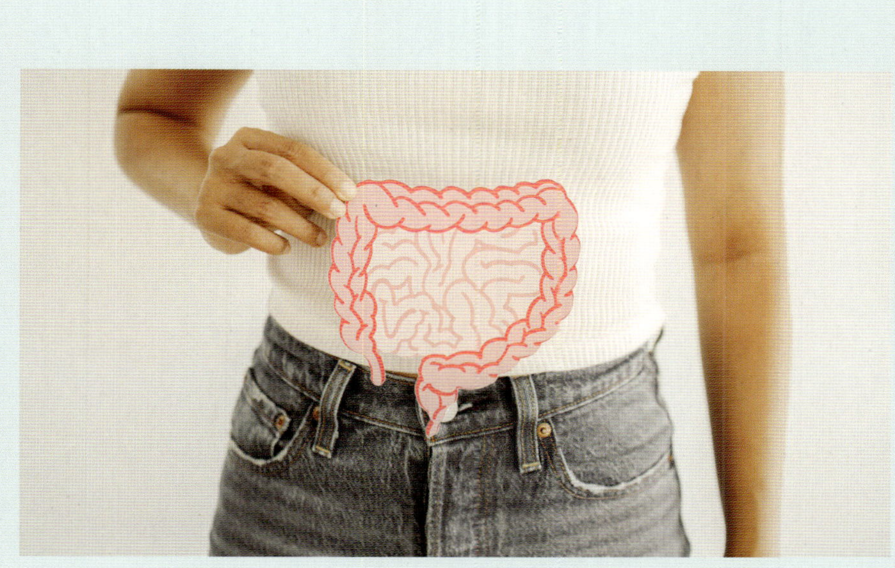

RESEARCH INTO THE GUT MICROBIOME

Scientists are currently exploring how eating more fibre and plant foods, probiotics and probiotic-rich foods, prebiotics, and even faecal transplantation could rebalance the microbiome, support blood glucose management and lower your diabetes risk. This area is still evolving, but it's so fascinating and positive.

The gut microbiome helps regulate the immune system, metabolism and inflammatory processes. Taking care of our gut is another important tool in managing type 2 diabetes.

SKIN AND DIABETES

People often forget about their skin, but our skin can tell us so much about our health. Type 2 diabetes has a significant relationship with skin health, resulting in many distinct skin changes and an increased risk of complications.

High blood glucose damages the small blood vessels and nerves supplying the skin. This reduces the amount of oxygen and nutrients reaching skin cells, but also impairs the skin's ability to detect injuries, regulate moisture and fight infections.

It's important to monitor the time it takes for minor wounds, blisters or cuts to heal. Poor wound healing increases the risk of serious skin infections and ulcers, especially on the feet. And it's a telltale sign of type 2 diabetes.

T2D can impact our immunity because of the constant high blood glucose. A weakened immune system, along with dry, cracked skin, allows bacteria and fungi to enter more easily. The result can be cellulitis, boils and sties (when bacterial) and yeast infections, ringworm and athlete's foot (when fungal). The better controlled the blood glucose, the less frequent these infections are.

CLASSIC DIABETIC SKIN CONDITIONS

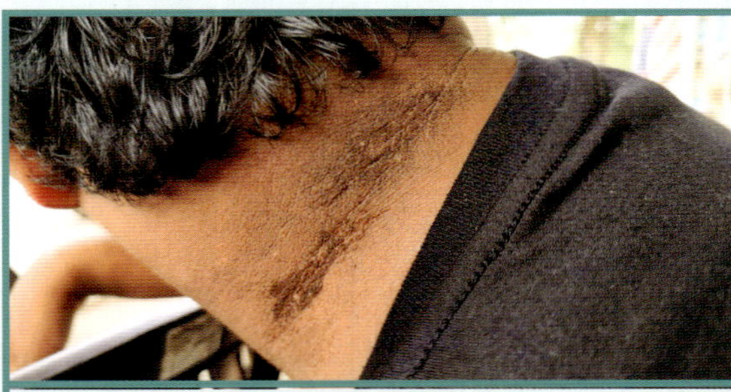

ACANTHOSIS NIGRICANS

Dark, slightly raised, velvety patches in skin folds such as the neck, armpits or groin. Linked to insulin resistance, they are often an early warning sign of type 2 diabetes.

NECROBIOSIS LIPOIDICA DIABETICORUM

Red-yellow shiny patches with a thin surface. While rarer, they are related to diabetes.

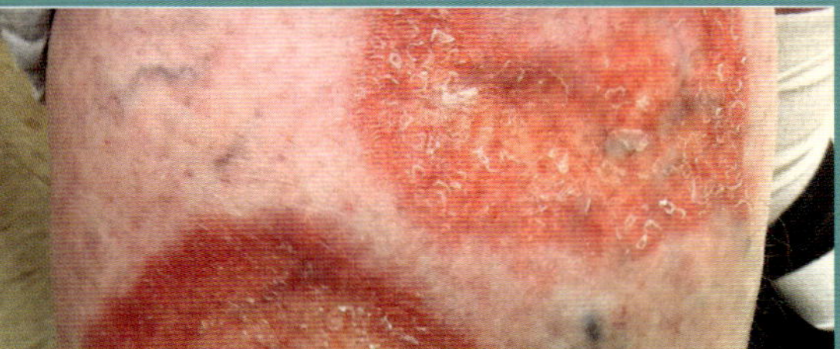

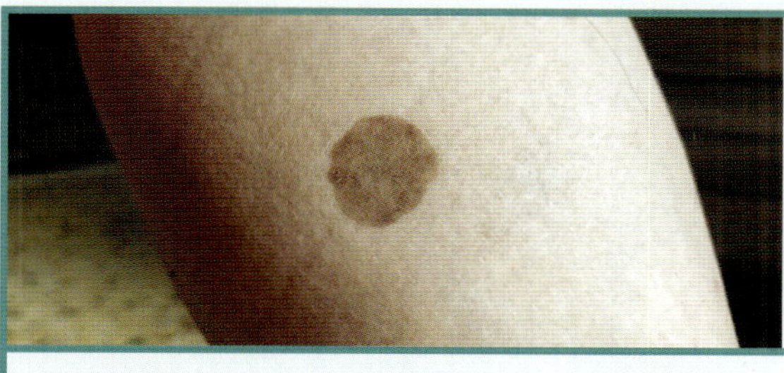

DIABETIC DERMOPATHY

Small, round or oval brown patches on the shins caused by changes in tiny blood vessels. While they are harmless, they indicate diabetes-related skin changes.

ITCHY, DRY AND THICK SKIN

When diabetes is not managed, you can get generalised itching (pruritus). Dry skin is a result of water loss from urinating way too much, and you see more cracks, flaking and roughness in the skin. Some people develop a hardening or thickening of the skin, particularly on the hands and joints.

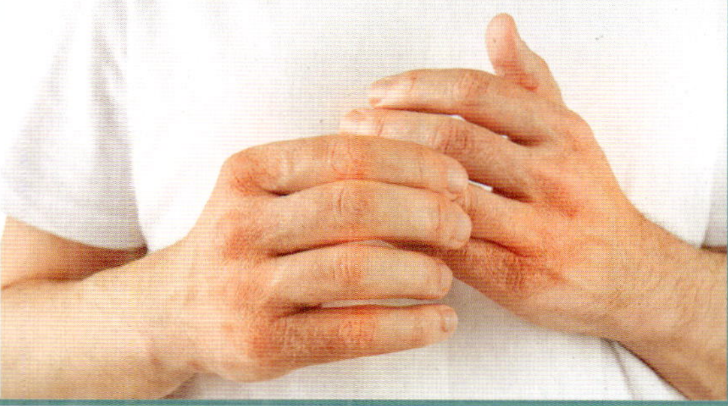

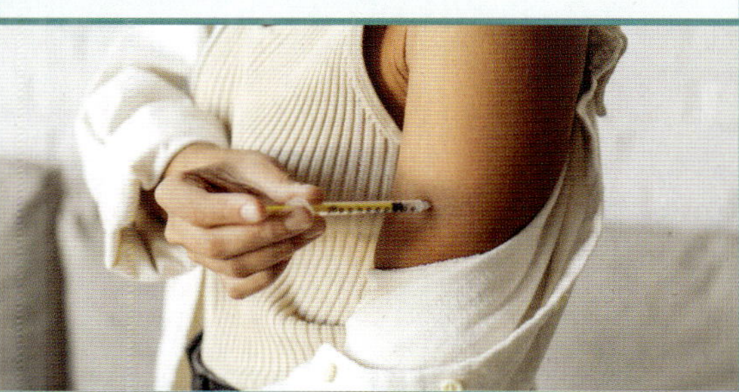

NERVE DAMAGE

Diabetic neuropathy damages the sensation in the skin, especially on the feet. People may not notice wounds, blisters or infections until they become severe.

SKIN CHANGES FROM MEDICATION

Insulin injection sites may develop lumps, bumps, redness or pigment changes if the same spot is used repeatedly. Plus new diabetes medications can sometimes cause rashes or allergic reactions.

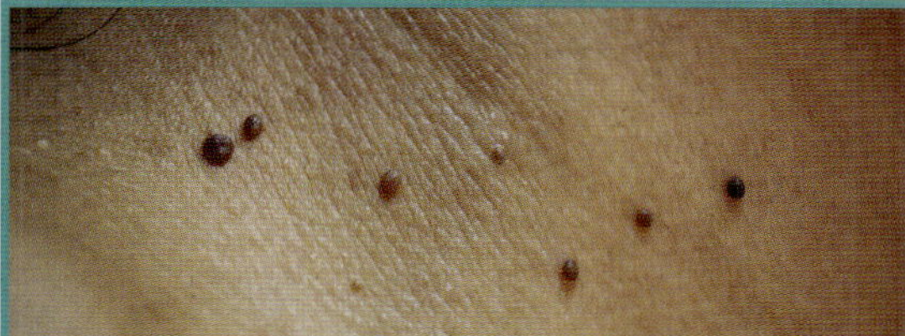

SKIN TAGS

Small, benign growths occur more often in people with insulin resistance. This is often one of the first signs I see.

Checking your skin and being aware of the relationship between skin and diabetes is really important. Skin problems are often an early or visible sign of underlying diabetes, and can indicate poor blood glucose control, increased risk of complications, and the need to take better care of yourself.

DIABETES AND YOUR SEX LIFE

Type 2 diabetes is strongly linked to changes in men and women's sexual behaviour as well as changes in libido and erectile functioning.

Having chronically high blood sugar damages the blood vessels and nerves, which you need for blood flow and to feel aroused. This is a contributing factor to men with erectile dysfunction. Women may experience reduced genital lubrication, less arousal and less sensation.

Diabetes can lower men's sex hormone levels. This disturbs the hypothalamus–pituitary–gonadal axis, reducing libido and the capacity for an erection. Men with T2D are more likely to have erectile dysfunction and develop it earlier than men without T2D, due to the damage to hormones, vascular system and nerves.

As well as feeling depressed, fatigued and self-conscious about body image, plus the fear of hypoglycaemia, the stress of being in a relationship while managing diabetes can reduce the desire for sex.

30% of men and 50% of women with T2D have low sexual desire and satisfaction.

Because of all this, people with T2D are having less sex, reduced spontaneity and in some cases avoiding sex when unwell.

If this is you, have open conversations with your partner and healthcare practitioner.

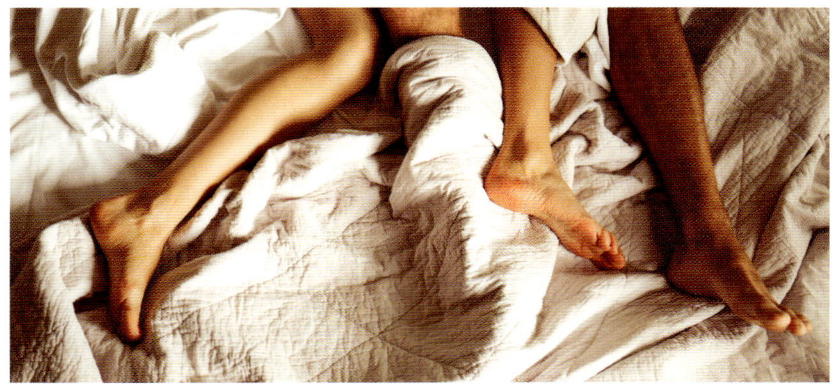

A FUNNY STORY ...

I recall a patient of mine who I treated many years ago. He was in his 40s and had been obese for a long time. But he lost around 50 kilograms and put his diabetes into remission. His wife often came to our consultations because she did all the family cooking.

When he had been in remission for a while, his wife (who had always been healthy and fit) mentioned in a consultation that he had regained the libido from when they were first married. 'Sarah, what have you done to my husband?' she said. 'He won't stop chasing me around the house!'

I had to laugh, but was so happy that he was a healthy, functioning male again.

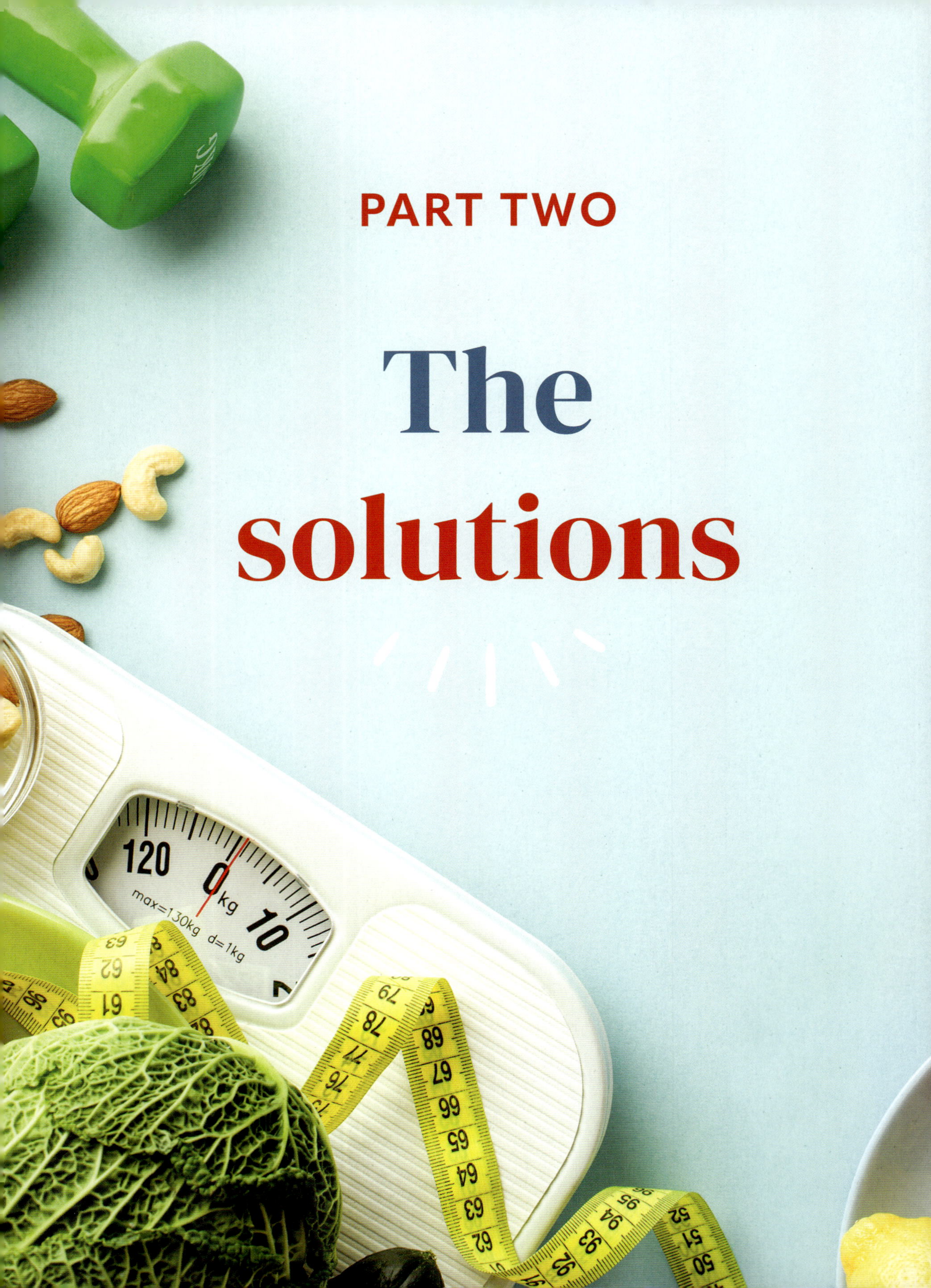

PART TWO

The
solutions

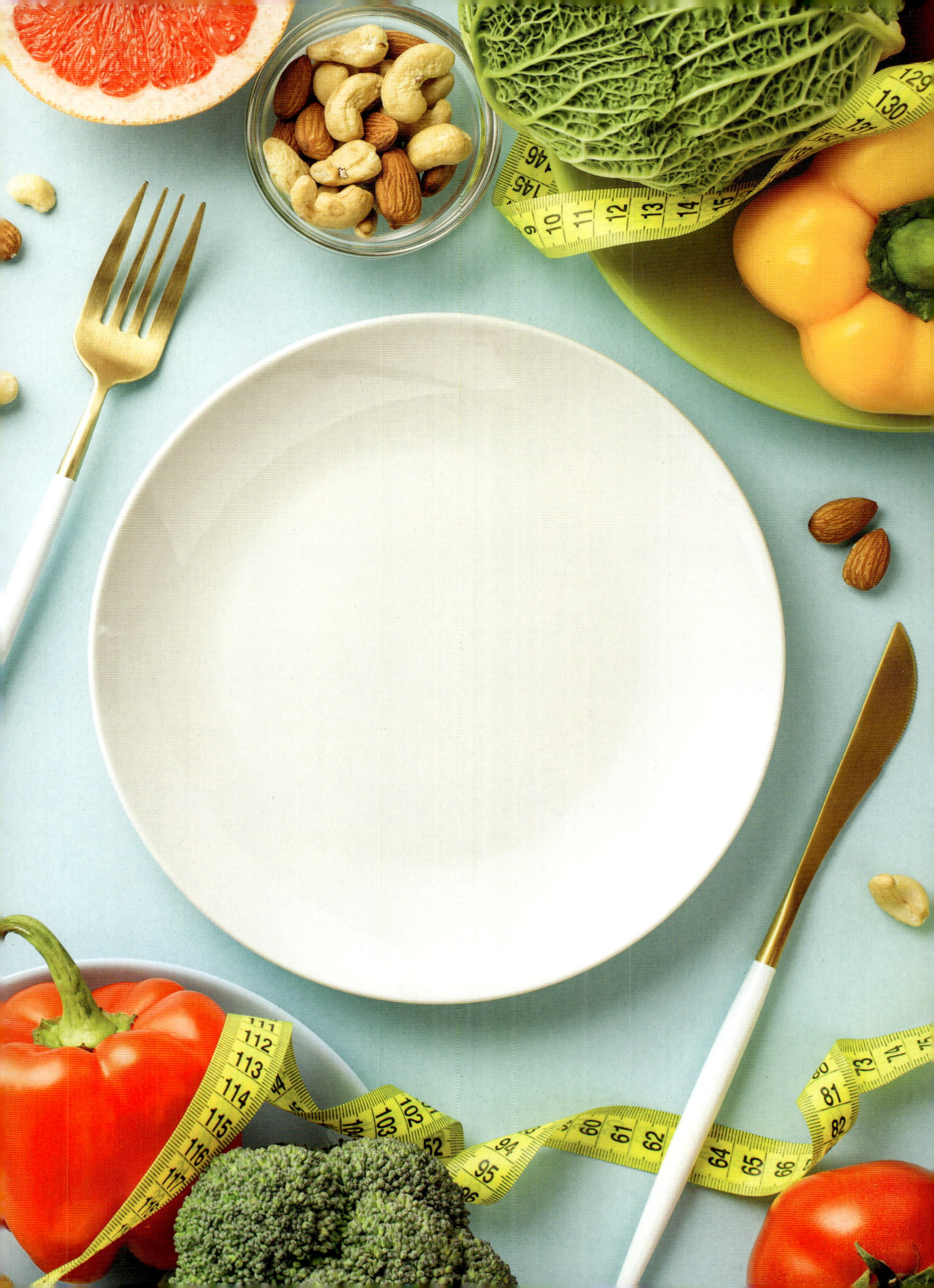

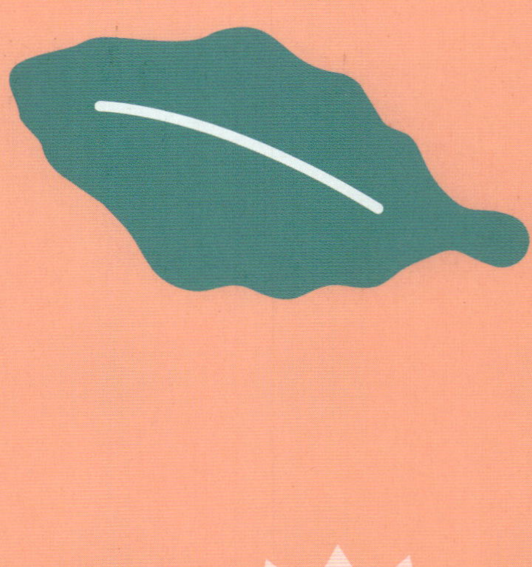

CHAPTER 9

Why nutrition matters

When it comes to type 2 diabetes, your diet needs to be focused on wholefoods, with high-fibre and low-GI carbohydrates, lean proteins, and healthy good fats. The diet needs to be anti-inflammatory, antioxidant rich, nutrient dense and well-balanced. Your goal is to stabilise your blood glucose, lower inflammation, improve metabolic health and keep your heart healthy.

A PLATEFUL OF NUTRITION

Don't skip meals and try and keep a consistent routine with meal times. Here's how to divide your plate for optimum health benefits:

- ½ plate = vegetables

- ¼ plate = protein

- ¼ plate = whole grains or legumes (when at healthy goal weight)

- Add a good fat (avocado or olive oil)

A note on diets … The incredible Mediterranean, low-carb and plant-based diets have all been shown to reduce diabetes complications, HbA1c and triglycerides.

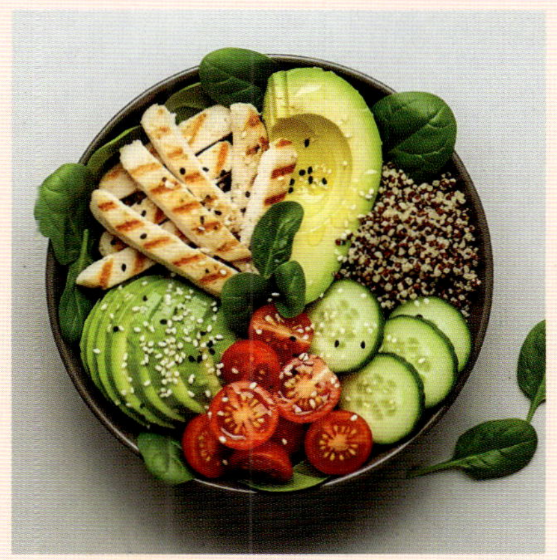

VEGETABLES

The best vegetables have a low GI. They should be high in fibre; non-starchy; and full of vitamins, minerals and antioxidants – these are heart-healthy, support overall metabolic health and regulate blood glucose levels.

My little hack for this with my patients is this: the darker the vegetable's colour, the lower the carbohydrate, higher the fibre and lower the calories. Think broccoli over potato, for instance.

LEAFY GREENS

All the wonderful leafy greens such as lettuce, spinach and kale have the lowest GI – around 10–15 – and are packed with folate, antioxidants, fibre, iron and magnesium. All these nutrients are amazing to stabilise our blood glucose. They are also rich in vitamin C and carotenoids, which are heart-healthy and keep blood glucose stable. Aim for 3 cups of leafy greens a day.

CRUCIFEROUS VEGETABLES

These include cabbage, brussels sprouts, broccoli and cauliflower. They lower inflammation and can improve insulin sensitivity. Some great research shows that people who eat these regularly have a reduced risk of diabetes and better regulated cholesterol and blood pressure. I'd also argue that people who eat like this are generally healthy, so again they're just a part of the bigger picture.

NON-STARCHY VEGETABLES

Cucumber, capsicum, asparagus, green beans, tomatoes, mushrooms, okra, radish, eggplant and zucchini are all low calorie, low GI, high fibre and hydrating. They also control blood glucose and are satiating. Think about the colours of these vegetables: other than the radish and possibly a red capsicum, they are all darker colours. Non-starchy vegetables will feature in Part 3: **The 9-week program**, and are the best options for healthy eating.

ROOT VEGETABLES

Carrots, pumpkin, turnips and beetroot are all high fibre and low GI. Now, they do have more carbs than leafy greens, but they still offer good nutrition and fibre. I tell my patients to keep root vegetables to a minimum, no more than once a day. A serving guideline would be ½ cup.

LEGUMES

This group includes beans, lentils, chickpeas and split peas. They are a good source of protein and excellent source of fibre, so good for our gut health. Try to consume them a couple of times a week. Plus, they are incredibly affordable. The key to enjoying legumes if you're new to embracing them is start slow and steady, and always soak overnight if using dried.

Always make sure half of your plate has salad or vegetables at lunch and dinner. You should grill, steam or sauté vegetables, or enjoy them raw, of course. When looking at your plate, imagine it as a rainbow. Get as many different colours on there as possible for the diversity our gut bacteria love and to get more nutrients into your diet.

WHOLE GRAINS

Choose whole grains such as brown rice, quinoa and oats, and avoid all refined (white) grains. Whole grains are high fibre and low GI plus minimally processed. They help slow down glucose absorption, provide energy, support insulin sensitivity and provide nutrients.

Note: whole grains are for when you are maintaining a healthy weight. While I do put them in the 9-week program, it's at a minimum only, so the body can be in ketosis. And save the whole grains for the end of each meal (for more on this, see 'What order you eat food matters' in Chapter 10).

- **Oats** (rolled, steel-cut or whole groats) are high in beta-glucan fibre that can improve blood glucose and cholesterol. (I always recommend oats for my high-cholesterol patients, and it works.) Oats have a low to moderate GI so can help glycaemic control.

- **Barley** consistently ranks among the best grains for diabetes. It has a very low GI (25–35), is rich in soluble fibre (beta-glucan), and helps regulate blood glucose and cholesterol.

- **Quinoa** is considered a 'pseudo grain' and has a moderate GI (50–53). It is high in protein, fibre and all the essential amino acids. Studies confirm its benefits for glucose stability and satiety.

- **Buckwheat** is gluten-free, and high in resistant starch and fibre, helping to stabilise blood glucose and improve cardiovascular health. Buckwheat flour is a good alternative for wheat flour.

- **Farro**, **spelt and other ancient grains** are high in protein, fibre and minerals, and have been linked to improving blood glucose and insulin sensitivity.

- **Brown rice** is a whole grain, so has more fibre and micronutrients in the bran and germ than white rice. This offers slower glucose release than white rice, especially when paired with vegetables or protein. Eat in moderation and always at the end of the meal.

- **Bulgur and whole rye** are both are low GI and high in fibre.

Many people ask me about grains when managing diabetes, and I'm always pointing out that it's the refined carbohydrates that we need to avoid – they are what spike blood glucose. These include cakes, white bread, doughnuts, biscuits, muffins, crumpets and crackers made with white flour.

Many long-term studies and meta-analyses show that whole grains are associated with lowering the risk for developing type 2 diabetes. I recommend only two serves per day (one serve is ½ cup cooked) at breakfast and lunch, never at dinner, and only when at a healthy goal weight. Less-processed grains such as steel-cut oats or hulled barley are better options.

LEAN PROTEINS

High-quality proteins support heart health, regulate blood glucose, are low in saturated fat, and can support muscle and metabolic function. Lean proteins include chicken, turkey, pork, fish, legumes, tofu, eggs, dairy, seeds and nuts.

- **Salmon, trout, sardines, mackerel and tuna** (oily fish for omega-3s) provide heart-protective fats. It's recommended to eat them at least twice a week, ideally four to five times. Other white fish are also excellent sources. The canned versions are affordable, plus portion controlled. Sardines are an excellent natural source of creatine – remember this next time you're consuming them. Try to make sardines a staple.

- **Skinless chicken and turkey** are lean, low in saturated fat and are great grilled, roasted or poached. Of all the meats, chicken has the highest protein content at 31 grams per 100 grams.

- **Lentils, chickpeas, black beans, split peas and kidney beans** are rich in protein and fibre, helping control your appetite and blood sugar. They also support heart and gut health.

- **Tofu, tempeh and edamame** are lean, plant-based protein alternatives that are associated with improved cardiovascular outcomes in diabetes.

- **Eggs** are affordable, plus they provide high-quality protein; vitamin B12; vitamins D, E and A; iron; and calcium. Eggs are best enjoyed poached or boiled.

- **Greek yoghurt, cottage cheese and cheese** supply calcium and protein for muscle and metabolic health. When choosing cheese for protein, the white cheeses are about 10 grams protein per 100 grams, but dry, hard cheeses such as pecorino are about 36 grams protein per 100 grams.

- **Almonds, walnuts, peanuts, sunflower seeds and seed/ nut butters** contain healthy fats, nutrients and plant protein. Just be mindful of portions due to calorie density. Your daily intake should be a cupped handful, or 30 grams. Because of their hard structure, when we consume nuts, we generally only utilise around 70% of the available calories. The other 30% is passed in the stool.

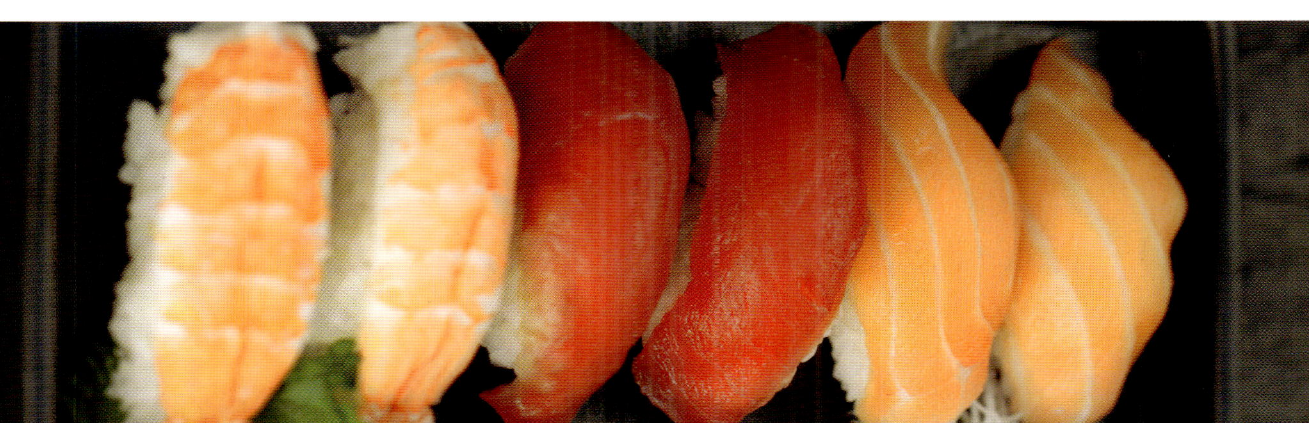

HEALTHY FATS

Monounsaturated and polyunsaturated fats are the healthiest choices for people with type 2 diabetes. They help control cholesterol and blood lipids, protecting against diabetic heart complications. They also support healthy insulin regulation and help flatten the blood sugar curve.

Healthy fats help keep you full and satiated, making it easier to manage your weight and blood glucose levels. Because they lower inflammation and improve blood vessel health, they help to prevent diabetes complications.

Healthy fats should feature in your diet daily.

What's the difference between monounsaturated and polyunsaturated fats? It's structural:

- **Monounsaturated fats** have one double bond in their fatty acid chain.
- **Polyunsaturated fats** have two or more double bonds per fatty acid chain.

ALL ABOUT FATS

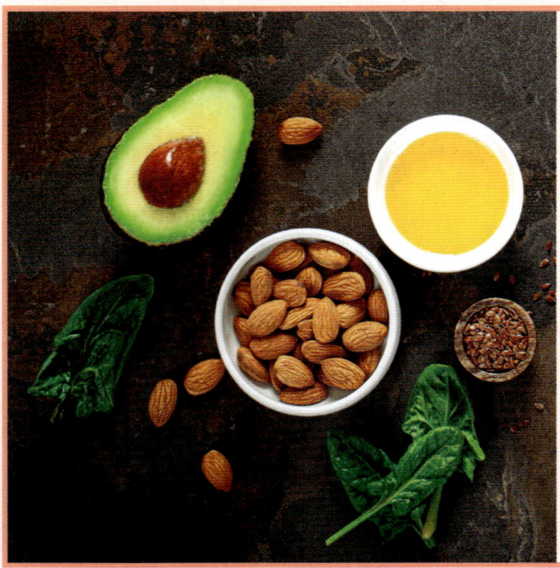

MONOUNSATURATED FATS

- Olive oil, avocado, most nuts (almonds, cashews, peanuts, macadamias), canola oil
- Help lower LDL ('bad') cholesterol while maintaining or raising HDL ('good') cholesterol
- Reduce heart disease risk
- Support cell membrane health
- May help control blood glucose
- The body can produce some monounsaturated fats, but they are also obtained from the diet.
- More stable than polyunsaturated fats, making them better for moderate-heat cooking

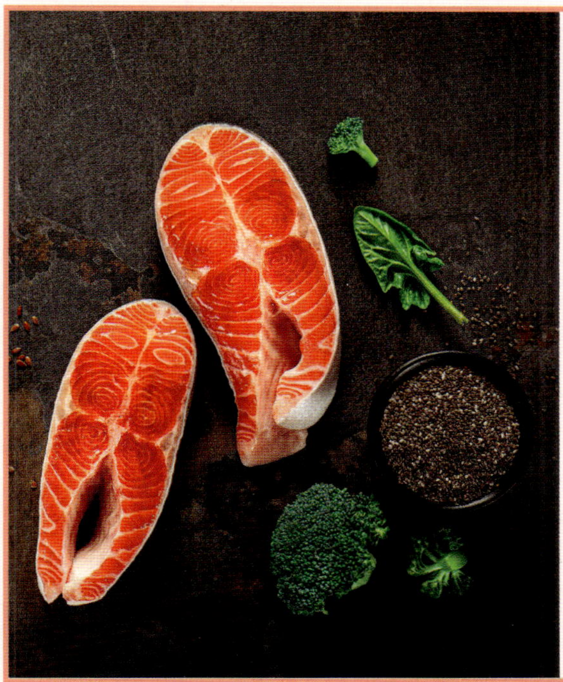

POLYUNSATURATED FATS

- Walnuts, sunflower seeds, linseeds (flaxseeds), fish (salmon, sardines, mackerel), corn oil, tofu, safflower oil, sunflower oil, chia seeds, soybean oil
- Essential fats (omega-3 and omega-6) that the body cannot synthesise and must get from food
- Crucial for brain function, building cell membranes, cell function, blood clotting and reducing inflammation
- Omega-3-rich foods such as fish and linseeds may further help with blood glucose control and lower cardiovascular risk
- Lower LDL cholesterol and support heart health
- Less stable and can be damaged by high-heat cooking – best used in dressings or lower heat applications.

SATURATED FATS

- Found in fatty meats, butter, cream and some processed foods
- Increase LDL cholesterol
- Worsen insulin resistance
- Coconut oil is a saturated fat, but it's not a bad saturated fat. It's a medium chain glyceride. I use coconut oil in some recipes, mostly for baked goods, but keep it to a minimum.

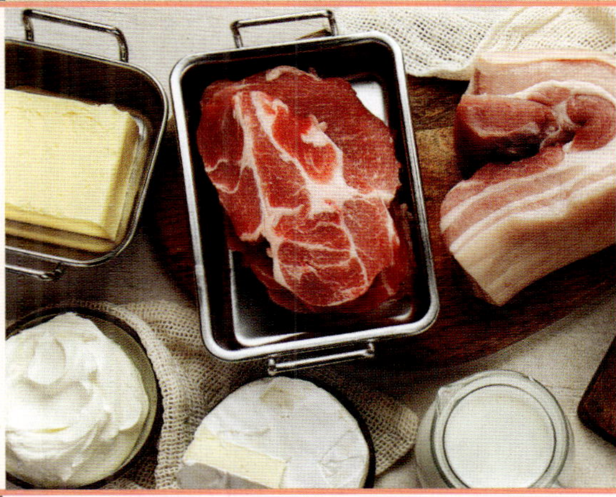

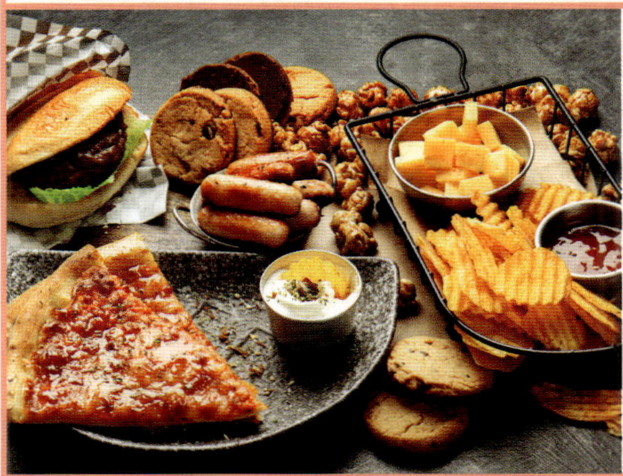

TRANS FATS

- Found in some margarines, some baked goods and in cheap deep-fried fast foods
- They just make everything worse for both heart health and diabetes.
- Trans fats are heavily regulated now, but still always check the label.

FIBRE

Have you noticed that fibre is having a moment, much like protein? Well, fibre is especially important for people with T2D because it can improve your blood glucose control, lower cholesterol, help with weight management and reduce the risk of diabetes complications.

Types of fibre:

- **Soluble fibre.** This is found in oats, barley, legumes, apples, citrus fruit, psyllium husk, and beta-glucan (found in the cell walls of various grains, mushrooms, yeast and some seaweeds). They form a gel in water and slow the absorption of glucose.

- **Insoluble fibre.** This is found in vegetables, whole grains, nuts, seeds and bran. It adds bulk, keeps the bowel regular and improves overall gut function.

It is best to enjoy both insoluble and soluble fibre for that broad spectrum of health benefits.

Adults should be having about 28 grams a day for women and 38 grams a day for men. Research shows that fibre can reduce premature mortality by up to 48% for people with diabetes. The key is to start gradually to avoid excessive flatulence, bloating and discomfort. And be sure to drink plenty of water.

The benefits of fibre:

- Soluble fibre slows digestion and reduces blood glucose spikes after eating, lowering demand for insulin.

- Fibre helps improve insulin sensitivity, helping cells use insulin more effectively as well reducing insulin resistance.

- You need fibre for heart health; it lowers LDL cholesterol, triglycerides and blood pressure – all risk factors for diabetes.

- Fibre helps manage weight by helping you keep full, thereby reducing calorie intake and curbing appetite, which is so important when managing diabetes.

Best sources of fibre for people with type 2 diabetes:

- oats and barley
- legumes
- whole grains
- fruit (especially berries and apples)
- vegetables (carrots and greens – always leave the skins on)
- nuts
- seeds.

One of my favourite sources of fibre is kiwifruit with the skin on. I have this daily. If you struggle to go to the bathroom and depend on fibre products, this is something you need to embrace. Finely dice the kiwifruit, add a tablespoon of Greek yoghurt, some chia seeds and sprinkle over psyllium husk. I promise, you will be forever grateful when armed with this hack. You could also add some cinnamon and ginger to the mixture to boost the nutrients.

FRUIT

Can you eat fruit if you have type 2 diabetes? I get asked about this a lot. Fruit is fine to consume. The key is to enjoy the appropriate serving size and *always* in the fruit form, never the juice. Eating the whole fruit is actually linked to improved insulin sensitivity, improved blood glucose levels and fewer diabetes complications.

Fruit is NOT the problem!

I would be hard pressed to find someone with T2D from eating too much fruit. Not only is fruit sweet and delicious, but it's rich in antioxidants, vitamins, minerals and fibre. It slows the absorption of glucose, is heart-healthy and a perfect snack, and can help with regulating hunger. But you do have to eat fruit in moderation.

The guidelines: have 2 whole pieces of fruit per day.

High-fibre fruits are the best choices for managing blood glucose:
apples, berries, pears, citrus and plums. Like everything in life,
too much fruit is not great. It can have a negative effect on your
blood glucose levels. Meta-analyses have found an association
with higher fresh fruit intake and improved insulin sensitivity,
plus lower risk of developing type 2 diabetes. This could also be
because fruit eaters are possibly healthy eaters all round.

FRUIT MYTHS AND TIPS

Myth: Fruit is bad for diabetics.

Fact: Fruit juice and dried fruit should be avoided or
significantly minimised. Also avoid canned or bottled fruit
packed in syrup or juice.

Tip: Pairing fruit with Greek yoghurt and nuts can slow the rise
of blood glucose.

Tip: Frozen fruit is also excellent in its whole form.

Tip: Berries are your new best fruity friend. How many berries
in a serve?

- blackberries: 1 cup
- blueberries: ¾ cup
- raspberries: 1 cup
- strawberries: 1 cup

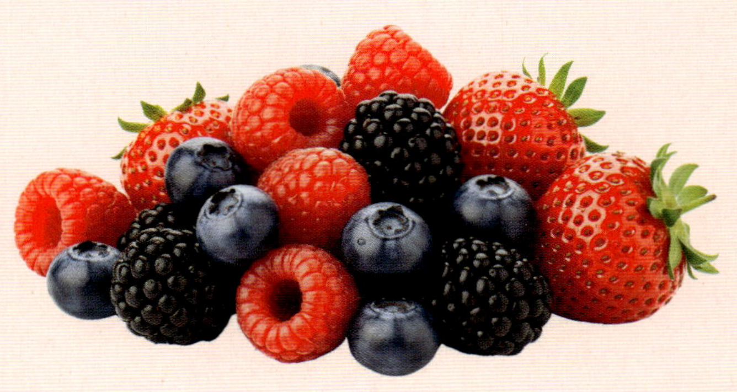

LOW-GI FRUITS FOR DIABETES

FRUIT	GI	WHY IT'S GOOD FOR YOU
APPLES	38	Good fibre content, supports gut and blood glucose health
APRICOTS	34	High in antioxidants and low sugar per serve
BLACKBERRIES	25	Rich in vitamins C and K and fibre
CHERRIES	22	High in fibre and antioxidants, with minimal glucose impact
GRAPEFRUIT	25	Very low GI, packed with vitamin C and fibre
KIWIFRUIT	50	Good vitamin C and fibre, helps with steady glucose absorption
LIMES/LEMONS	20–32	Very low sugar, best for flavouring and low impact on blood glucose
ORANGES	35–43	High vitamin C, fibre, hydrating and lower GI than orange juice
PEACHES	28–42	Nutrient-rich, helps with satiety and blood glucose regulation
PEARS	38	High in fibre, supports digestion and blood glucose control
PLUMS	35	Antioxidants and fibre for glucose regulation
RASPBERRIES	32	Fibre-rich, supports gut health and lowers glycaemic load
STRAWBERRIES	41	Excellent for immune health and blood glucose management

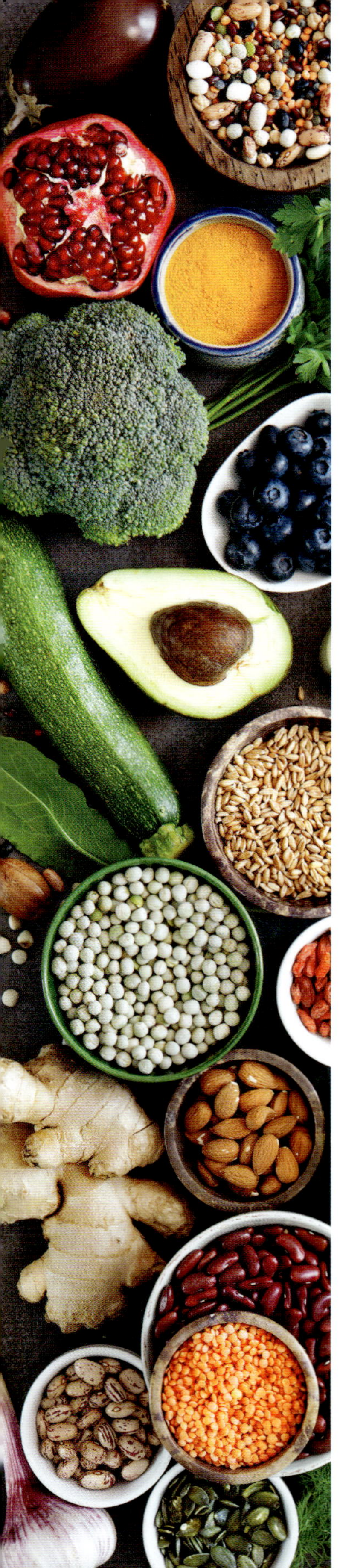

ANTIOXIDANTS

To manage type 2 diabetes, antioxidants are extremely important because they can support insulin sensitivity, lower inflammation and counteract oxidative stress. These include:

- Vitamins
  - vitamin C (ascorbic acid)
  - vitamin E (tocopherol)
  - vitamin A (retinol and carotenoids such as beta-carotene, lycopene).

- Minerals and cofactors
  - selenium, zinc, magnesium, manganese.

Note: these minerals support the action of antioxidant enzymes such as superoxide dismutase and glutathione peroxidase.

- Phytochemicals
  - flavonoids (found in berries, citrus, tea, dark chocolate)
  - polyphenols (berries, cocoa, coffee, spinach, green tea)
  - anthocyanins (blue or red fruits and vegetables)
  - lutein, lycopene, zeaxanthin (leafy greens, tomatoes, eggplants).

- Non-enzymatic antioxidants (These are found in foods and within the body. They protect cells from oxidative damage, but are not enzymes themselves.)
  - glutathione (produced by the body and found in some vegetables)
  - alpha-lipoic acid (spinach, broccoli)
  - coenzyme Q10 (CoQ10) (meat, fish, some grains and vegetables).

- Omega-3 polyunsaturated fatty acids
  - walnuts, linseeds (flaxseeds), fatty fish (have both antioxidant and anti-inflammatory roles).

WHY ARE ANTIOXIDANTS IMPORTANT?

Antioxidants neutralise free radicals and reactive oxygen species, reducing oxidative stress and cellular damage related to diabetes. Antioxidants such as vitamins C and E, flavonoids and polyphenols help prevent diabetes complications such as neuropathy, retinopathy and cardiovascular disease, and support insulin sensitivity.

A diet rich in these antioxidants improves metabolic health, lowers inflammation and helps control blood sugar in people with type 2 diabetes.

TOP ANTIOXIDANT-RICH FOODS

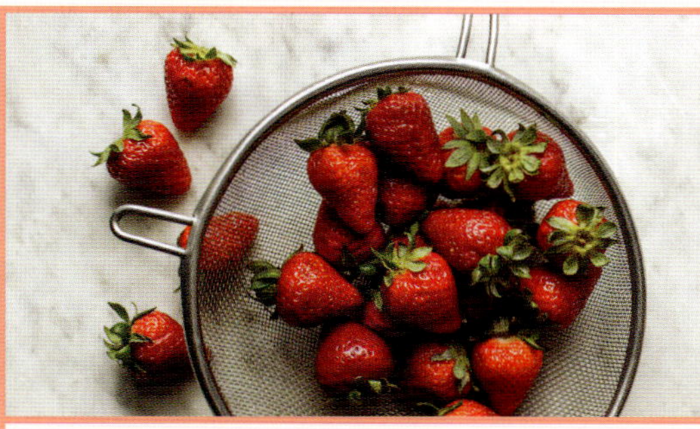

BERRIES

Blueberries, raspberries, strawberries and blackberries are rich in anthocyanins and vitamin C, which improve insulin sensitivity and fight cell damage.

Eating berries regularly can help to lower post-meal glucose spikes and support heart health in diabetes.

CITRUS

Limes, oranges, grapefruit and lemons are rich in vitamin C and flavonoids such as hesperidin. These are linked to better insulin action and lower diabetes risk.

Reminder: always eat the whole fruit, not the juice.

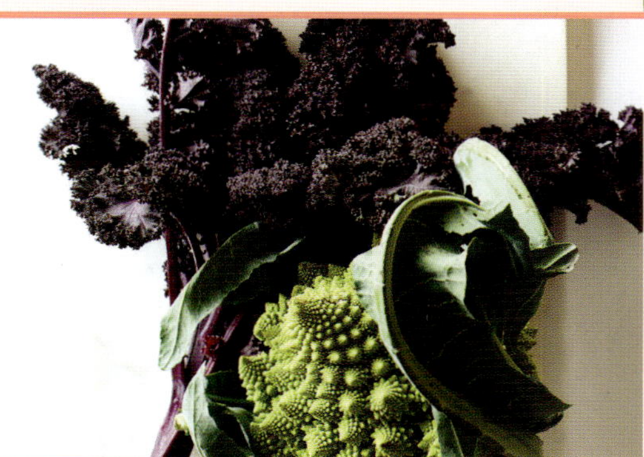

LEAFY GREENS AND CRUCIFEROUS VEGETABLES

Spinach, kale, broccoli, cauliflower and brussels sprouts offer a wide spectrum of antioxidants (vitamins A, C and E, lutein and sulforaphane).

These vegetables are amazing because they lower inflammation, improve blood vessel health and help regulate blood glucose. They should be a part of your daily diet.

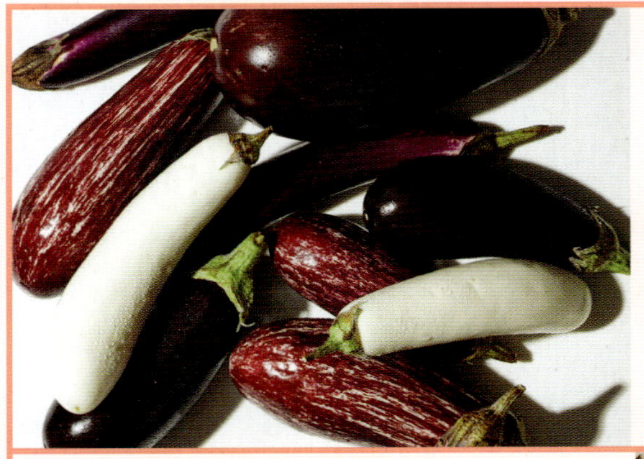

TOMATOES AND EGGPLANTS

Tomatoes provide lycopene and vitamin C, protecting against vascular damage and improving metabolic health. To get the most out of tomatoes and get all that extra lycopene, make sure you cook them.

Eggplants are high in anthocyanins, which help to slow carbohydrate absorption and fight oxidative damage. Eggplants are incredibly versatile and so delicious. Two of my favourite recipes are miso eggplant and ratatouille.

SEEDS AND NUTS

Nuts need to feature in your diet every day. Walnuts and linseeds (flaxseeds) are rich in vitamin E, ellagic acid and omega-3s, which lower inflammation and blood lipids. This further supports blood glucose control.

Aim to have 30 grams, or 1 cupped handful, per day. I personally love cashews and find them incredibly filling. I usually have a handful before the gym in the morning.

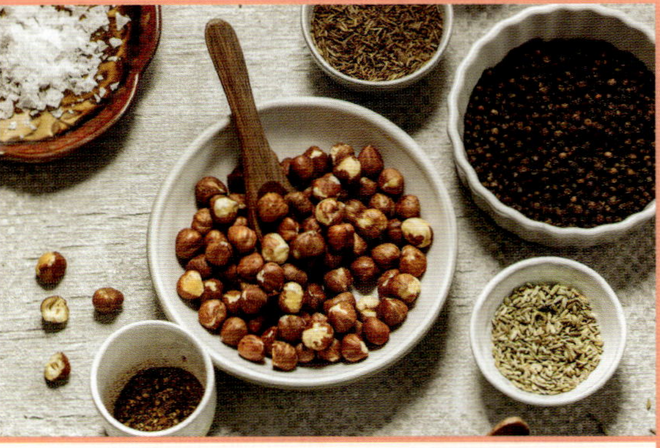

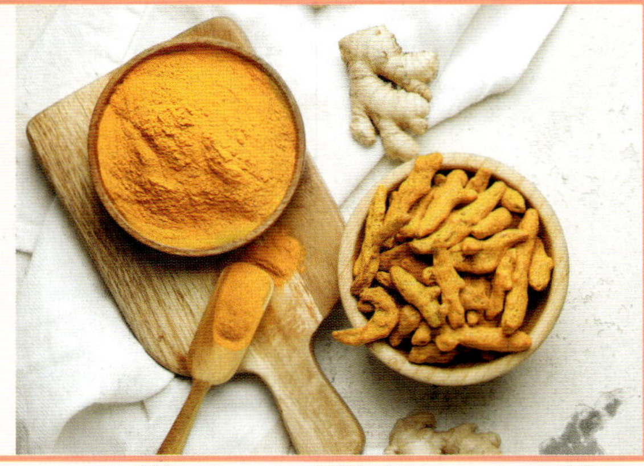

LEGUMES – BEANS AND LENTILS

Beans and lentils are full of fibre and polyphenols. They slow glucose absorption and provide protection for pancreatic beta cells – how good is this!

Eating beans is also linked to improved blood glucose control and less risk of complications. And beans are so affordable! If you buy dried beans, soak them overnight before cooking.

TURMERIC

The active compound in turmeric is curcumin, a strong antioxidant and anti-inflammatory compound. Curcumin has been shown to lower blood glucose and improve insulin sensitivity. It's amazing for lowering inflammation and helping to treat inflammatory conditions such as arthritis.

When you add black pepper to turmeric, it increases the curcumin's activity by 2000%.

ANTI-INFLAMMATORY FOODS

Reducing inflammation is important for people with type 2 diabetes. Chronic inflammation is linked to insulin resistance, high blood glucose and heart disease. I love herbs and spices, and add ginger and turmeric to my yoghurt every day.

- Anti-inflammatory foods reduce inflammation; chronic inflammation can harm beta cells in the pancreas, making the body less insulin sensitive.

- Many anti-inflammatory foods are full of fibre, omega-3s and antioxidants that can lower inflammation. Anti-inflammatory nutrients improve how cells respond to insulin, therefore stabilising blood sugar levels.

- A diet rich in anti-inflammatory foods is linked to a lower risk of heart disease and diabetes.

Note: every year, make sure you're getting your C-reactive protein tested to stay on top of it. This is an inflammation marker.

BEST ANTI-INFLAMMATORY FOODS FOR DIABETES

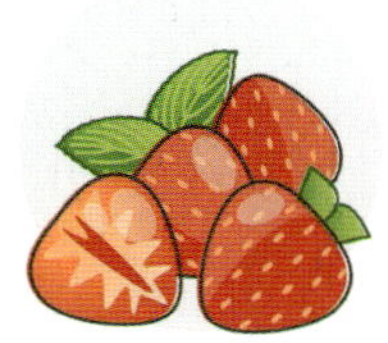

Berries, including blueberries, strawberries, raspberries and cherries

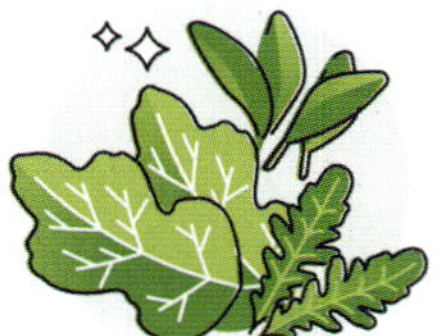

Leafy greens (spinach, kale, rocket)

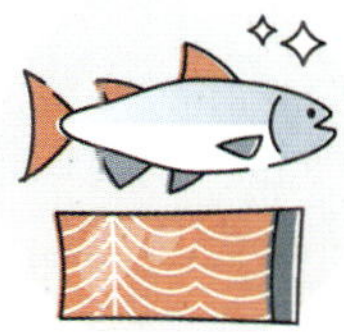

Fatty fish (salmon, mackerel, sardines)

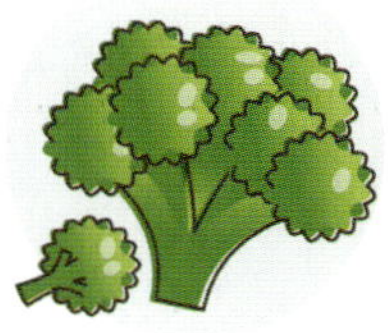

Cruciferous vegetables (broccoli, cauliflower, brussels sprouts)

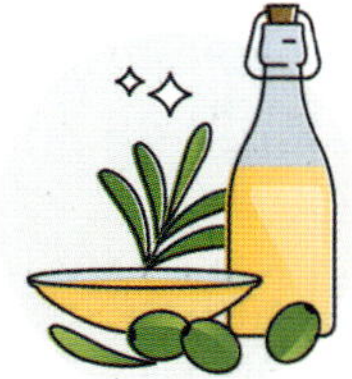

Extra-virgin olive oil, avocados, nuts, seeds

Tomatoes, capsicum, squash

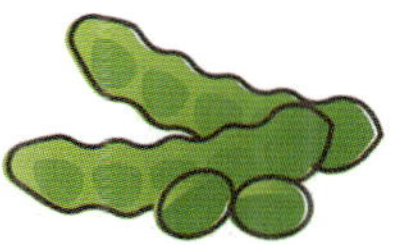

Beans, entils, chickpeas

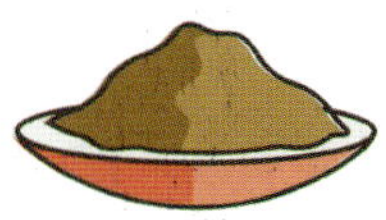

Spices (turmeric, ginger, cinnamon)

WHAT'S RECOMMENDED DAILY

- Vegetables: minimum of ½ plate per meal – aim for six serves per day
- Fruit: two serves per day
- Fatty fish: two to three times per week
- Nuts: 30 grams daily
- Extra-virgin olive oil: 2 tablespoons daily
- Whole grains and legumes: daily at breakfast or lunch

DAIRY PRODUCTS

Cheese can be included within serving recommendations. Fermented dairy (yoghurt, kefir, some cheeses) may have extra metabolic and gut health benefits. For those who avoid dairy, plant-based alternatives (soy, almond, pea milks) should be unsweetened and fortified with calcium.

Top cheese choices:

- cottage cheese: very low fat, source of protein, and low in carbohydrates and salt

- ricotta cheese: lower fat, low-salt, good source of protein

- mozzarella: high-protein, low-fat and among the lowest-sodium cheeses

- swiss cheese: lower in sodium and lactose, high in protein

- parmesan: excellent protein source, low carbohydrate (just keep to a minimum)

- aged cheddar

- feta and goat's cheese: lower in calories per serve and moderately salty. Feta is often made from goat's or sheep's milk, which can be easier to digest than cow's milk.

- best source of protein is Parmigiano Reggiano.

Serving size is about 60 grams per day, as part of getting enough dairy, calcium and protein. Note: this is when maintaining a healthy goal weight.

WHAT'S RECOMMENDED DAILY

The current guidelines are two to three serves of dairy daily, more for adults over 65 – around four serves to get optimum calcium. Don't forget, calcium needs vitamin D for absorption.

A serve is:

- 1 slice hard cheese
- ¾ cup yoghurt – always choose Greek
- 1 cup milk
- ½ cup ricotta cheese.

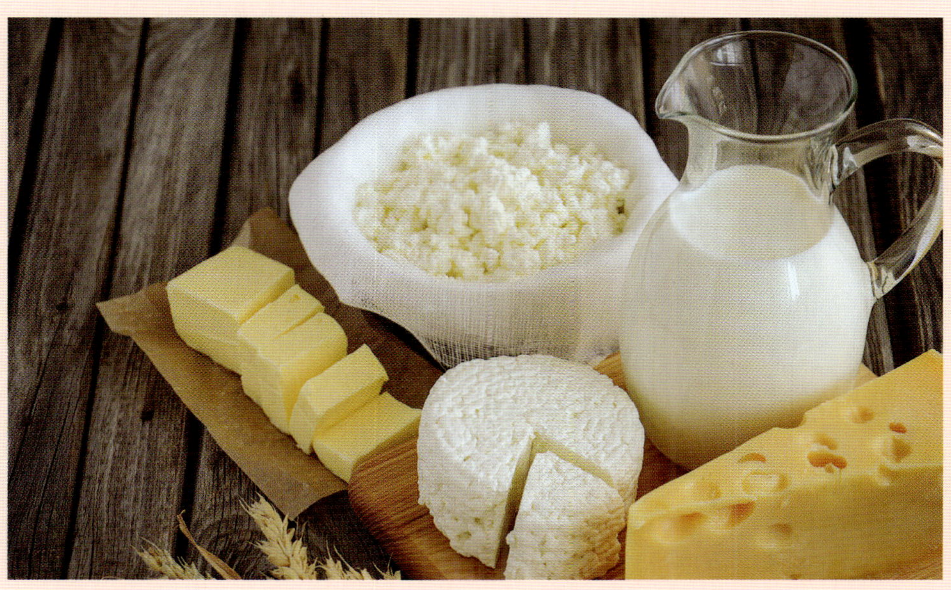

STAR FOODS FOR LIVING WITH TYPE 2 DIABETES

APPLE CIDER VINEGAR

Clinically, I have talked to many people who find apple cider vinegar helps them curb their appetite, especially when used regularly in foods such as salad dressings or diluted in water. Emerging research suggests vinegar and apple cider vinegar can modestly reduce appetite and support weight management when combined with a healthy diet, and it may improve fasting and post-meal blood glucose and insulin sensitivity in some people. It should be used as an adjunct rather than a primary treatment. I just recommend people to be mindful of their teeth if drinking it diluted – use a straw.

WHAT'S THE DEAL WITH APPLE CIDER VINEGAR?

Some people swear by apple cider vinegar (ACV) for lowering blood glucose after a meal by consuming it before a meal. So after a deep dive, several clinical studies and meta-analyses do indicate people taking ACV before or with a meal can lower blood glucose, especially those with type 2 diabetes. When ACV was taken with a high-carb meal, it significantly reduced postprandial (after-meal) blood glucose at the 30–60-minute mark. The protocol was 30 ml diluted in water before eating.

So how does it work? ACV slows gastric emptying, which blunts the glucose spike after eating. It also inhibits enzymes involved in carbohydrate digestion and improves insulin sensitivity in insulin-resistant people.

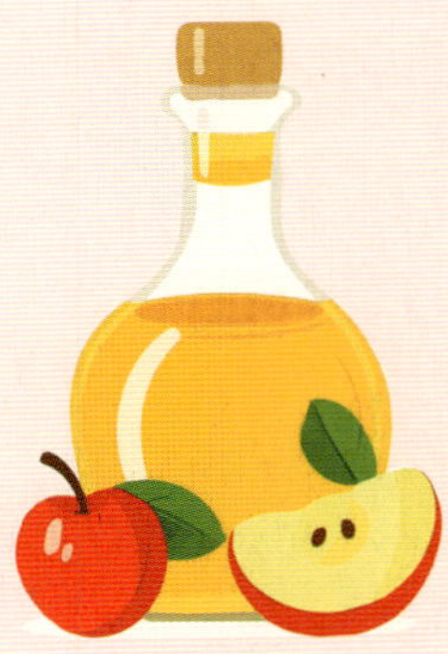

In general, ACV before a meal can only modestly reduce blood glucose levels, especially in people with T2D and insulin resistance.

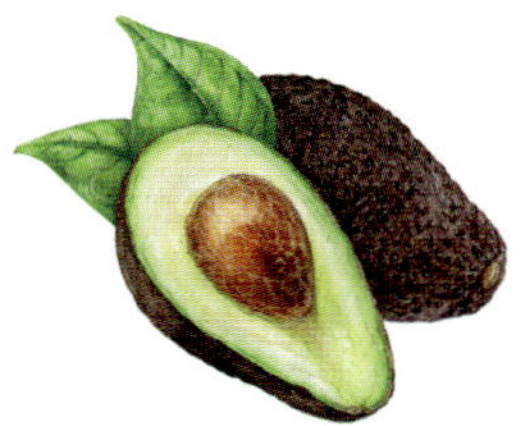

AVOCADOS

High in fibre and healthy fats, very low sugar and minimal carbohydrates, avocados have no impact on our blood glucose levels. Avocado lowers our risk of heart disease and can help us get to a healthy weight. I like to refer to avocado as natural butter, but they can be so much more than that because they're so easy to add to your diet.

BEANS

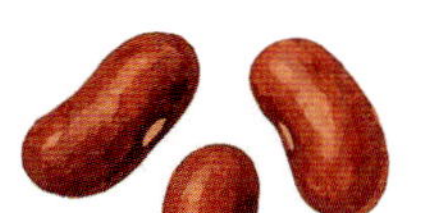

It can be tricky to get people to start eating beans because about 10% of people have irritable bowel syndrome and sometimes when they start to eat them, they eat too many and end up with digestive problems. The key is to start small, about 2 tablespoons per meal, and slowly build up over weeks. Easing into eating beans allows your gut bacteria and digestive system to adjust. Beans are high in fibre, B vitamins, calcium, magnesium and potassium, and have a low GI. And they're so versatile!

BROCCOLI

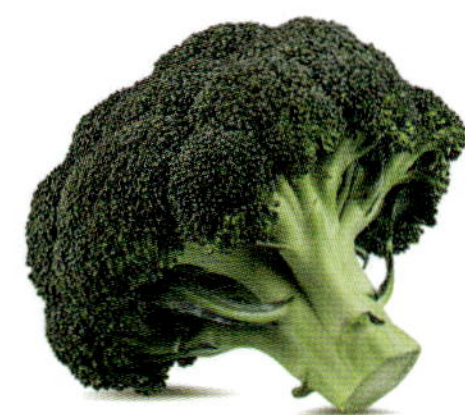

Another superfood and so versatile to cook with. I love lightly cooking broccoli in a pan with olive oil, garlic and chilli, but also as a pizza base and soup. A serve of broccoli is only 27 calories and 3 grams digestible carbs, along with important nutrients such as vitamin C and magnesium.

Some research links lower blood sugar with eating broccoli. This could be due to the sulforaphane in the broccoli. Our body converts glucosinolates found in broccoli to sulforaphane then utilises it.

CHIA SEEDS

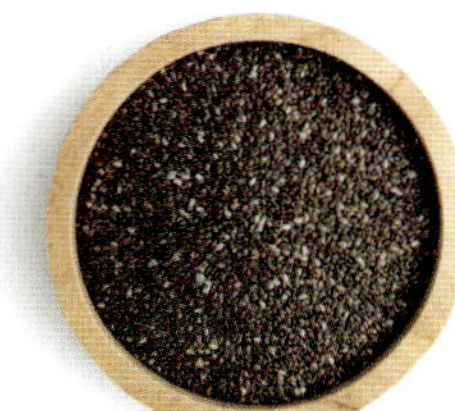

I love chia and eat it every day. Chia is an excellent source of omega-3s and good for our gut health. Chia seeds are high in fibre and low in digestible carbs, so they're good for people with type 2 diabetes, plus they are an excellent source of calcium, so great for bones. The viscous fibre in chia seeds can lower blood glucose. Chia seeds are great for weight loss, and help reduce blood pressure and inflammatory markers. I don't soak my chia if I'm adding it to fruit and yoghurt in the morning. The only time I would is if I was making chia pudding (which is delicious).

EGGS

Not only are eggs extremely affordable and versatile – you can
have them for breakfast, lunch and dinner – they may reduce
your risk of heart disease. Eggs increase HDL cholesterol, lower
inflammation and improve insulin sensitivity. Breakfast egg-
eaters have also been shown to have lower blood pressure as well.
Eggs can help keep you feeling full, regulating blood glucose and
protecting eye health. Another plus: they are good for healthy hair.

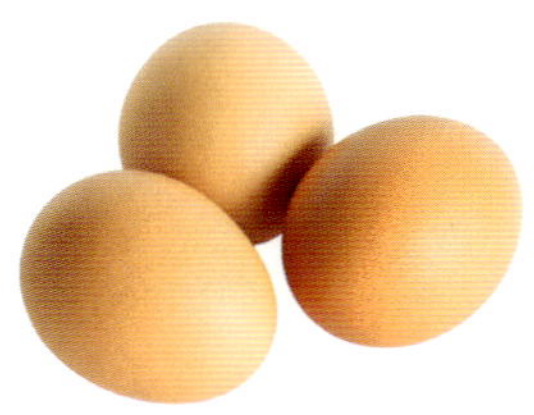

EXTRA-VIRGIN OLIVE OIL

This contains oleic acid, a type of monounsaturated fat that reduces
inflammation and is linked to improved glycaemic management,
reducing fasting and post-meal triglyceride levels. It also has
antioxidant properties.

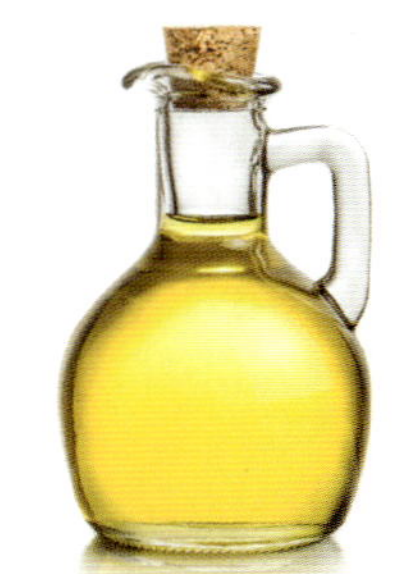

Olive oil is essential for people with type 2 diabetes to help manage
triglycerides and blood sugar. Oleic acid may stimulate the fullness
hormone GLP-1. Olive oil can also reduce heart disease risk. An
antioxidant called polyphenol also reduces inflammation, lowers
blood pressure and protects blood vessels.

Always make sure you are consuming extra-virgin olive oil, and
just olive oil, not olive oil mixed with other, cheaper oils.

Try and aim for around 2 tablespoons per day.

Add it to smoothies, drizzle over lunch or dinner, and have it
readily available next to the salt and pepper in your kitchen.

FATTY FISH

Think salmon, herring, anchovies, mackerel and sardines – they
are excellent sources of heart-healthy and anti-inflammatory
omega-3 fatty acids (eicosatetraenoic acid [EPA] and
docosahexaenoic acid [DHA]). EPA and DHA protect the cells
that line our blood vessels and can improve how our arteries
function. They also lower your risk of stroke and heart disease.

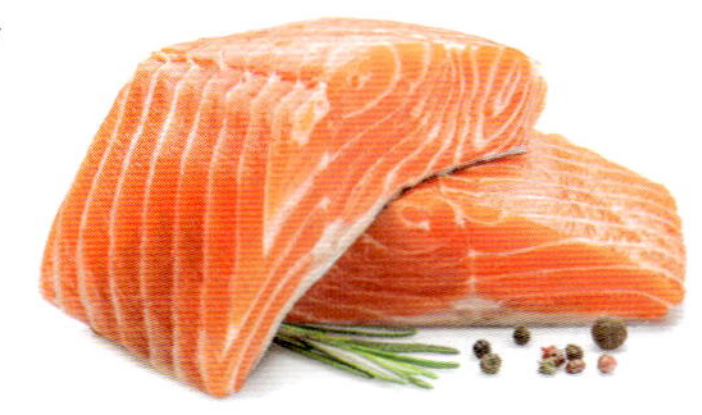

Consuming fish regularly can also help with managing weight
because it's a good source of lean protein and may help manage
blood pressure. Protein helps us stay full and keeps blood glucose
levels stable, therefore helping prevent or lower the risk of diabetes.

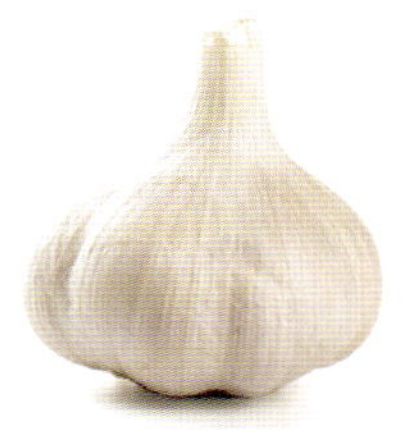

GARLIC

Try to embrace garlic as much as you can because it's just so nutritious. Garlic is a good source of vitamins and minerals, plus it can improve cholesterol levels and manage blood sugar. I recommend adding garlic to as many recipes as possible. Try making a garlic confit or roasting garlic.

GREEK YOGHURT

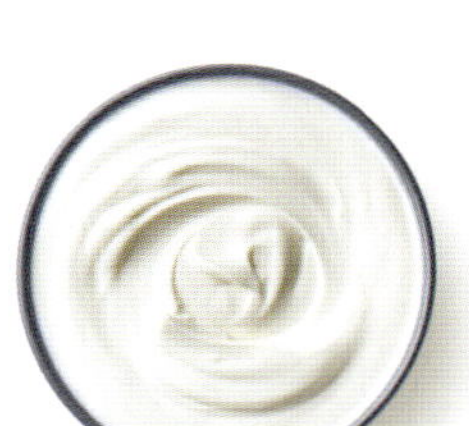

This is another food I make sure to have daily. Greek yoghurt has 1½ times the amount of protein as regular plain yoghurt. It's a good source of calcium and great for gut health.

Greek yoghurt can help with weight loss because it's so high in protein and has a special type of fat called conjugated linoleic acid that helps keep you full. Greek yoghurt is also lower in carbohydrates than other plain yoghurts.

LEAFY GREENS

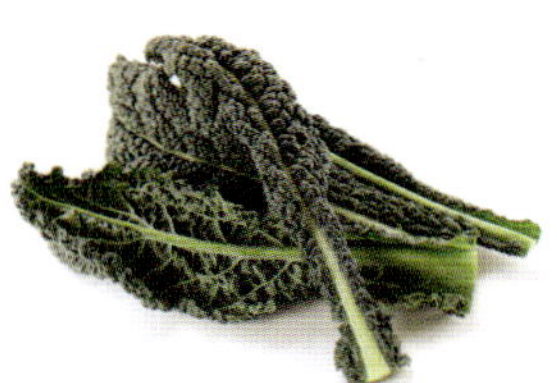

Not only are leafy greens such as spinach and kale nutrient dense and full of vitamins and minerals, but they are also low in calories and easily digested. Leafy greens have a minimal impact on blood glucose levels. They are an excellent source of vitamin C, an antioxidant and anti-inflammatory, so are excellent for diabetes.

LINSEEDS (FLAXSEEDS)

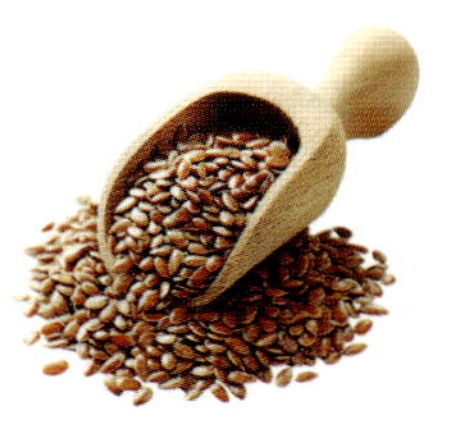

Garnish meals with linseeds or add them to smoothies or baked goods. They are a good source of heart-healthy fibre and omega-3s. The fibre content helps with managing blood glucose.

NUTS

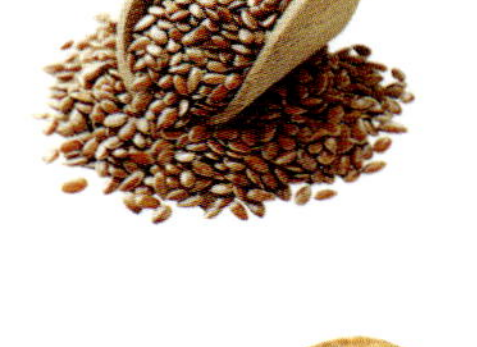

In all my programs, I recommend nuts daily, either as a snack or as a garnish on a salad. Eating nuts regularly can help manage weight as well lower inflammation. Nuts improve heart health and can help people with diabetes by improving blood glucose levels.

PUMPKIN

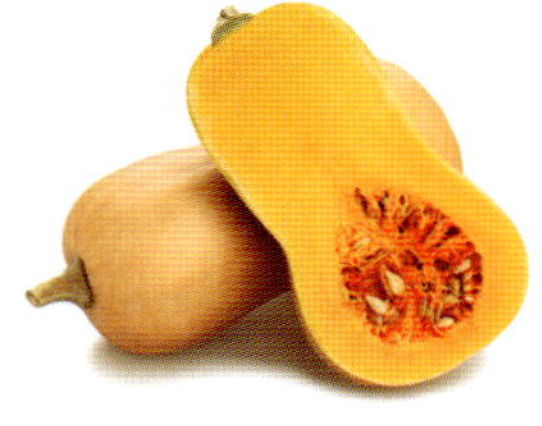

I love squash as a replacement for potatoes in recipes. Research shows that pumpkin can improve insulin sensitivity, helping to lower blood glucose.

STRAWBERRIES

I love strawberries for the taste. They are high in vitamin C and low in calories. Just 1 cup strawberries will give you your recommended daily amount of vitamin C, plus they're an excellent source of fibre. I eat them fresh most mornings with Greek yoghurt.

Strawberries are high in antioxidants known as anthocyanins, which gives them their red colour. They are also rich in other antioxidants called polyphenols. Polyphenols are linked to improving insulin sensitivity.

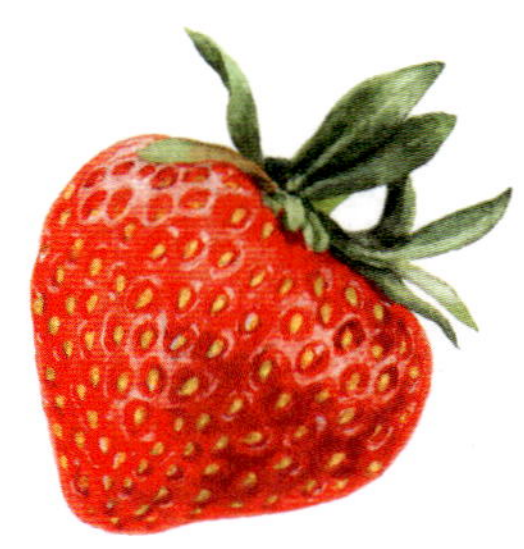

ARE SATURATED FATS REALLY THE BAD GUY?

It depends. Diets high in total saturated fat increase inflammation, raise LDL cholesterol and may heighten insulin resistance. Saturated fats from processed meats and baked goods can worsen insulin resistance, and increase metabolic and heart disease risk for people with type 2 diabetes. But some saturated fats from wholefoods such as dairy or yoghurt may be less harmful or even neutral. You need to know the difference. I don't want you to be scared of eating foods such as yoghurt or dairy, which also come with protein, probiotics and calcium.

TYPES OF SATURATED FAT

PALMITIC ACID	The most abundant saturated fat in palm oil, red meat and dairy. Consuming too much palmitic acid is strongly linked with raising LDL cholesterol and promoting insulin resistance.
STEARIC ACID	Found in cocoa and some meats, this has a lesser effect on LDL cholesterol and may be less harmful than palmitic acid.
LAURIC ACID	Mainly from coconut oil, there's some evidence for neutral to mildly beneficial effects on cholesterol. Like all fats, keep your intake moderate.
SHORT-CHAIN SATURATED FATS	Produced in the gut via fibre fermentation – these are amazing because they benefit our all-over metabolic health.

As a general guideline, avoid saturated fats from processed meats, chicken skin, sausages, cream, pastries and junk foods. Unsaturated fats such as olive oil, nuts, seeds, avocado and fatty fish, and fermented dairy such as yoghurt, are a better choice.

GLP-1 BOOSTING FOODS

Given the rise of glucagon-like peptide-1 (GLP-1) medications for weight loss, I thought it only fitting to highlight foods that can support GLP-1.

WHAT IS GLP-1?

GLP-1 is a hormone produced in the gut that helps regulate blood glucose by increasing insulin, decreasing glucagon, slowing stomach emptying and increasing feelings of satiety. GLP-1 is really important for controlling glucose and appetite, which is why GLP-1 medications are used for weight loss and to treat T2D.

In the last two years of treating people with T2D who are on these medications, I can honestly say I haven't seen the success you would hope for. So many of my patients have complications, while other patients are looking for short cuts and not addressing the core of why they have T2D in the first place. Many haven't lost weight; others who have lost weight regain it and more when coming off the medication. Sadly, the weight is regained as fat, putting them in a worse place than when they started. Recall, muscle is extremely important for regulating blood glucose and these medications cause about 40% muscle loss. People need to change their relationship with food when on these medications. If you do choose to take them, then you must get a decent amount of protein in your diet and start a weight-training program.

Bringing foods into the diet that help increase GLP-1 is an excellent start to naturally boost your GLP-1. Your diet needs to be high in healthy fats, fibre and lean protein – these all slow down digestion and help trigger the release of GLP-1 from gut cells. Consuming fibre helps the good bacteria in your gut produce short-chain fatty acids that also stimulate the production of GLP-1.

Here are the best natural GLP-1 boosters:

- **Eggs.** Rich in protein and healthy fats, studies show a meal with eggs can boost GLP-1 and keep blood glucose stable after eating.

- **Nuts.** These are the perfect snack, especially almonds, pistachios, walnuts and peanuts, thanks to their high fibre and monounsaturated fats.

- **Whole grains.** Oats, barley and other fibre-rich grains stimulate GLP-1 by promoting gut fermentation, which creates short-chain fatty acids.

- **Avocado and extra-virgin olive oil.** They have monounsaturated fats and fibre.

- **Legumes.** Beans, lentils, edamame and split peas are high in protein and fibre.

- **Lean proteins.** Fish, chicken, turkey, tofu and Greek yoghurt help increase GLP-1 response at meals.

- **High-fibre fruit and vegetables.** Artichokes, asparagus, brussels sprouts, carrots, apples, pears, citrus and all types of berries promote fibre fermentation in the gut.

- **Fermented foods.** Yoghurt, kefir, sauerkraut, kimchi, miso and tempeh promote gut health, influencing GLP-1 activity. They're a daily essential.

- **Dark chocolate 70+%.** While rich in flavanols, which may support GLP-1 activity, dark chocolate is an occasional treat and only ever a couple of squares.

- **Cinnamon and turmeric.** Studies show these spices can improve insulin sensitivity and support blood glucose balance, and may help stimulate GLP-1 release in the gut.

HOW FOODS IMPACT BLOOD GLUCOSE LEVELS

Foods and how they impact blood glucose levels are best ranked by their GI and glycaemic load. This basically indicates what blood glucose levels are once you have eaten. This is important to educate yourself about for long-term success – knowledge is key.

LOW GI: 1–55 = SLOW BLOOD GLUCOSE RISE

- Whole grains, including rolled oats, steel-cut oats, barley, quinoa, wholegrain pasta, and brown and wild rice

- Legumes, including lentils, beans, chickpeas and split peas

- Non-starchy vegetables, including leafy greens, broccoli, cauliflower and carrots

- Most fruits (always when whole, and with skin on) such as apples, oranges, berries, pears, citrus and stone fruit

- Nuts and seeds, including almonds, walnuts, chia seeds, linseeds (flaxseeds) and pepitas

- Dairy, including yoghurt and kefir

- Fermented foods, including kimchi and sauerkraut

- Lean protein – very low GI, if at all.

MODERATE GI: 56–69 = MODERATE BLOOD GLUCOSE RISE

- Starchy vegetables, such as green peas, parsnips, beetroot and edamame

- Sweet potato (only ever in small portions), pumpkin and corn (portion controlled to just one cob)

- Medium-grain brown rice and basmati rice

- All sweetened dairy (I never recommend these).

HIGH GI: 70+ = RAPID SPIKE IN BLOOD GLUCOSE

- Processed/refined grains, such as white bread, white pasta, ramen noodles, bagels, baguettes, white rice, jasmine rice, sushi rice, rice cakes, cornflakes, pretzels and so many commercial breakfast cereals

- Potatoes: baked or mashed white potatoes, fries and potato chips

- All sweet foods, such as regular soft drinks, lollies, biscuits, desserts, cakes and pastries

- Tropical fruits, such as watermelon and pineapple.

BEST FOODS FOR LOWERING BLOOD GLUCOSE

These foods can help lower blood glucose as part of a healthy, balanced diet:

- all berries (raspberries, strawberries, blueberries)
- leafy greens
- fatty fish
- eggs
- fermented foods.

Remember — add the carbs to protein and fat to help keep your glucose spikes low.

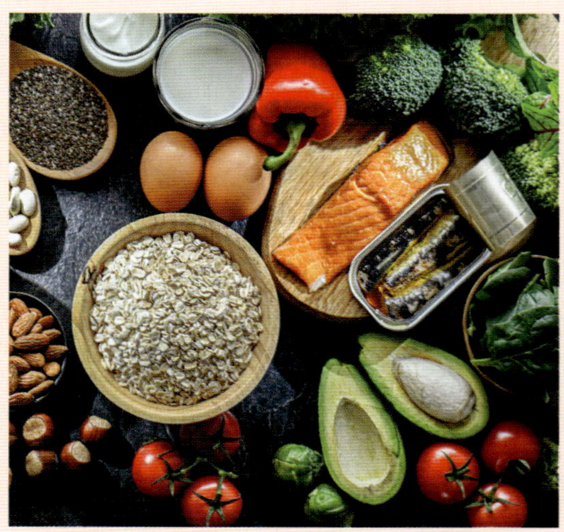

HOW TO READ FOOD LABELS WITH TYPE 2 DIABETES

Learning how to read food labels is all part of having diabetes. You need to have full autonomy when managing your diabetes, after being fully educated about the disease and how to manage it. Understanding food labels will help you manage your blood sugar levels and make healthier choices.

Here is a guideline on how to read food labels:

- **Check the serving size and number of servings per package.** All nutrition information on the label is based on this amount. You'll have to adjust your calculations if you eat more or less than this serving.

- **Look at total carbohydrates.** This is the most important value for managing blood glucose. This figure includes fibre, sugars (both added and natural) and starches. Both sugar and starch impact blood glucose, so always use the total carb amount.

- **Check for added sugars.** Added sugars increase blood glucose more quickly, so scan the ingredient list for words such as 'sucrose', 'glucose', 'fructose', 'corn syrup', 'honey' and 'maltose'. The closer to the start of the ingredient list sugar is listed, the more sugar the product contains.

- **Choose high-fibre foods.** Higher fibre foods are healthier for everyone, but especially when you have diabetes. Aim for foods with more than 3 grams fibre per serving, or at least 10% of the daily value. Fibre helps slow sugar absorption and stabilises blood glucose.

- **Avoid fat and sodium.** Choose items lower in saturated fat (less than 3 grams per 100 grams) and sodium (less than 120 mg per 100 grams) to support heart health.

- **Compare per 100 grams values.** For easy comparison between products, use the 'per 100 grams' column rather than 'per serve' – this helps you spot healthier options.

- **Key tip!** Focus on total carbs, fibre, serving size, added sugars, unhealthy fats and sodium when comparing packaged foods. If needed, consult with a clinical nutritionist or dietician to tailor choices to your specific needs and meal plan.

By understanding these numbers, you can choose foods that support good blood glucose control and overall health. If this is new to you, have a look at what is in your pantry now. You may be shocked at what you find!

SUPPLEMENTS

I take supplements and feel they can really help to support an already healthy diet. The effectiveness of supplements depends on the individual, their current medication and any nutrient deficiencies. Some supplements can interfere with diabetes medication or blood glucose control.

Always check with your doctor first before taking any supplements to make sure there are no contraindications with any medications you are taking.

BEST SUPPLEMENTS FOR T2D

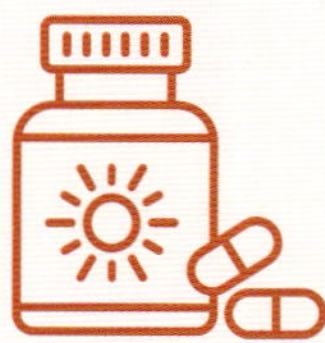

VITAMIN D

I am obsessed with vitamin D. Most people I see have extremely low vitamin D. We need vitamin D for bone health, energy, mental health and insulin sensitivity. Vitamin D deficiency worsens insulin resistance, so correcting low vitamin D can help improve insulin sensitivity and support better blood glucose control.

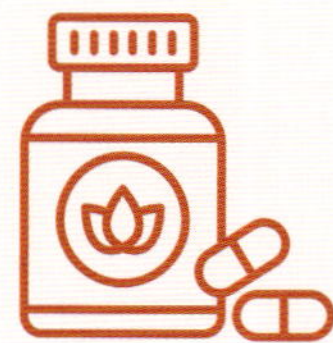

MAGNESIUM

Magnesium deficiency is common in most people I see but also those with diabetes. Supplementation can improve insulin sensitivity, fasting glucose and blood pressure for those low in magnesium.

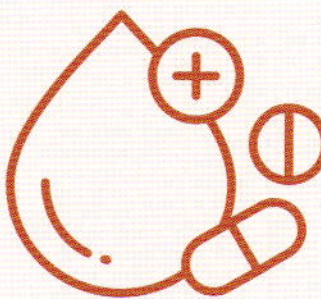

VITAMIN B12

Supplements for vitamin B12 are often needed for people taking long-term metformin, which can lower B12 levels and increase your risk of neuropathy. Always check your levels first.

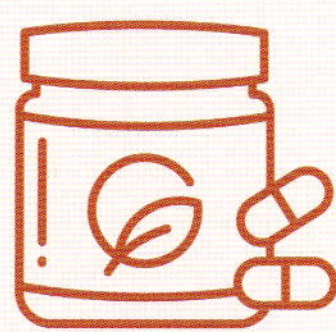

ALPHA-LIPOIC ACID

This may help with diabetic neuropathy symptoms (nerve pain).

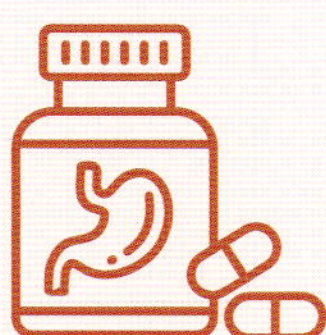

PROBIOTICS

Taking care of your gut health is key. Probiotics are so good for our gut and can modestly improve glucose control.

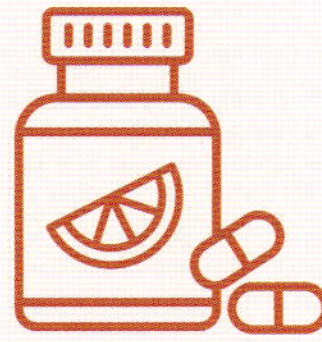

VITAMIN C

Interesting emerging research shows people taking vitamin C have some improvement in post-meal blood glucose.

In general, supplements should never replace food. Rather, they should support an already healthy diet and lifestyle. Always discuss with your healthcare provider, especially if you're on medication, and monitor your symptoms.

I only ever take good-quality supplements. If you're interested in what I take, please email me: contact@sarahdilorenzo.com

THE WORST FOODS FOR BLOOD GLUCOSE

I feel that much of this is obvious, but you should avoid all refined and processed foods, sugary drinks and foods full of saturated fats. Not only do these have a negative effect on heart health, but they also worsen your diabetes and cause weight gain.

When it comes to beverages, soft drinks are obviously bad, but energy drinks and sweetened teas are too. Also avoid all those additions to coffees and smoothies, such as sugar, cream and syrups.

FRIED FOODS

Fried foods are bad for managing blood glucose as they are often high in unhealthy fats such as trans fats, which are linked to an increased risk of heart disease. They are also high in calories and carbohydrates causing rapid blood sugar spikes.

SUGARY BREAKFAST CEREALS

Sugary breakfast cereals can have as many empty calories as desserts. When looking for a breakfast cereal, always opt for one made with oats and sweeten it with fresh fruit. Whole fruit is nature's sweetener.

FRUIT JUICES

I've never been a fan of fruit juices. They have as much sugar as a can of soft drink. Fruit is best enjoyed in its true form, where the sugar is released slowly due to being coupled with the fibre.

LOLLIES

This is obvious, but lollies have so much sugar. Just a single 'red frog' lolly can have about 10 grams of sugar. One jelly snake can have 3 teaspoons of sugar. Of course, this means blood sugar highs and lows.

PROCESSED MEATS

This includes salami, bacon, hot dogs and cold cuts. Not only are they processed, but they're also high in sodium, additives and preservatives, increasing your risk of heart disease.

SOFT DRINKS

Both artificially and sugar-sweetened soft drinks are an absolute NO go. I have zero tolerance in my programs for these in any human diet. Both are linked to a significantly higher risk of type 2 diabetes. Both are linked to blood glucose spikes, hidden calories, weight gain and increased risk of insulin resistance, while artificial sweeteners also have adverse metabolic effects.

Regular soft drinks contain large doses of rapidly absorbed sugars (glucose, fructose, sucrose), causing immediate blood sugar surges and putting stress on insulin production and action. They can lead to increased weight and visceral fat, and are dangerous liquid calories that many of us forget about, worsening diabetes and complications.

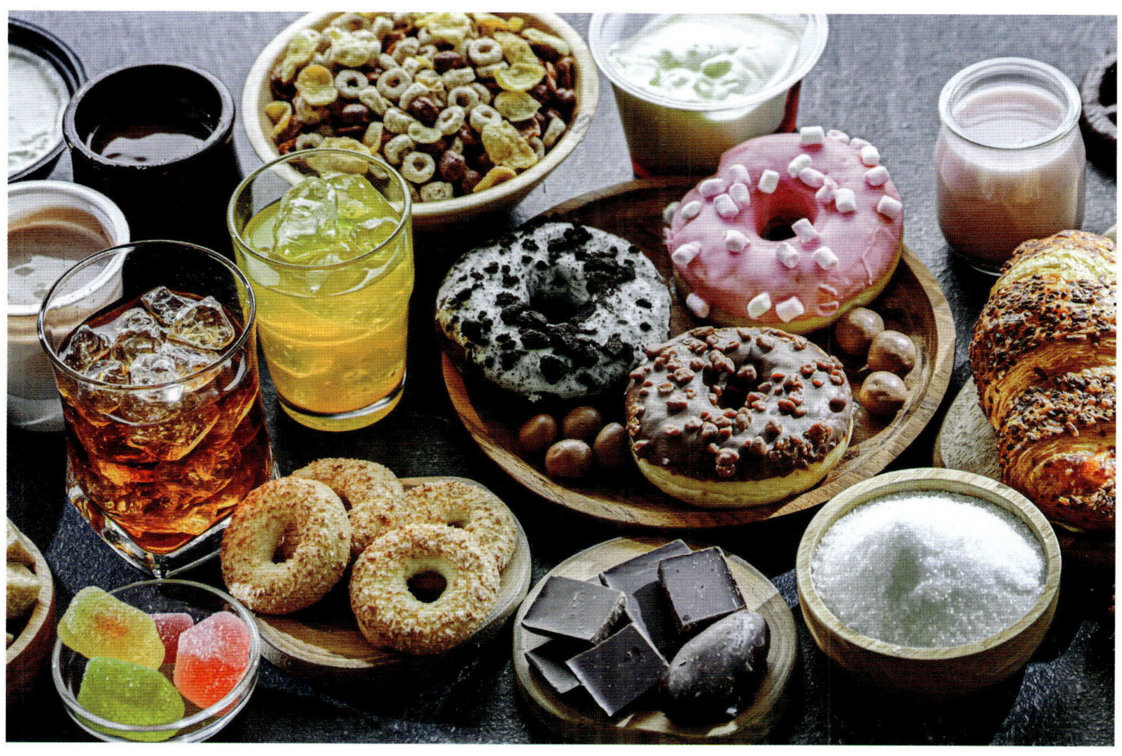

Instead, add some fresh lemon, mint, ginger and lime to mineral water; drink herbal teas and kombucha; and always choose water.

FOODS THAT ARE 'ZERO', 'DIET', 'LITE' AND 'SUGAR FREE'

Over my years as a practitioner, so many of my diabetic patients consume these products. I insist that they're removed in all my programs. Consuming them has no upside whatsoever for your health.

Many are full of artificial sweeteners, artificial flavours and have absolutely *zero* nutritional value. Often you can get sweet cravings due to the intense artificial sweeteners. These foods and beverages are also highly acidic, so consuming them regularly can erode your tooth enamel and cause dental cavities.

Consuming large amounts of artificial sweeteners has been linked to disrupted gut health, increased appetite for high-calorie foods, and weight gain. These sweeteners may also confuse the body's insulin response. Having a daily diet soft drink potentially increases your risk for metabolic syndrome, type 2 diabetes, heart disease, high blood pressure and even chronic kidney disease. An Australian study found people who drank a daily diet soft drink had a 38% higher risk of diabetes.

While diet drinks may not cause blood glucose spikes directly, the overall evidence suggests it's best to avoid them for optimal health, focusing instead on water, milk, herbal teas and mineral water.

ALCOHOL

The recommended amount of alcohol is a maximum of 2 units a week. That said, according to the latest research on alcohol consumption, it's best to avoid alcohol completely.

When it comes to T2D and alcohol, much depends on your current health status. If you drink heavily, you increase your risk of developing T2D and making managing blood glucose harder. Alcohol causes fluctuations in blood glucose, rising after drinking and then dropping several hours later. Too much alcohol will make the body more insulin resistant, increasing weight gain and worsening type T2D. If you have diabetes, excessive drinking can increase the risk of any complications in your pancreas and liver function.

The alcohol guidelines for T2D are that you can have it in moderation but ideally avoid it. If you do choose to drink, then make sure you're eating as well, to manage blood glucose better. If you have diabetes complications such as eye, nerve, kidney and liver disease, then the best advice is to avoid alcohol all together.

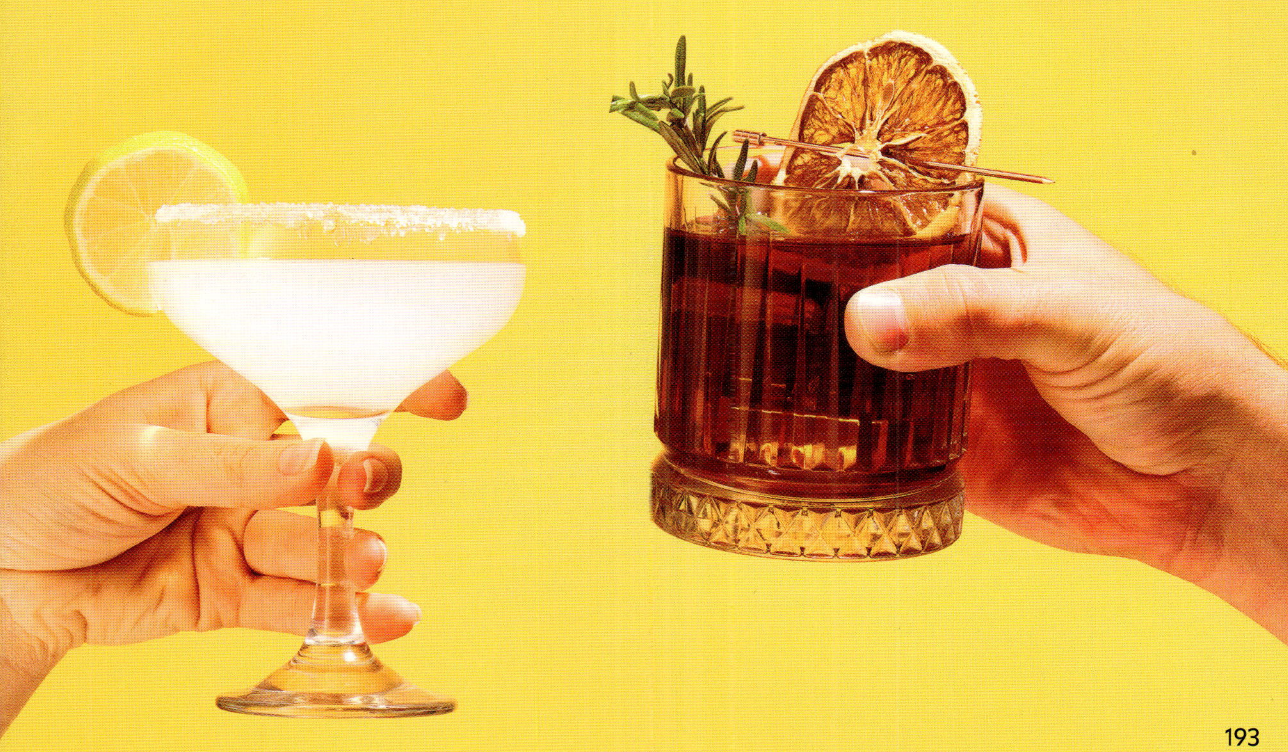

CHAPTER 10

Losing weight with type 2 diabetes

Weight loss is critical and essential when treating most people with type 2 diabetes. The thing is, most people with insulin resistance, prediabetes and type 2 diabetes are overweight. The best way to lose weight with type 2 diabetes is holistically and in a measured way. You need to make both diet and lifestyle changes: eating portion-controlled meals, doing regular exercise, sleeping well, managing stress and keeping well hydrated.

WEIGHT AND DIABETES RISK

	OVERWEIGHT OR OBESE?	PREVALENCE AND RISK
INSULIN RESISTANCE	90%	About 90% of people with insulin resistance are overweight or obese. Obesity is the strongest modifiable risk factor. Abdominal fat is associated with insulin resistance.
PREDIABETES	>80%	More than 80% of people with prediabetes are overweight or obese. Even if you have a 'healthy' BMI, your prediabetes risk will increase if you are sedentary and have abdominal obesity.
TYPE 2 DIABETES	80% to 90%	About 80% to 90% of people with T2D are overweight or obese. The higher your body weight, the higher your risk of developing T2D. If you are already obese, you have a 70% lifetime risk of diabetes compared to those at a normal weight, who have a 10% risk.

Carrying excess weight, especially around the abdomen (visceral fat), is the single largest risk factor for insulin resistance, prediabetes and type 2 diabetes across most populations.

KEY STRATEGIES TO LOSE WEIGHT WITH T2D

You need to start with a reduced-calorie, nutrient-dense diet. The focus is lots of non-starchy vegetables, lean protein, nuts, some fruit, dairy and healthy fats. Whole grains and legumes are included but minimal.

- **Portion control is essential.** I suggest eating using a plate that is 23 cm diameter, not the current oversized 32 cm plates.

- **Don't skip meals.** This really can help with blood sugar stability and reduce overeating.

- **Exercise is essential.** Aim for at least 150 minutes per week of cardiovascular exercise (walking, cycling, power walking, cross trainer, swimming, dancing) plus resistance or strength training to build that all-important muscle.

- **Treat the weight-loss journey like a job.** Do your prep, keep a diary of your journey, and find support groups or additional support if you need it.

- **Get professional help.** Consider guidance from a diabetes educator, dietitian or clinical nutritionist. This is really important to manage hypoglycaemia or 'hypos'.

- **Monitor your blood glucose.** Consider purchasing a glucose monitor if you don't already have one, to help you manage your blood glucose.

- **Don't follow fads.** I don't recommend intermittent fasting and you need to be careful when doing extremely low-carb diets, such as the classic keto diet.

The safest and most effective way to lose weight is with healthy eating, exercise, portion control, regular meals and behavioural support. You should avoid:

- crash dieting

- diet fads or fad supplements

- skipping meals.

THE EVIDENCE

Mediterranean-style diets, reduced-calorie diets and moderate-to low-carb diets have been demonstrated to be successful for weight loss. I find in my clinic that when people lose anywhere from 5% to 10% of their starting weight, they see significant improvements in their blood glucose and T2D. This of course depends on each individual's starting weight and health status.

5% to 10% less weight and you'll start seeing your diabetes improve.

Once you start losing weight and your blood glucose stabilises, your risk of hypoglycaemia reduces.

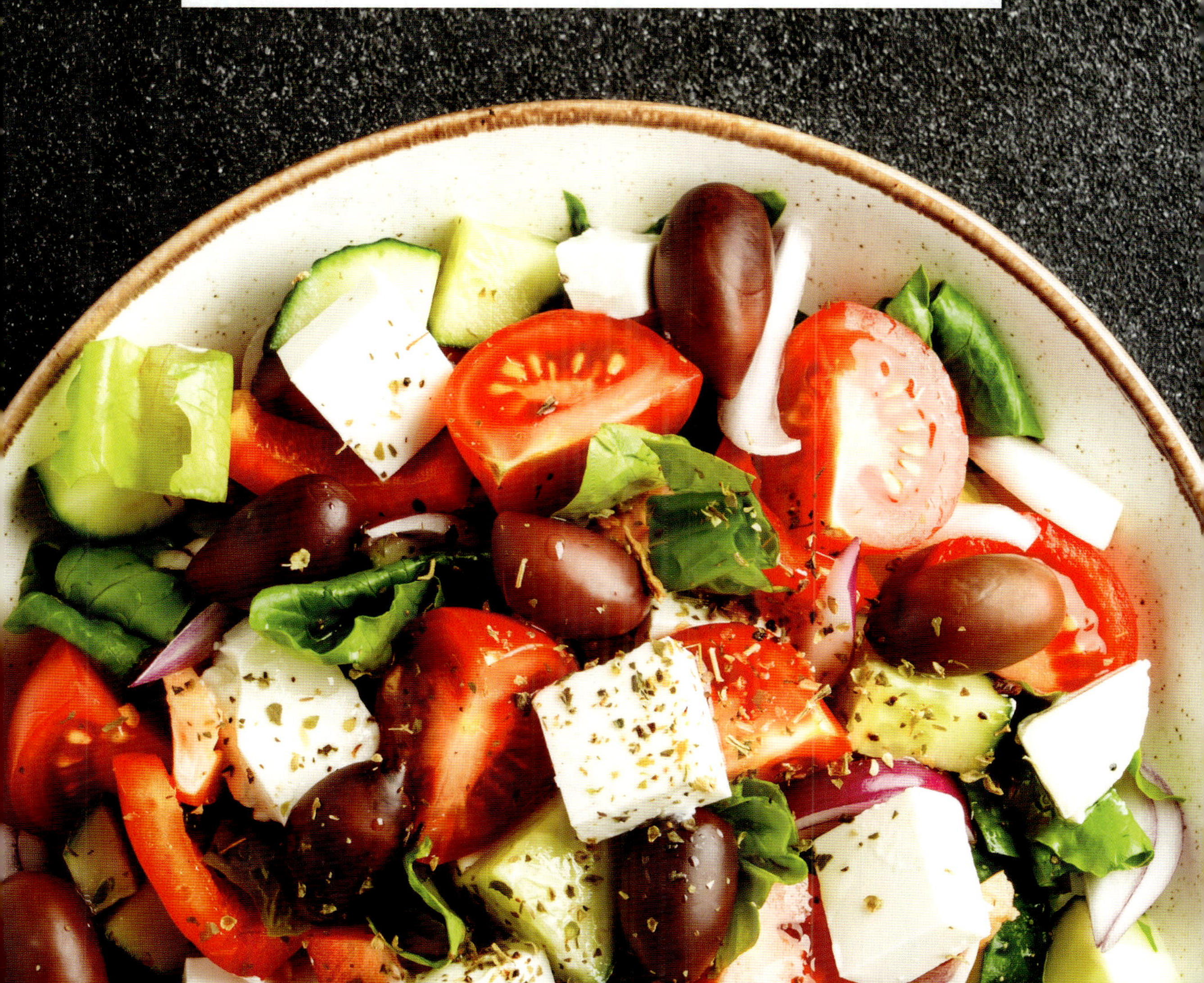

FOOD CHOICES WHEN MANAGING DIABETES

What you choose to eat is essential to managing diabetes as what you eat directly impacts blood sugar levels.

- **Always choose low-GI foods and avoid refined carbohydrates.** You need to understand how carbohydrates can affect blood glucose.

- **Eat vegetables, lean proteins, healthy fats, nuts, wholegrains and legumes.** This will improve cholesterol and blood pressure, and reduce the risk of heart disease as well.

- **Lower calorie, nutrient-dense foods are key to a healthy weight.** By eating well you can avoid gaining weight, which drives insulin resistance and diabetes.

- **Stay hydrated.** 80% of people don't drink enough water.

A healthy diet will reduce the risk of diabetic complications. When planning meals, always pair a carb with protein and good fats, e.g. an apple with nut butter, or wholegrain sourdough toast with eggs.

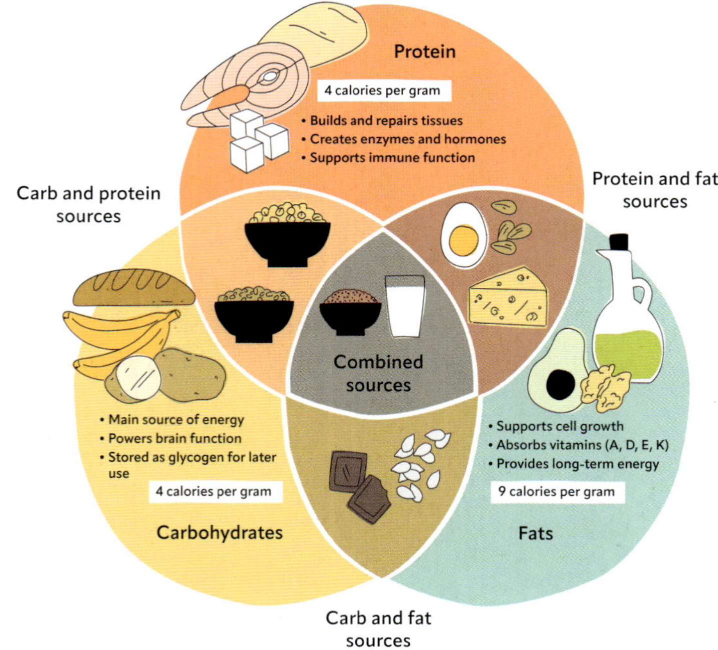

MACRONUTRIENTS AND TYPE 2 DIABETES

NUTRIENT GROUP	WHAT TO LOOK FOR	EFFECTS ON DIABETES
CARBOHYDRATES	Carbs should be high fibre and low GI to support blood glucose.	Strongest immediate impact on blood glucose, but a lot depends on the timing and type
FIBRE (SOLUBLE/ INSOLUBLE)	Fibre, both soluble and insoluble, is really important for managing diabetes to improve your insulin sensitivity.	Lowers blood glucose, supports gut and heart, supports weight control, lowers cholesterol and regulates appetite
PROTEIN (LEAN SOURCES)	Protein can help keep you full and not spike blood glucose, plus preserve muscle. All meals need to include protein to slow down carbohydrate absorption.	Satiety, muscle health, slows carb absorption
HEALTHY FATS (MONO UNSATURATED AND POLYUNSATURATED)	Fat is really important – choose unsaturated fats such as nuts, seeds, avocado, fatty fish and extra-virgin olive oil.	Improves cholesterol and insulin sensitivity, lowers inflammation and heart disease risk
MICRONUTRIENTS	Essential micronutrients include chromium, vitamin D, magnesium and potassium.	Support metabolic pathways, reduce complications, help support the action of insulin and keep your heart healthy

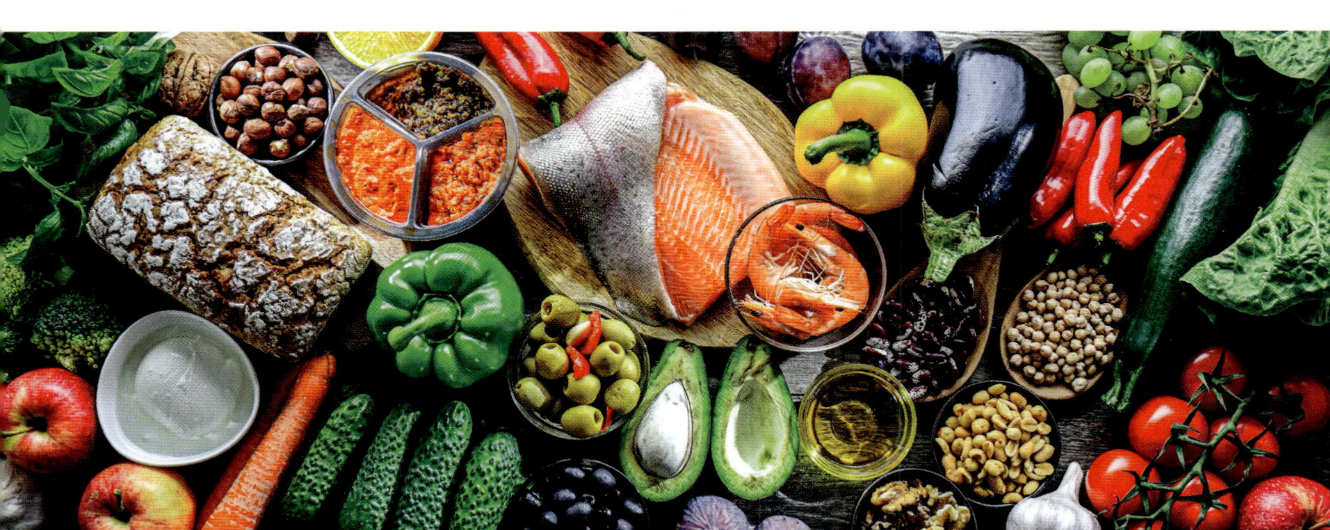

THE HEALTHY PLATE METHOD

I always tell my patients their hand is their plate, but understanding the plate method is also really important. Today's popular large dinner plates can hold about 1800 calories of food, so a great way of portion controlling your meals is to use a bread-and-butter plate for your main meals instead.

A small bowl is another good option. One reason we all love nourish bowls, acai bowls and salad bowls is that they're filled to the brim with goodness. Psychologically, we love to see a full plate of food, even if it's small. Just avoid the big plates.

I love the plate method because it means you learn to measure food by eye and don't need to be tracking or weighing food, which can be a real deterrent for many. Simply fill half of your plate with non-starchy vegetables such as broccoli, leafy greens, cauliflower and zucchini; one-quarter should be a lean protein; and the remaining quarter should be legumes, fruit, dairy or complex carbohydrate such as brown rice (for those maintaining a healthy weight).

In my weight-loss programs, I reduce complex carbohydrates but still keep fibre intake high with vegetables, salad and fibre-rich snacks (such as a kiwifruit with the skin on and nuts).

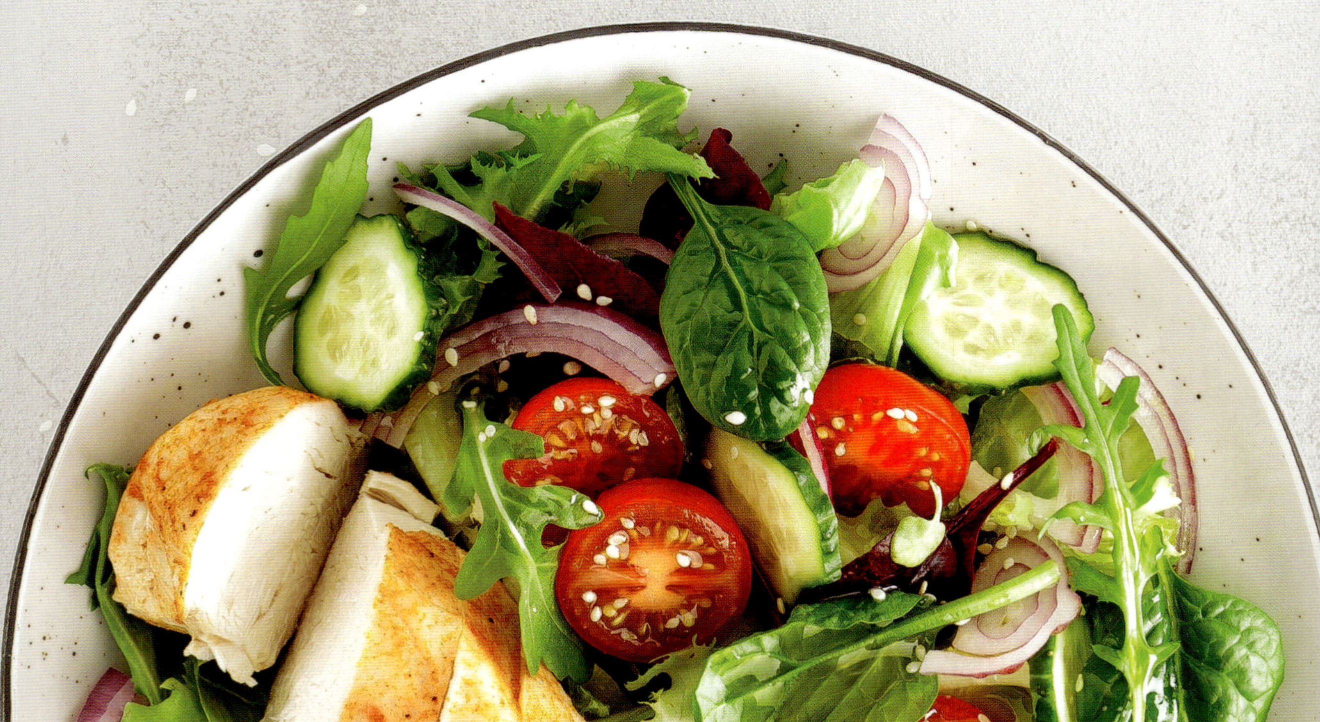

CARBOHYDRATE COUNTING

Many people with diabetes understand carbohydrates very well. Carbohydrate counting is literally counting grams of carbohydrates to manage blood sugar levels. If taking insulin, you'll adjust your dose of insulin based on the carbs you consume.

The amount of carbohydrates you should have depends on your age, activity level, weight and health goals.

DAY ON A PLATE FOR T2D

BREAKFAST	MID-MORNING	LUNCH	MID-AFTERNOON	DINNER
Omelette with spinach and mushrooms	10 almonds	Greek salad with grilled chicken and ¼ cup cooked quinoa	Berries and Greek yoghurt	Baked salmon with steamed greens

Remember your portions, stay hydrated and stick to mealtimes.

WHAT ORDER YOU EAT FOOD MATTERS!

Did you know the order in which you eat foods during a meal profoundly impacts your blood glucose levels? I really love this as a hack! The key is to eat vegetables and protein before carbohydrates. This has been shown consistently to lower post-meal blood glucose spikes.

Here is the best order for eating:

1. Vegetables – have to be high fibre (above ground)

2. Fat – avocado or fatty fish

3. Lean protein

4. Carbohydrates – complex carbs, including starchy vegetables.

Facts and physiological mechanisms:

- Eating carbs last (after vegetables and proteins) results in a lower and more gradual increase in blood glucose after meals, compared to eating them first. Studies show reductions of 17% to 37% in post-meal (postprandial) glucose levels at various time points.

- Eating fibre, protein or fat before or together with carbohydrates slows down digestion and the absorption of glucose. These nutrients delay gastric emptying and 'buffer' the body's glycaemic response, so blood sugar rises more slowly and less sharply.

- You need less insulin when you eat carbs last, reducing strain on the pancreas and supporting better long-term diabetes control – and it is so easy to do!

- Eating carbohydrates alone or first means they are quickly absorbed, causing rapid rises followed by quicker drops in blood glucose.

Consider when you go to a restaurant – the first thing many of us eat is bread. Now think of that initial blood glucose spike. You then eat your meal and by the time the blood glucose drops you are craving sweets – so you end up ordering the dessert. Seems like a pretty clever trick to get you to order more, right?

MEAL TIMING

As I have mentioned before, meal timing is crucial with type 2 diabetes. This is because what you eat influences your sensitivity to insulin, blood glucose levels, metabolic health and the body's circadian rhythm.

With consistent and well-timed meals, you'll manage your weight, reduce the risk of complications of diabetes and improve blood glucose.

- **You'll prevent blood glucose fluctuations.** Having big gaps and eating inconsistently can cause hypoglycaemia; however, having many large meals can cause blood glucose to spike.

- **You'll align your mealtimes with the body's circadian clock.** This means you eat during the daylight – no night-time eating. Eating this way supports your metabolic functioning and improves your sensitivity to insulin.

- **Don't have late-night snacks or skip breakfast.** This is linked to having much better blood glucose control, lower HbA1c and losing weight.

- **You'll avoid big swings in appetite.** When you're consistent with meal times, you're more satiated, less inclined to overeat, and can lose and maintain weight. These are all essential when reversing insulin resistance in diabetes.

- **Preparation and planning is key.** The key to success is preparation: write a meal schedule, do your shopping and plan your meals. Try and organise family dinners to be earlier in the evening or late afternoon. Most days, my family eat at around 5–6 p.m. Always aim to stop eating at least 3 hours before going to bed.

- **It's a new way of life.** You'll optimise insulin function, support metabolic health, lose weight and keep blood glucose stable. The time of your meal will influence your appetite, how your body manages blood glucose and sensitivity to insulin.

I am a big believer in living aligned with the body's circadian rhythms. If you do so, you can enhance glycaemic control, manage weight and blood glucose.

YOUR MEAL-TIMING CHEAT SHEET

APPROACH	GLYCAEMIC IMPACT	WHAT IT DOES
Regular, consistent meal schedule	More stable blood glucose	Eases medication matching, reduces fatigue
Not skipping breakfast	Lower HbA1c, better weight management	Supports circadian rhythm, reduces spikes
Avoid late-night eating or snacking	Less glycaemic variability	Supports fasting state, better sleep

SLOW DOWN!

This is another free and easy habit to get into. Chewing your food slowly! We've all been told time and time again to chew our food well. Eating quickly can lead to higher and sharper increases in post-meal blood glucose than eating slowly. Eating too fast is linked to less stable blood glucose levels. Over time, this can raise your risk of developing insulin resistance, type 2 diabetes and metabolic syndrome.

I remember my mum telling me to chew each bite 20 times.

Taking your time to eat supports better digestion, slows the absorption of sugars and improves satiety. This all helps maintain steadier blood glucose levels and lower insulin demands.

My tip is to consciously slow down your meals. Make sure you are chewing slowly. Pause between bites. Listen to your body and try to work out when you are feeling full.

CIRCADIAN RHYTHMS

It's no secret that I am obsessed with living aligned with our circadian rhythms. I've been doing my best to live by them for most of my adult life. Understanding how our hormones stack up against our circadian rhythms is so interesting, and it really does make sense to align your diet to them.

Think about cortisol, which wakes us up in the morning and dips in the afternoon, and melatonin, which helps us sleep at night. How does this impact our blood sugar? Well, cortisol helps us be more sensitive to insulin in the morning and melatonin makes us relatively resistant to insulin at night. It makes sense.

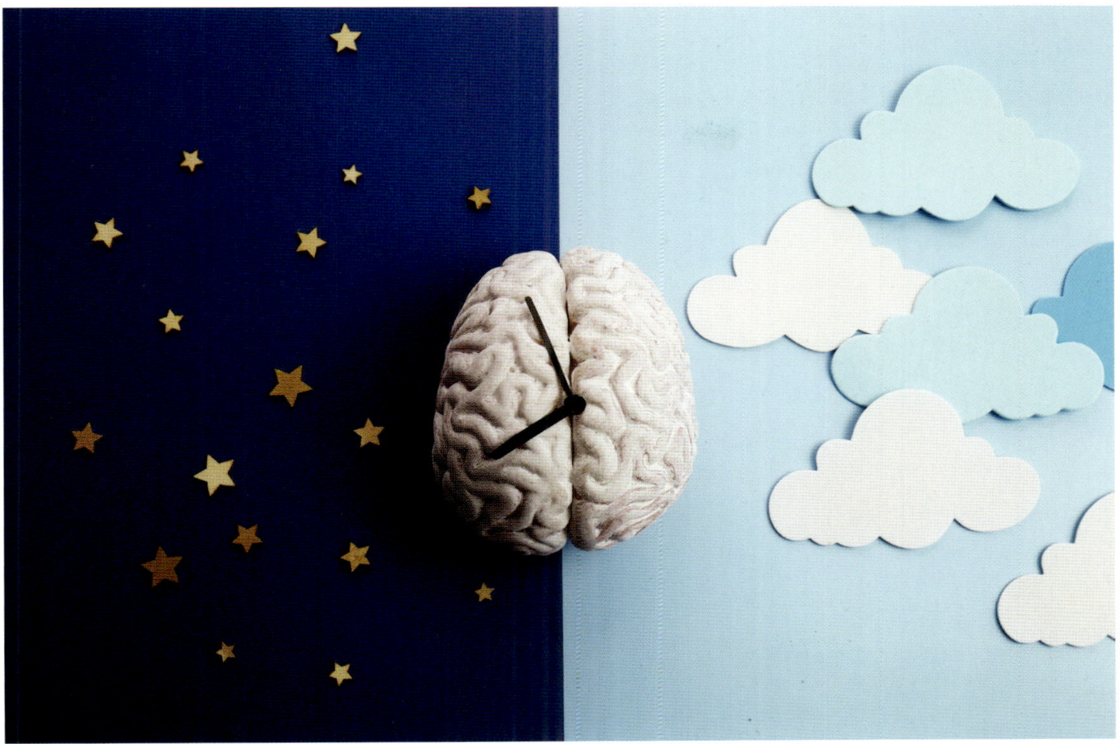

We don't need energy at night when we're trying to go to sleep with melatonin release so we're resistant to insulin. Our bodies are not designed to eat at night. This is why I only recommend carbohydrates in the morning, because it's when we are most sensitive to insulin.

The best way to eat to in alignment with your circadian rhythms and hormones (cortisol, melatonin, insulin) is to have breakfast with a later lunch around 2–3 p.m. This a combination of lunch and dinner that you could call 'linner'. Then at night-time have something small with an extremely low GI, such as a bowl of green soup, some protein or a snack such as pickles and cheese.

2–3 p.m. is when your body tells you it's lunchtime.

Think about it: your body is starting to release melatonin late afternoon to help you settle into a good night's sleep and then you go and eat something high-GI such as chips, spaghetti bolognaise or a big stir-fry with lots of white rice. Your blood is full of glucose, triggering insulin to move it to the cells. And guess what? You can't fall asleep, you struggle to stay asleep, you get more inflammation, an increased risk of disease and poor quality of life. The melatonin and insulin are clashing.

If you look back over the history of dinner, hunter-gatherers just ate based on what was available. The ancient Greeks and Romans ate their biggest meal mid-afternoon, and in medieval Europe they had 'dinner' at noon and a light supper at night. It was not until the 18th–19th centuries that a late dinner became a family meal. This was because of the industrial revolution and the start of the 9–5 working day. It was the industrial revolution that formatted our 'traditional' breakfast, lunch and dinner.

I started to eat aligned with my circadian rhythms about twenty-five years ago and swear this is one of the reasons why I've not had weight fluctuations during my adult life. As a parent, I did my best to feed my daughters this way and have seen the same results with them. I always kept dinner to 5 p.m. and made their breakfast and lunch filling, healthy and abundant. Dinner needs to be protein, healthy fats, salad and veg – avoid those carb-heavy meals!

5 p.m. is time for your low-carb, non-starchy vegetable and protein dinner.

When it comes to type 2 diabetes, you can see how aligning our meals with our circadian rhythms is so important – how closely linked they are. The timing of our meals and meal composition influence glucose management and insulin sensitivity. When circadian rhythms are disrupted with irregular meal timing, poor sleep and shift work, this impairs our insulin sensitivity and glucose response, increasing the risk of diabetes. Also avoid late-night snacking, to help regulate metabolic rhythms and improve glycaemic outcomes for those with type 2 diabetes.

Avoid the temptation of late-night snacks!

When your meals are well-timed and aligned with our circadian clock, you can reduce inflammation, improve your gut microbiome, help maintain a healthy weight, and prevent or even reverse type 2 diabetes.

FASTING AND TYPE 2 DIABETES

There is a lot of research and conversation around fasting and type 2 diabetes. Human bodies are designed to feast and fast. It's only in modern times, where food is so accessible, that we constantly have food.

The evidence behind fasting and diabetes is solid. Fasting brings down insulin and is good for the immune system, growth hormone and mitochondria.

Fasting can also help with weight loss, insulin sensitivity, blood glucose and HbA1c, and visceral fat loss, decreasing your need for medications and improving blood pressure and blood lipids. Plus it reduces the long-term risk factors for diabetes.

During fasting, the body first uses stored glycogen for energy then turns to fat stores, reducing harmful fat in the liver, pancreas and abdomen. Hormones also shift: insulin is lowered, and more glucagon and growth hormone are produced, which encourages cellular repair, reduces inflammation and resets the metabolism.

Fasting is generally safe for people with type 2 diabetes, but those taking medications need medical supervision to avoid hypoglycaemia. You need to monitor your blood glucose closely and adjust medication as needed.

There are many different types of fasts, including 16/8 and 12/12, while some can go for days. During the fast, you can have black coffee, tea and water.

In my program, I recommend a 12/12 fast. This is where you have 12 hours without food. This is why I get my patients to have their dinner at around 6 p.m. and fast until breakfast the next day.

THE LOW-CARB APPROACH

The low-carb diet is widely known, with a lot of evidence to support it for managing T2D. Evidence shows it improves blood glucose control, lowers HbA1c and promotes weight loss, and some people can even stop their diabetes medication.

This diet involves consuming less than 130 grams carbohydrates per day. This amount of carbohydrates will lower blood glucose and can help with weight loss, but the quality of the diet really does matter.

It is always important to ensure a low-carb diet is nutritious, to avoid becoming malnourished. If you have kidney issues, please speak to a healthcare provider first to make sure you're a candidate for a low-carb diet.

I do believe in low-carb diets for weight loss, but feel people should have breaks along the way and have a healthy relationship with complex carbohydrates.

Teaching and coaching many patients who have been on low-carb diets for years to embrace carbohydrates can be a struggle because carbs have got such a bad reputation. But once they understand the times of day to eat carbs, as well as which complex carbs to enjoy and in what portions, they actually enjoy them again.

It should have lean protein, seeds, nuts, high-fibre fruit and vegetables, and healthy fats.

KETOSIS AND MANAGING DIABETES

The best way to lose weight is through ketosis. As you know by now, muscle is so important for managing our blood sugar, so it would be criminal to be on a diet where muscle was lost. But this is what we see in a lot of low-calorie diets.

Ketosis is not only important for weight loss but also improving blood glucose control for people with T2D. But you need to manage it carefully, and know the difference between ketosis and ketoacidosis.

WHAT IS KETOSIS?

Ketosis is a natural metabolic state that is triggered when our intake of carbohydrates is very low. Instead of the body using glucose from carbs for energy, the body breaks down fat into molecules called ketones. These become the body's fuel source for the brain and body.

I do have to say, there is something magical about being in ketosis. I love it! I feel energised, sleep better, my thinking is clearer and I feel motivated.

When it comes to ketosis, weight loss and type 2 diabetes:

- Very low-carb diets reduce blood glucose and insulin levels, making it easier for the body to burn stored fat and lose weight. This is a huge benefit for type 2 diabetes management and even remission.

- Low-carb intake means fewer blood glucose spikes after eating. This will lower your average blood glucose (HbA1c) and reduce the need for diabetes medication.

- Ketosis often leads to reduced hunger, making calorie restriction and weight loss easier to maintain. I do find it so effective – people have fewer cravings, much more success and stay in the program longer.

- It also improves insulin sensitivity. Poor insulin sensitivity (or insulin resistance) is the driver of type 2 diabetes.

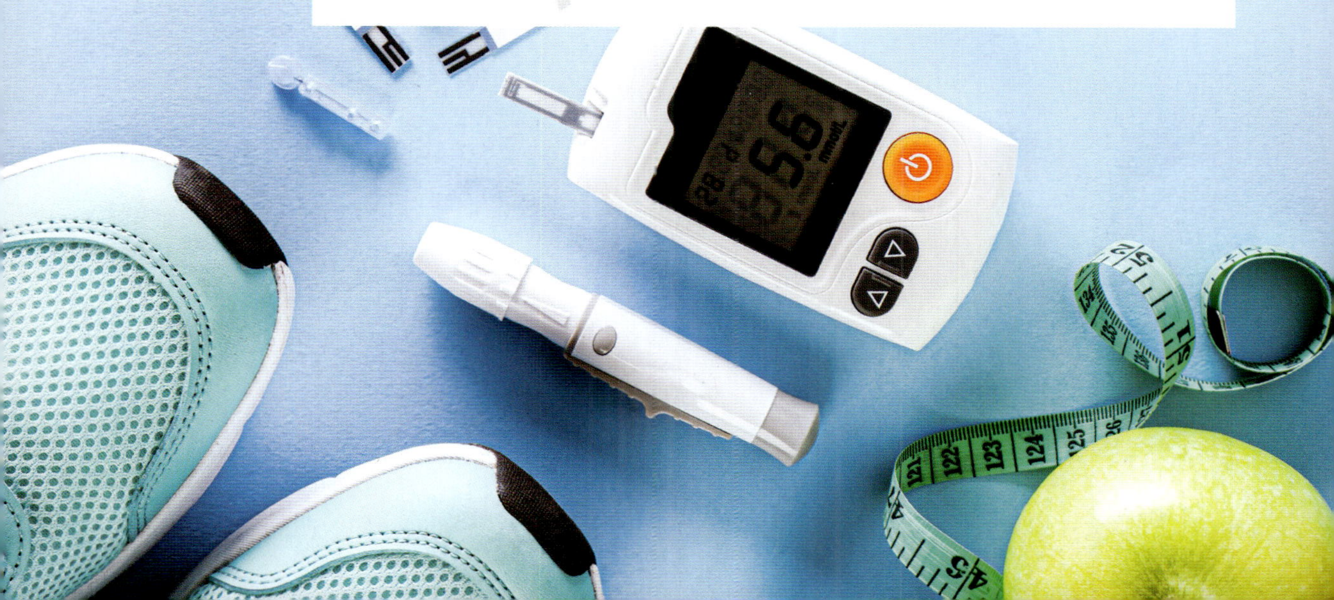

WHAT ARE THE DANGERS?

Ketosis is not without its risks. Here are some of them:

- **Diabetic ketoacidosis (DKA).** This is different from ketosis and is a dangerous emergency. DKA occurs when ketones build up to very high levels and the blood becomes acidic. It occurs most often in people with type 1 diabetes but is also possible in type 2 diabetes.

- **Electrolyte imbalance.** In some cases, low-carb diets can upset sodium, potassium and magnesium balance. This raises the risk for cramps, palpitations or more severe issues. In my program, I recommend daily electrolytes in the first 3 weeks to help manage this.

- **Micronutrient deficiency.** Restrictive diets can leave gaps in fibre, vitamins and minerals, affecting your gut and overall health. Always make sure the program you are doing is a healthy one.

- **Sustainability and long-term effects.** I don't recommend low-carb diets for long periods of time and am always trying to make sure people are still having a lot of non-starchy, high-fibre vegetables. Very low-carb diets are hard to maintain long term, and they come with an increase in cholesterol or cardiovascular risk for some patients who have been on low-carb diets for decades. This is individual but still a risk.

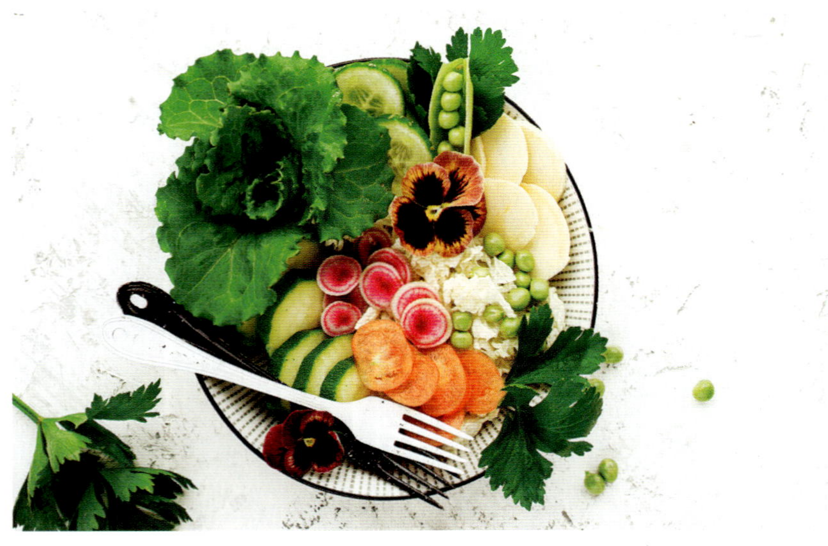

KETOSIS OR KETOACIDOSIS?

SYMPTOM	KETOSIS (NUTRITIONAL)	DIABETIC KETOACIDOSIS (DKA)
Breath odour	Mild, fruity 'keto' breath	Strong fruity breath
Thirst/urination	Mild dehydration	Extreme thirst, frequent urination, severe dehydration
Nausea/vomiting	Mild, temporary	Severe, persistent
Stomach pain	Rare	Severe, common
Energy	Mild fatigue, improvement over time	Extreme tiredness, possible confusion
Breathing	Normal	Rapid, deep, laboured
Mental status	Clear, alert	Confusion, impaired, may become unconscious
Need for medical care	No (with proper management)	Yes – emergency

This is so important if you have insulin resistance, prediabetes or T2D, especially if you're on diabetic medications.

- Always monitor your blood glucose and ketones.

- Stay hydrated and consider taking electrolytes.

- Your diet needs to be full of low-carb veggies, healthy fats and protein.

Going into ketosis is never pleasant. You can get headaches or the 'keto flu' where you actually do feel like you have the flu. The good news is that this passes quickly. Once in ketosis, you feel great. If you're really sick, vomiting, unwell and unable to eat, however, you could be at risk of ketoacidosis.

Ketosis promotes fat-burning, especially that dangerous abdominal fat. It improves insulin sensitivity, lowers blood glucose spikes and lowers insulin demands. Always inform your healthcare practitioner about what you are doing if you are managing T2D with medication. Consider wearing a continuous glucose monitor at the start of this program – it's what I recommend for all my patients.

EATING OUT

Eating out is part of life – just because you have type 2 diabetes and you're doing something about it, it doesn't mean you have to avoid it. You just need to learn some strategies. The focus needs to be on knowing your non-starchy vegetables, lean proteins and portion sizes. Obviously, you need to avoid refined carbohydrates, added sugars, fast food, junk food and desserts too.

The key to success comes in the planning. For starters, I tell my patients to google the menu first. You can even contact the restaurant, let them know you have T2D and ask for a special request. When you're ordering, you can ask the restaurant for a tweak, have dressings on the side, and to serve the meal without chips or carbs. Alternatively ask for extra veggies and salad.

Look at the plate and decide to have half the plate full of non-starchy vegetables, a quarter of the plate with protein such as grilled fish or chicken and the other quarter whole grains (for those maintaining weight). If you're still needing to lose weight, leave out the whole grains.

POINTS TO REMEMBER WHEN EATING OUT

- **Eat the whole grains last.** Always eat vegetables, fat and protein first.

- **Mindfulness is key.** You can choose the entree size as your main to manage portions.

- **Drink water.** You could choose sparkling, or, if you're having alcohol, choose wine or a spirit with no mixers.

- **Avoid the bread at the start of the meal.** This is a strategy to get you to order dessert. When you eat bread, your blood glucose spikes then drops. By the time your blood glucose drops, it's time for dessert and of course you end up ordering it.

- **Try to eat at your usual mealtimes.** This helps avoid blood glucose fluctuations and if a meal is late for reasons out of your control, then have a healthy snack to adjust your meal time.

- **Get that after-dinner walk in.** Try to park your car further away from the restaurant or walk to the restaurant to help with blood glucose management.

- **Be assertive.** Ask how the food is made, and consider telling the place you have type 2 diabetes.

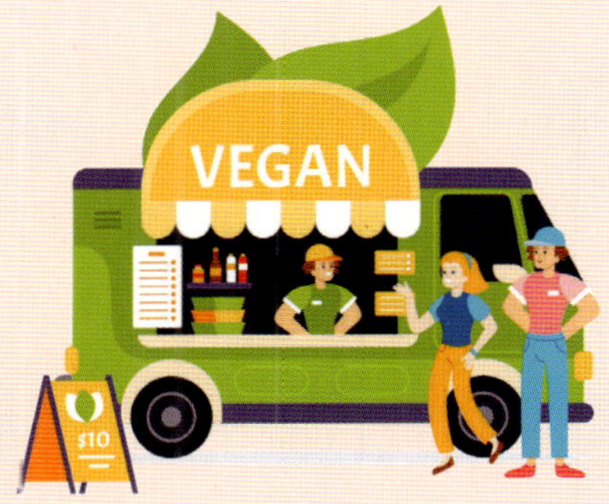

Choose a restaurant where you know you can decipher the food. Avoid Thai, Chinese and Indian cuisine, which have a lot of sauces. I tell my patients they need to be able to see the ingredients they're choosing. When people ask me where I want to eat, I mostly suggest Greek or Japanese places.

You will need to be mindful in the beginning when making these changes, but over time they will become automatic. Remember, taking care of your health is like a job.

SOCIAL SITUATIONS

Holidays, work functions and parties can be tricky for many with insulin resistance or type 2 diabetes. Social events can include birthdays, weddings, anniversaries and catching up with friends.

Managing social situations is the same as when you go to restaurants: you need to plan ahead. Many of my patients feel disgruntled, like they are missing out. My response is, 'It's only food, nothing new; you've been there and eaten this before. You are here for the person or people, not the food. The food is just part of the event and your health is way more important.'

Try to rewire your thoughts around food.

It is the same with what I call 'the buffet mentality'. Why is it that when we see a buffet, we feel the need to overeat, gorge ourselves and be wasteful? Do we feel the food is 'free' (which of course it isn't) or want to feel like we are getting food for free?

- **Stop, be mindful, remember your goals.** Look all the way along the buffet to find what you can put on your one and only serve.

- **Remember the importance of good health.** Think about the effect the food will have on your blood glucose, weight, mental health and the rest of your day.

- **Have 2 glasses of water before the buffet.** If you're hungry, drink first to take the sting out of your hunger. Sparkling water is best, because the bubbles make it seem more filling.

- **Eat a small snack before you go to an event.** Snack on a boiled egg to curb your impulse to eat and support your blood sugar control.

If you're invited to an event where you need to 'bring a plate', take something diabetes-friendly that you can eat. Again, divide your plate into quarters: ½ salad and non-starchy veg, ¼ lean protein and ¼ complex carbohydrate.

- Always survey the food table, as with a buffet, and decide what you are going to eat first. Stick to normal eating as much as you possibly can, stay hydrated, and avoid grazing or picking.

- Avoid chips, dips and fatty party foods. Know that sometimes when you just 'taste', it can make you want more, with the sugar high, which could derail you from your health goal.

- Sit more than an arm's length away from the food and snacks down the centre of the table, where there can be bowls of nuts or chocolates.

- Be the person who helps clean up after the meal. This is a great way to get your walking in after a social meal. I do this all the time.

If people ask you about your dietary choices, be honest. They'll then get off your back with pressuring you to eat. Consider contacting the host before an event to let them know. This way, you're not offending the host by not eating their food or drinking their cocktails. Be a communicator.

What is really important is being prepared, focused and mindful, and putting yourself and your health first.

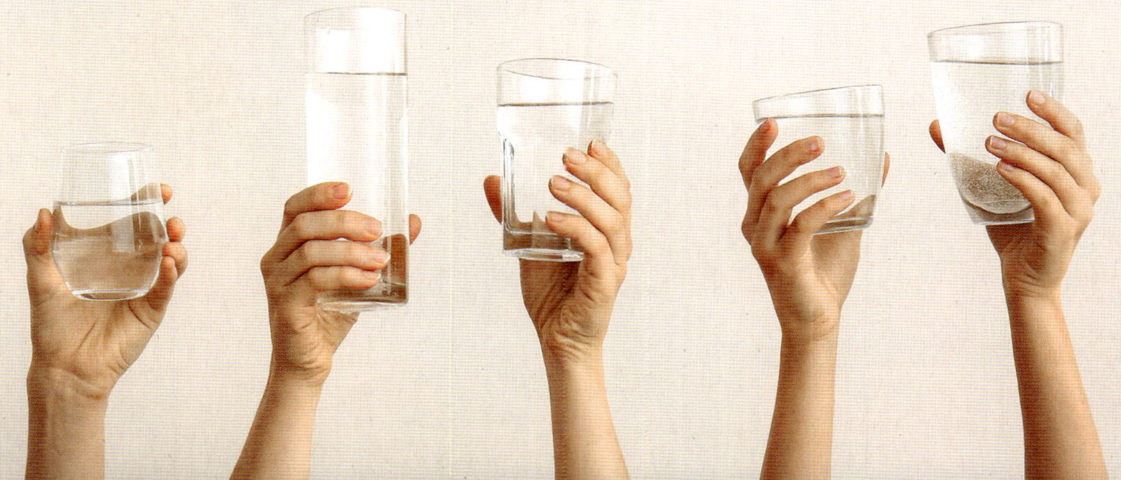

WHERE ARE YOU GETTING YOUR DOPAMINE FROM?

As a practitioner, I go right to the core of disease, just like with writing this book to help people understand why they ended up diabetic and what we can do about it. Treating from the core is what works, not just treating symptoms, which I call the 'band-aid approach'. It never works, and this is why so many people end up yo-yo dieters.

For many of us, when we go back the root of our problems with weight gain, it starts with an unhealthy relationship with food. I write about this a lot in my book *The 10:10 Plan*, which explains how to lose weight and keep it off for life.

1 million kilograms – that's how much weight Australians have lost with The 10:10 Plan!

This is why quick fixes such as weight-loss medications don't work. The core of the problem hasn't been resolved – that is, the learned relationship with food – and it starts right back when we were babies and children.

Food can be a dopamine fix for many people.

Dopamine is a neurotransmitter and hormone in our brain and body. It plays a key role in transmitting signals between nerve cells; regulating mood, reward and movement; and giving us feelings of pleasure, satisfaction and motivation. Dopamine can also influence learning, attention, mood, memory, sleep and hormone regulation.

The pleasurable effects of dopamine are linked to addiction to food but also sex and drugs, which boost dopamine release in the brain. For instance, some people may feel sad and emotional, then reach for the chocolate and ice cream. They may be stressed and eat to calm themselves, or feel bored and eat for entertainment.

My strategy to break this cycle is to write down what I call my 'list of six'. Write down six things that make you feel good, then when

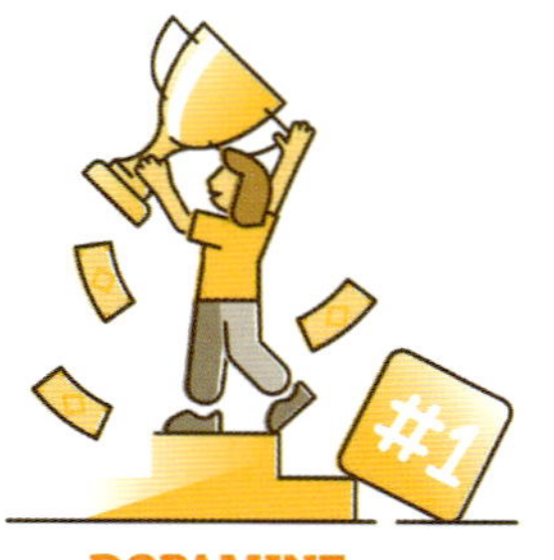

you're feeling sad, emotional, stressed or bored, pick something to do from that list. This is where you get your dopamine hit from.

I remember writing this list around 10 years ago for myself, really to see if it was a tool that I could use in my clinic. Here's what's on my list:

- shopping
- swimming in the ocean
- massage
- manicure
- a few hours phone free
- a big walk listening to my favourite podcast.

Once you start using your list of six proactively, you'll end the dopamine relationship with food and, like me, see food purely as nutrition.

Think about what could go on your list. Write it down somewhere you can reflect on it and start to apply it to your life. I promise you, there is something very rewarding about self-care and self-love.

MANAGING FOOD CRAVINGS

A food craving is an intense and persistent craving for a specific food. In most cases, foods craved are high in salt, calories or sugar. They are not related to hunger sensations. Hunger sensations come from the hormone ghrelin, which we get when we need food.

Cravings are triggered by dopamine, hormonal fluctuations (ghrelin, leptin, cortisol), emotions and comfort eating. They can be caused by poor sleep, deficiencies, the menstrual cycle, bad habits, disturbances in the microbiome, impulsive personality traits and pregnancy.

So how do we manage cravings?

Getting to the core of the problem is so important for long-term success with health and wellness. First, make sure you are eating balanced meals that include protein, a good fat, salad or veggies, and a complex carbohydrate. Keep your protein intake high, stay hydrated, manage stress, be mindful and always have something on hand as an alternative.

When a craving hits …

- **Drink a glass of water.** Interestingly, cravings and hunger can actually mean you are thirsty.

- **Always plan your meals** and have nutritious snacks handy, such as nuts, hummus, vegetable sticks, boiled eggs, cheese and pickles, a protein bar (mine are amazing – 10:10 SDL protein bar), a protein shake, piece of fruit, nut butter, some avocado, seeds, cottage cheese or Greek yoghurt.

- **Don't allow yourself to get extremely hungry.** Extreme hunger can lead to bad food choices and overindulging.

- **Be mindful, acknowledge the craving,** have a glass of water and wait about 20 minutes. Assess why you are having the craving.

- **Look for distractions** such as exercise, a walk, calling a friend, having a shower – just shift your focus away from the craving.

Don't let the craving control you, but stay in control of the craving. Like all things, it will pass.

CRAVINGS WHEN YOU HAVE TYPE 2 DIABETES

When blood glucose is poorly controlled, you have cravings for carbohydrates, so stick to your diabetes-friendly snacks. Aim to keep your blood glucose in the target range, keep monitoring your levels. For those with diabetes who are stressed, obese and using alcohol, all of this will make cravings worse.

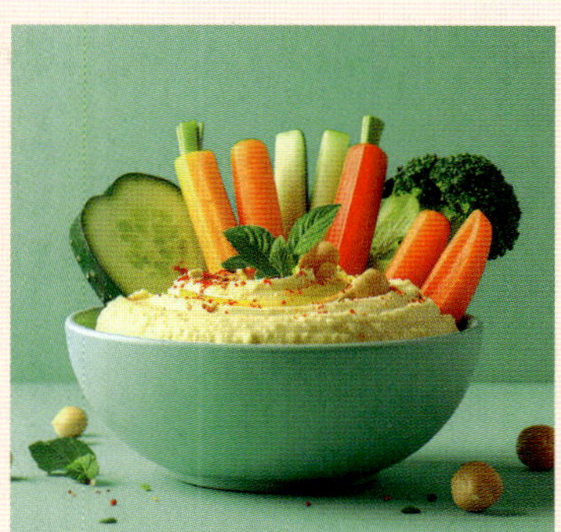

OZEMPIC AND GLP-1 MEDICATIONS

I always say medications have a place for those that need them. But many medications come with side effects. In my opinion, Ozempic and GLP-1 medications are only for those who are seriously ill with T2D. The plusses of taking these medications then outweigh the side effects they cause.

Over the past few years in my clinic, I've seen many people on these medications. I have never seen anything good come from them. I've seen chronic diarrhoea, nausea, unwanted pregnancy, gut dysbiosis, mood swings, depression, weight regain, malnutrition, hair loss, loss in quality of life, chronic constipation, depression and in many cases no weight loss. The most distressing side effect for me are people who have osteoporosis at age 50 after taking these medications for 6 months.

I currently have four patients who are seriously ill with type 2 diabetes. They have been on these medications for 2 years without any weight loss, but they are still prescribed the medication. I have done more for these patients in 1 month than this medication has done for them in 2 years.

Many people who take these medications have not addressed the root cause of the problem that made them need these medications – which is poor diet and lifestyle. Rather, they see it as a quick fix for the short term. Once they stop the medication, they regain the weight.

What alarms me the most about Ozempic is the muscle loss. As you know by now from reading this book, muscle is sooooo important to regulate blood glucose. It's like a glucose disposal unit. Think of the state of someone's health now that their muscle is lost. Just worse than when they started.

SERIOUS SIDE EFFECTS OF GLP-1 MEDICATIONS:

- **Gastrointestinal problems.** Nausea, vomiting, diarrhoea, constipation, bloating and stomach pain are frequent – these symptoms can be uncomfortable and sometimes severe.

- **Muscle loss.** Rapid weight loss from Ozempic can cause loss of muscle mass, not just fat, leading to frailty. This is what leads to the famed Hollywood 'Ozempic face'.

- **Stomach paralysis (gastroparesis).** Ozempic slows stomach emptying, which can result in prolonged nausea, vomiting and even dangerous intestinal blockages in rare cases.

- **Pancreatitis.** Inflammation of the pancreas is a rare but serious complication, potentially requiring hospitalisation.

- **Gallbladder and kidney problems.** Increased risk of gallstones, kidney injury and reduced kidney function, especially if dehydration results from severe vomiting or diarrhoea.

- **Thyroid tumours.** Animal studies have linked Ozempic and similar medications to thyroid cancer, although direct risk in humans is still under investigation.

- **Vision changes and retinopathy.** In people with diabetes, Ozempic can increase the risk of vision-related complications.

My conclusion is that medication has its place for those that really need it, who are on the cusp of blindness or being an amputee due to T2D; otherwise, my advice is to treat a disease caused by diet with a healthy diet and lifestyle choices.

ARTIFICIAL SWEETENERS AND GLP-1 MEDICATIONS

I have never been backward in my thoughts on artificial sweeteners (such as aspartame, sucralose and saccharin). They come with risks and aren't effective in what they set out to do.

There is NO place for artificial sweeteners in anyone's diet.

Many people on GLP-1 medications drink diet products. Taking artificial sweeteners and GLP-1 medications together is generally not known to cause direct, dangerous interactions – but both have their own risks, and combining them may compromise your gut health, metabolism and overall health.

Regular use of artificial sweeteners has been linked to increases in appetite, cravings and weight gain, which could undermine the appetite-suppressing effects of GLP-1 drugs for some people.

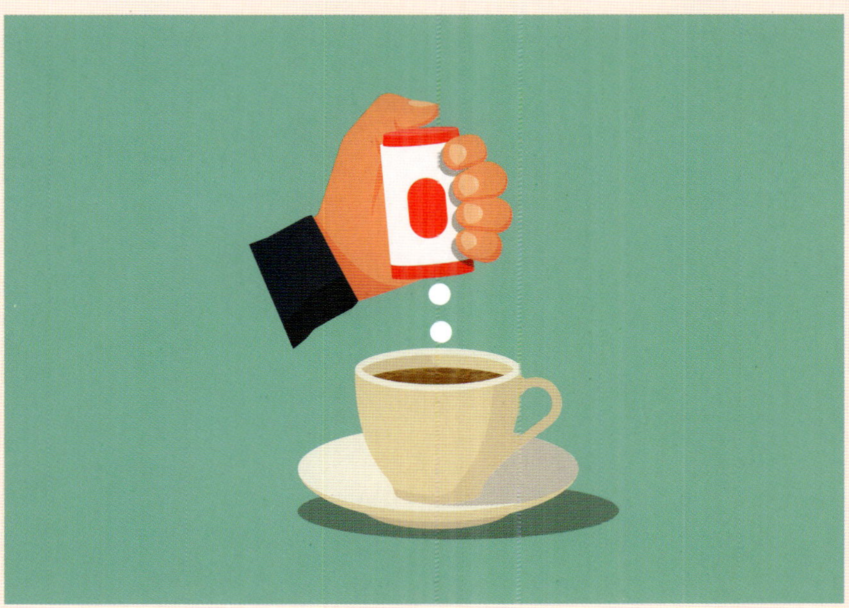

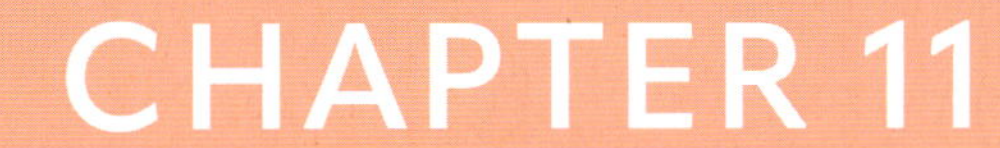

CHAPTER 11

Lifestyle – what it means for type 2 diabetes

EXERCISE

Exercise is the best medicine – it's as simple as that. Everyone needs to exercise. Not exercising creates disease; being sedentary is a disease. Find what you love doing and do something daily.

Doing exercise is essential when you have type 2 diabetes. This includes both cardio and resistance training. Remember when we talked about the importance of muscle? Muscle is active tissue so can help regulate blood glucose.

It is essential that all my diabetes patients are doing exercise. For those who haven't exercised before, I start them exercising in stages:

1. **Take a walk every morning and build from there.** Walk out your front door and walk 20 minutes in one direction, then turn around and come back.

2. **Choose something you love doing.** It could be dancing, hiking, cycling, Pilates, jogging, power walking, cross training, group training or swimming ... the key is to find something and embrace it.

3. **Start resistance training.** This is just so important for managing type 2 diabetes.

Exercise improves insulin sensitivity, lowers cardiovascular risks, supports weight management and helps control blood glucose levels.

So you can see why I insist on it when treating diabetes.

Physical activity helps insulin work more effectively, allowing muscle cells to take up glucose from the bloodstream directly, lowering blood sugar and countering insulin resistance. When you exercise regularly, haemoglobin A1c (HbA1c) is reduced. HbA1c measures blood glucose over a 3-month period.

- **Focus on aerobic activity and resistance training.** These have the strongest effects on metabolic health and blood glucose.

- **Exercise reduces fat mass.** It improves lipid profiles, lowers blood pressure, strengthens the heart, and can help or manage the complications of diabetes such as stroke and heart disease.

- **Resistance training and weights builds muscle.** Muscle, as we know, boosts the uptake of glucose and can counter the muscle loss associated with diabetes and aging.

- **Exercise is so good for your emotional wellbeing!** It can reduce anxiety and depression and really does improve the quality of life for people with type 2 diabetes. I love this part so much!

- **Exercise needs to be regular.** Consistency is key. Exercise is essential for survival and longevity in those with type 2 diabetes.

Consistent physical activity is the most powerful evidence-based way to control type 2 diabetes and help prevent complications. So much exercise is free. It makes you feel amazing, is the best way to start your day, supports healthy metabolism and significantly improves your quality of life.

MY EXERCISE GUIDELINES

EXERCISE TYPE	FREQUENCY
Resistance training	3 x per week
Cardiovascular training	5 x per week at least
HIIT training	2 x week

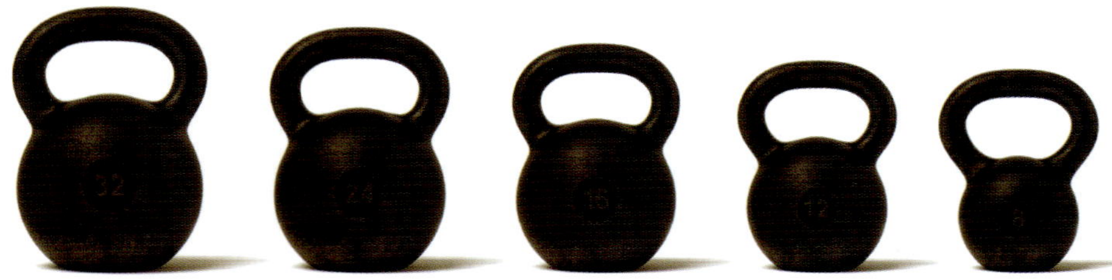

HIIT TRAINING

One of the best forms of exercise is high-intensity interval training (HIIT). HIIT is intense training alternating bursts of high effort (such as brisk walking, running, cycling or bodyweight movements) with short rest or easy intervals. Research has proven it outperforms moderate-intensity exercise in delivering health benefits.

HIIT is great for people with type 2 diabetes, insulin resistance and prediabetes because it significantly improves your blood glucose control and insulin sensitivity in less time than traditional exercise.

Exercise is the elixir of life – embrace it!

THE BENEFITS OF HIIT

BOOSTS INSULIN SENSITIVITY	HIIT rapidly increases the muscles' capacity to take up and store glucose. This improves your sensitivity to insulin for 24–48 hours after a session. About 2 weeks after starting HIIT training, your insulin resistance will measurably drop.
LOWERS BLOOD GLUCOSE	HIIT significantly reduces fasting glucose and post-meal glucose spikes. HIIT lowers your HbA1c more effectively than moderate-intensity continuous training such as long runs.
PROMOTES FAT LOSS AND MUSCLE GAIN	This is so important! HIIT reduces visceral fat and improves muscle mass and your overall metabolic health. This is essential for reversing insulin resistance.
IMPROVES CARDIORESPIRATORY FITNESS AND HEART HEALTH	HIIT strengthens the heart and lungs with shorter workouts, lowering risks of the complications associated with T2D.

HOW DOES HIIT WORK?

HIIT triggers rapid muscle glycogen depletion and builds more muscle fibres. This stimulates the body to quickly replace that fuel by absorbing more glucose from our blood and making our body's cells respond better to insulin.

Combined with the metabolic boost and increased post-exercise calorie burn, HIIT is especially effective for people who struggle with blood glucose control.

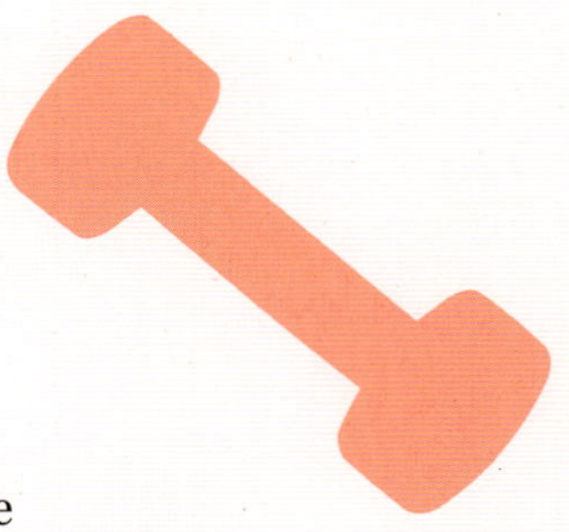

HOW TO DO HIIT

BASELINE PROTOCOL

30 seconds to 1 minute of high-intensity activity, such as brisk walking, sprinting, running, cycling, mountain climbers or squat jumps at 70% to 90% maximum effort

Followed by:

1–2 minutes of low-intensity recovery (slow walking, gentle cycling).

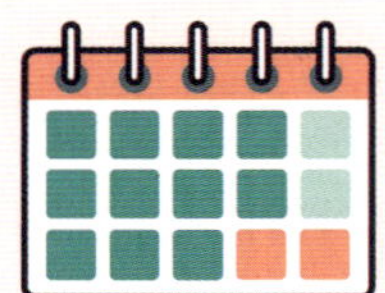

SESSION DURATION

15–30 minutes in total

My suggestion is 2–3 times per week.

GETTING STARTED

Begin with four rounds – 30 seconds hard, 1–2 minutes easy. Add on more intervals as your fitness improves.

When I do HIIT, I sprint hard, then walk or light jog for the easy.

Be sure to warm up and cool down.

STAYING SAFE

Monitor your blood glucose before and after meals.

Stay hydrated and be aware of feeling hypoglycaemic.

Buddy up with someone in the beginning or enlist a personal trainer to get you started.

HIIT is scientifically proven to reverse and help control prediabetes, insulin resistance and T2D.

It's so worth doing! It's not much time out of your day and just a few sessions are effective for blood glucose control.

Where there is a will, there is a way!

CALF RAISES – A QUICK HACK

You can do calf raises literally anywhere: at your dinner table, on the train, at work – anywhere. In this exercise, you repeatedly lift your heels off the ground while keeping your toes down, which activates the soleus muscle. This is a way of circulating glucose for energy and something you should do after a meal outside of walking.

Some research shows that calf raises for several minutes after eating can flatten or reduce post-meal glucose spikes by 52%, improving blood glucose management and insulin sensitivity. The exercise increases circulation in the lower body, which can help counteract the effects of prolonged sitting (a risk factor for poor diabetes outcomes) by keeping glucose and oxygen moving through the legs.

Calf raises can help build muscle and improve your metabolic health.

This is important for people with diabetes when they have reduced lower limb strength and increased risk of nerve and circulatory problems.

How to do calf raises:

1. Sit or stand with your feet flat on the ground.

2. Push down on the balls of your feet and lift up your heels as high as possible.

3. Lower your heels back to the ground.

4. Repeat steadily for 3–10 minutes, ideally after meals for best results.

Calf raises are for anyone of any fitness level. They are low impact, a great place to start, a fantastic habit to get into and ideal for people with T2D who have issues with mobility concerns.

I suggest doing calf raises along with walking after each meal; they're easy, practical and something everyone can do.

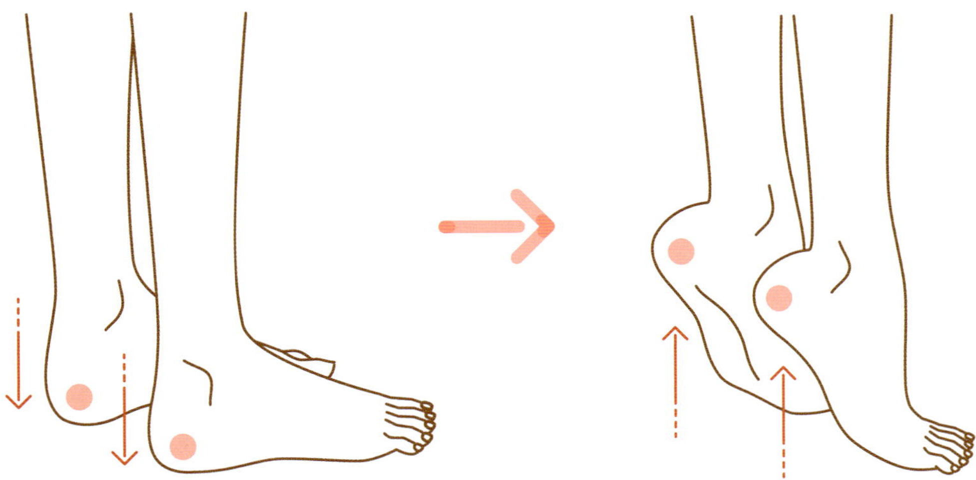

WALKING AFTER MEALS

Now, this is something I've been talking about a lot in this book. I love this so much – it is free, simple, convenient and works!

Walking after meals is an important tool for treating type 2 diabetes because it helps to lower blood glucose levels, enhances insulin sensitivity and reduces the risk of blood glucose spikes after eating.

So how does it work? Well, walking after eating activates our muscles, thus increasing their demand for glucose in the blood, which helps move glucose out of the bloodstream and into muscle cells for energy. The result is a more gradual rise and fall in blood sugar levels, reducing the risk of those harsh spikes and drops that are linked to cardiovascular risks, inflammation and diabetes progression.

Some recent research shows that walking for 2–10 minutes within 30–90 minutes after a meal can significantly lower your post-meal blood glucose levels. For people with diabetes, starting to walk within about 30 minutes (yes, before you wash up and stack the dishes) is especially recommended for better control.

Studies comparing walking after meals versus once-daily exercise found that timing walks after meals improved participants' blood glucose control by 12% to 22%, especially after dinner, when carbohydrate intake and sedentary time are highest. How easy is this to incorporate! I love this.

2–10 minutes: your daily walking prescription for better blood glucose.

Walking has some amazing additional benefits:

- It improves long-term glycaemic control, supporting the management of T2D.

- It encourages you to be consistent and mindful with physical activity, and gets you into a healthy mindset.

- It improves your circulation, mood and digestion, and regulates appetite, all of which benefit your overall wellbeing.

STRESS

Diabetes and stress have a bidirectional relationship. When you have diabetes, your stress can increase, and stress can worsen your metabolic health and diabetes management.

Having type 2 diabetes comes with demands. It's like having another job. Your day involves managing medication, glucose monitoring, meal planning, exercise, and maybe feeling anxious or overwhelmed. You worry about the future, stigma, social pressures and anxiety.

Diabetes can also impair the body's stress response systems, in particular regulating cortisol. Chronic stress triggers the release of hormones such as cortisol and adrenaline, which will lead to and increase insulin resistance and make blood glucose harder to control.

This can become a vicious cycle. The more stressed you are, often the poorer the lifestyle choices you make, and the less physical activity you do. You may neglect yourself or fall into emotional eating and all this can make the diabetes worse. Research shows that those with type 2 diabetes are at higher risk of anxiety and depression.

Diabetes distress is a specific type of stress linked to the burden of care and stress about outcomes.

There is the fear of heart disease, amputations, kidney problems or loss of vision – and this worry can result in depression, isolation and psychological stress.

People with diabetes can also have a heightened emotional response and lower ability to recover from stress due to the hormone imbalance.

So it's really important to manage your stress well. Type 2 diabetes and chronic stress reinforce each other, creating a cycle that – if not managed – will worsen overall psychological wellbeing.

TIPS TO MANAGE STRESS

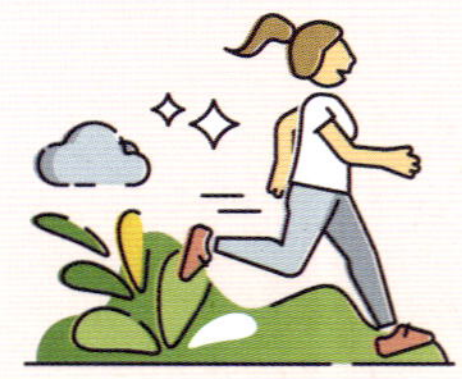

EXERCISE

Exercise is the top of my list when it comes to managing stress. Physical exercise boosts mood, improves sleep and reduces stress hormones.

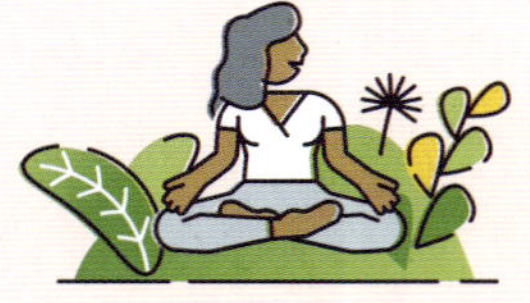

MEDITATION

Try meditation, yoga, deep breathing, massage or tai chi.

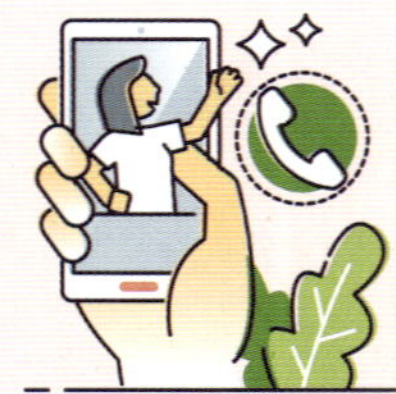

BE SOCIAL

Stay socially connected – this is really important to protect against stress.

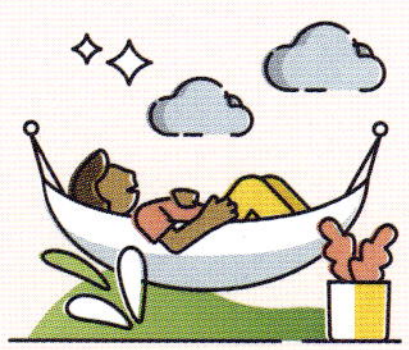

SLEEP

Focus on good sleep – create a beautiful sleep routine. This builds resilience.

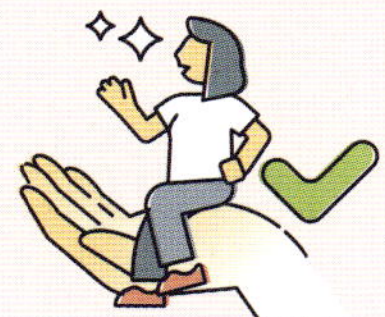

ME TIME

Set boundaries – learn to say 'no', delegate and schedule breaks for 'me' time. (I'm getting better at this – it takes practice.)

EAT WELL

A healthy diet is a given. Eating well, especially protein, helps keep blood glucose stable and improves melatonin production.

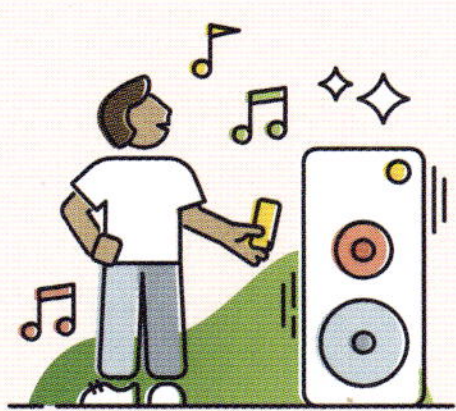

SELF-CARE

Remember self-care and enjoyment. Make sure you are doing things you love, such as a hobby, art, big walks, listening to music – things that can lower stress.

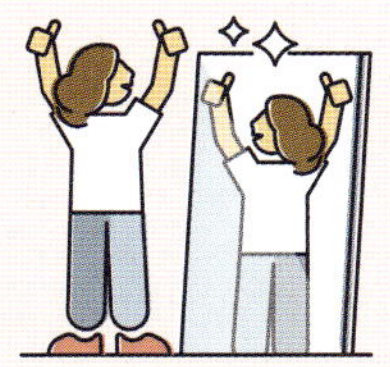

BE POSITIVE

Manage negative self-talk. This is so important. Try to find the silver lining, accept who you are, look at solutions. Negative talk is toxic to us. What we think is what we start to believe.

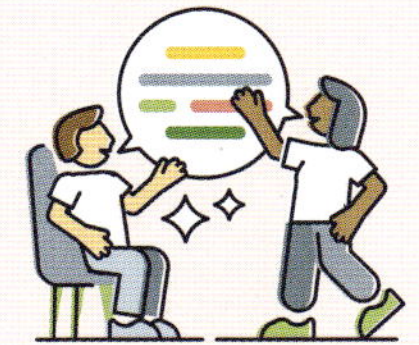

GRATITUDE

Practice gratitude – this can boost your mood.

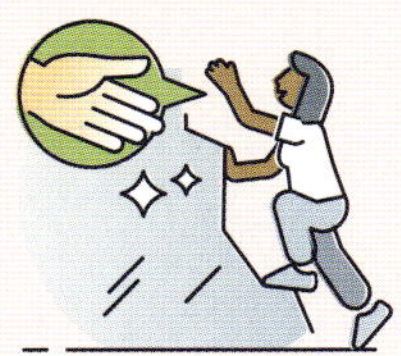

SEEK HELP IF NEEDED

Of course, seek professional help. Don't be ashamed – it's so important for growth.

SLEEP

Sleep is so incredibly important for your overall health, wellness, mood, quality of life and blood glucose. Lack of sleep disrupts blood glucose by increasing insulin resistance, raising stress hormones such as cortisol. Plus it drives inflammation and can impact your hunger hormones ghrelin and leptin, which combine to raise both fasting and post-meal glucose, even after a single night of poor sleep.

HOW DOES LACK OF SLEEP IMPACT US?

REDUCES INSULIN SENSITIVITY	Lack of sleep makes cells less responsive to insulin, so more glucose is in our bloodstream.
INCREASES CORTISOL AND STRESS	Poor sleep elevates our stress hormones, which promote glucose release from the liver and worsen insulin resistance.
DRIVES INFLAMMATION	Not enough sleep drives inflammation, further impairing the uptake of glucose and worsening disease.
APPETITE	Poor sleep lowers leptin (our feeling-full hormone) and raises ghrelin (our hunger hormone). The cravings we get aren't for healthy food – rather, we crave refined carbohydrates and sugars that raise blood glucose.

The cycle of poor sleep just worsens blood glucose control. It's not only bad for people who are insulin resistant, prediabetic or type 2 diabetic; it worsens this for everyone.

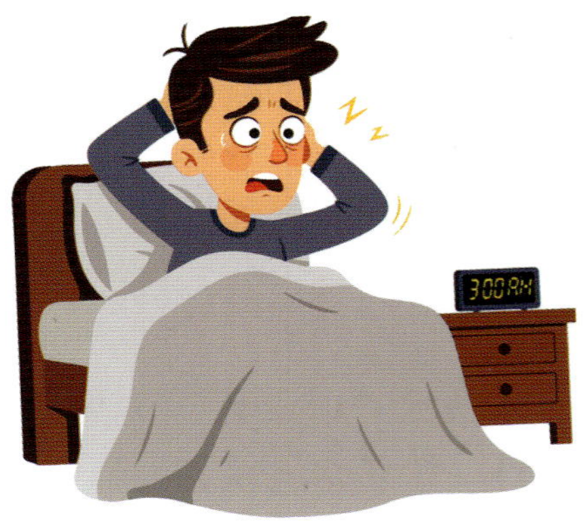

TIPS FOR GOOD SLEEP

Poor sleep increases blood glucose, impairing the body's ability to use insulin effectively, raising stress hormones and increasing inflammation – all making it harder to regulate your blood glucose and appetite.

- Maintain a regular routine – go to bed and wake up at the same time every day.

- Push your bedtime earlier. I found going to bed around 8–9 p.m. much more effective for falling asleep faster. Much of this is linked to our alignment with our circadian rhythms.

- Avoid caffeine later in the day, and alcohol. They both affect our sleep and regulation of glucose.

- Limit screen time; the blue light suppresses melatonin, keeping our brain alert, so try to avoid devices a minimum of 1 hour before bedtime.

- Make your sleep environment restful, dark, quiet and cool (the ideal room temperature is 19°C), and always sleep with a window open.

- Exercise daily: even walking can improve your sleep quality and insulin sensitivity.

- Avoid night-time eating.

- Your last meal should be 3 hours before bedtime.

- Try relaxation techniques such as meditation, breathing exercises and reading.

- Stick to that healthy diet, including protein with each meal. Plus stay well hydrated.

Sleep is so important for our blood glucose, just as much as exercising and a healthy diet. When we're sleeping well, we have better energy, glucose regulation, appetite and quality of life.

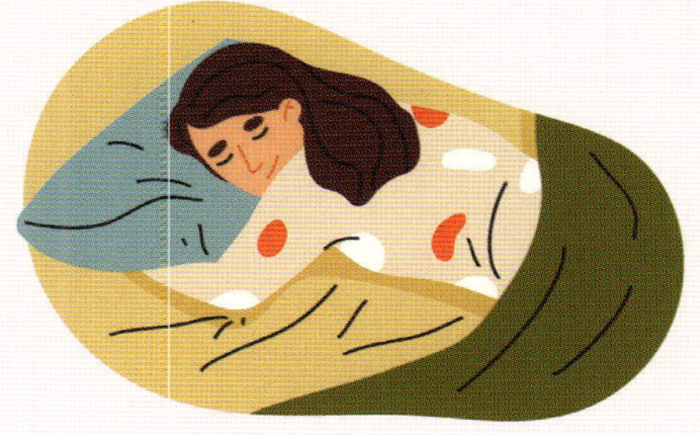

BUILDING HEALTHY DAILY HABITS

For long-term success, you need to build healthy daily habits. I always tell people to look at their health like a job. In the beginning, you need to be proactive, plan and prepare. Over time, it will become second nature.

Getting to a health goal is just one stage of your journey. Staying at your health goal is what is so incredibly important. Creating healthy daily habits is an important strategy for long-term success.

The consistent routine of exercise, meal prep, healthy food choices, sleep, stress management and regular meals is proven to help stabilise your blood sugar, improve insulin sensitivity, prevent complications and support long-term disease management.

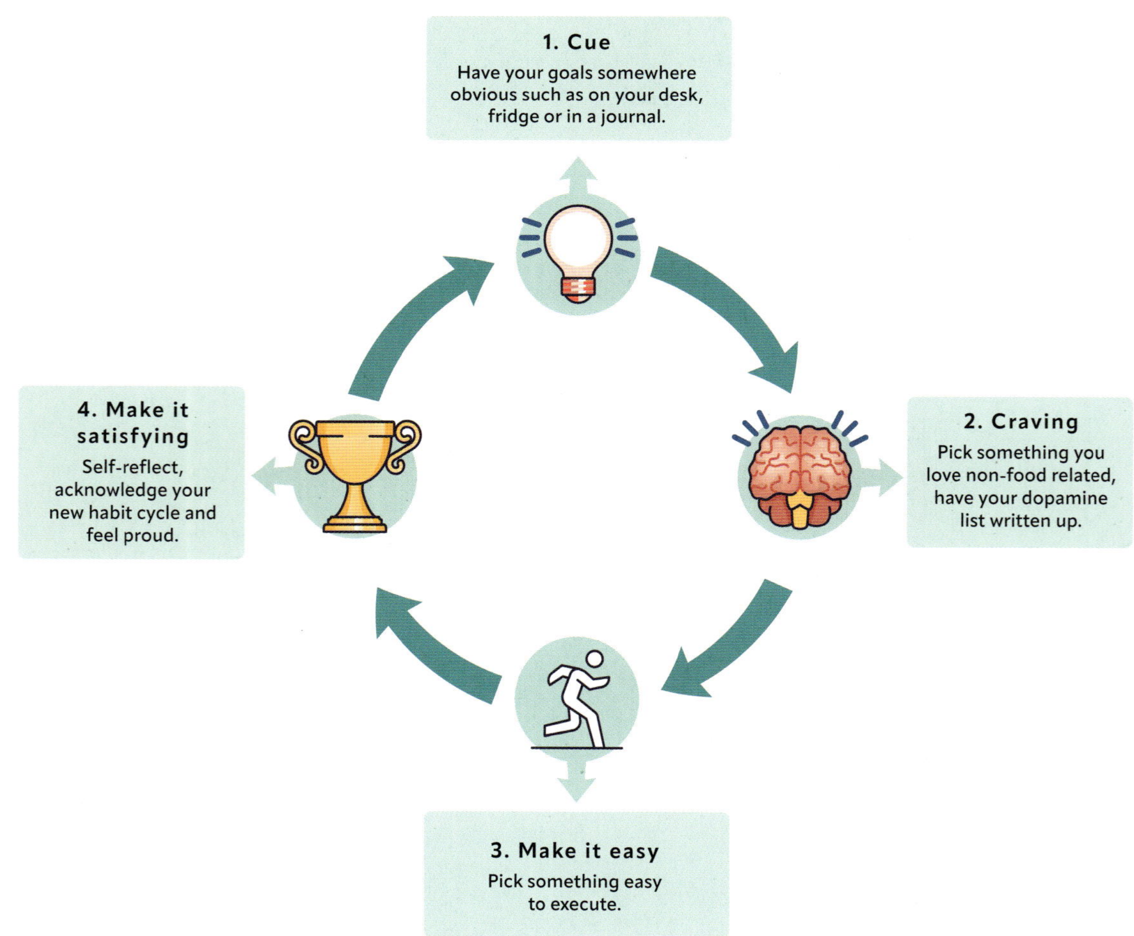

It's important to make habits effective. Try habit stacking – drink water with your coffee or meal, or listen to your favourite podcast while exercising. I love habit stacking. It makes you feel like you're accomplishing more and achieving something.

Start with small achievable changes to make them habits, such as walking after dinner, meal prepping or checking blood glucose at the same time every day. This helps you avoid disappointment – if you try to achieve too much too soon, you can end up feeling overwhelmed.

WHY DO HEALTHY HABITS MATTER?

BLOOD GLUCOSE STABILITY	Regular meal timing, healthy eating, good nutrition and structured activity prevent extreme fluctuations in blood glucose. This lowers your risk of hypo- or hyperglycaemia, improves energy, and protects against organ damage.
BEING CONSISTENT REDUCES COGNITIVE BURDEN	Make important rituals such as testing glucose, taking medications, walking after meals, good sleep, staying hydrated and calf raises into daily habits. This reduces the mental effort needed for disease management and lessens 'diabetes burnout'.
PREVENTING COMPLICATIONS	Daily healthy behaviours such as exercise, eating healthy and managing blood glucose all lower your risk of nerve damage, heart disease, eye problems and kidney failure.
FEELING EMPOWERED	Habit formation is so good for our mental health. It gives us confidence, better resilience, good mental health, better self-care and better diabetes management.
WEIGHT AND INSULIN SENSITIVITY BENEFITS	When you are consistently eating healthy and exercising you are improving how your body responds to insulin. You are also managing your weight. Two major pillars of diabetes management.

Celebrate your progress with something non-food related, such as going to a movie or buying a new outfit. This is positive reinforcement to sustain changes over time.

Remember, building healthy habits is empowering when you have type 2 diabetes. They can reduce complications and give you a better quality of life. Embrace your self-care and enjoy the success and confidence that comes with it.

PLATEAUS AND SETBACKS

Plateaus and setbacks are part of any health journey. I always tell my patients the health journey is a line that goes up and down.

Common plateaus and setbacks in type 2 diabetes involve periods when your blood glucose control stalls, weight loss plateaus, you lose motivation, or the complications are depressing and make management so much harder. These setbacks can result from changes in routine, poor sleep, less exercise, stress, illness, aging and medication issues, or they can be as simple as the body adapting.

Always be positive and patient as they can be managed with targeted strategies and support.

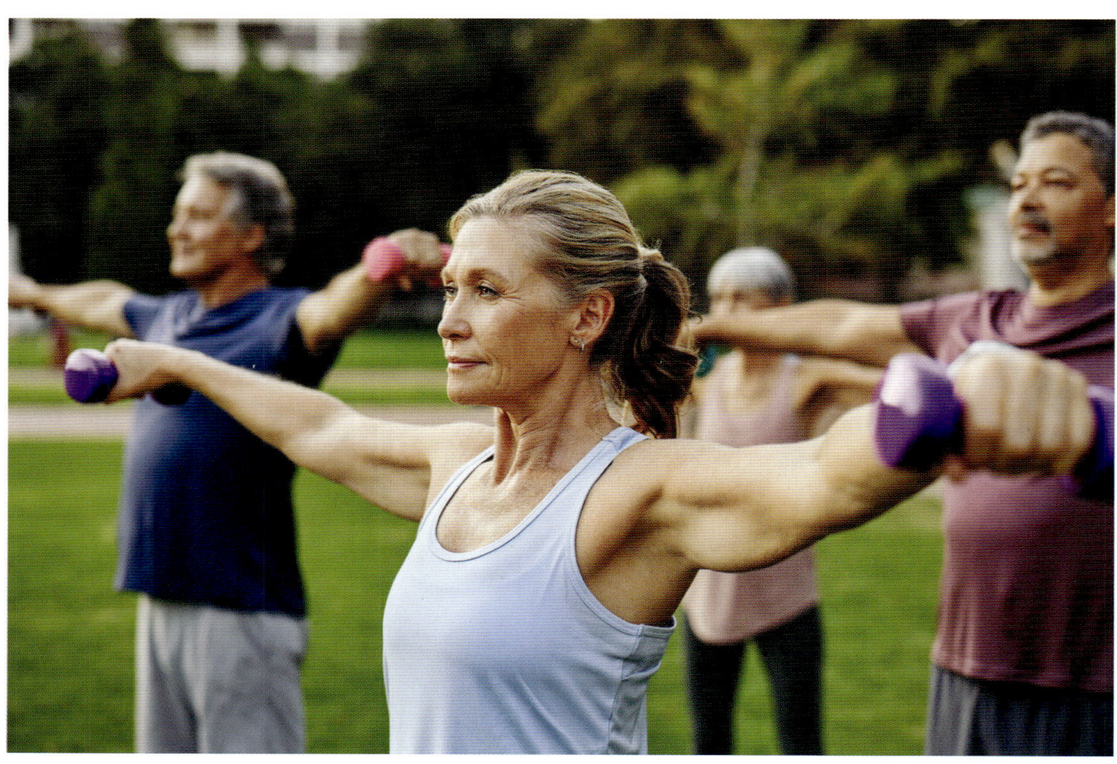

COMMON SETBACKS

BLOOD GLUCOSE PLATEAUS	Even when doing your best to manage blood glucose, the plateau can be for many reasons, such as aging, hormonal changes, medication adjustments, or being sick or stressed.
WEIGHT LOSS PLATEAUS	This can be so frustrating, especially when you feel you've been amazing on your program. A weight-loss plateau can be when you're picking more than usual, your portions could be getting bigger, you're drinking more liquid calories, you're exercising less, or your body is just adjusting to the weight loss with a pause. Be honest with yourself. Keep a really strict diet diary and find out where you have gone wrong.
LOSS OF MOTIVATION	Diabetes burnout is a real challenge. I see so many people grow tired of the relentless self-monitoring, dietary restrictions and constant appointments, which can lead to setbacks in healthy habits and blood glucose control.
HEALTH COMPLICATIONS AND STRESS	The stress of life, being sick, getting infections, injuries or diabetes complications can disrupt your daily routine and blood glucose.
HIDDEN FACTORS	Changes in sleep, snacking and picking, change in diet and possible hidden sugars in foods, drinking alcohol, late-night eating, or lack of physical activity can quietly erode your progress.

STRATEGIES TO COMBAT SETBACKS

Plateaus and setbacks are normal in lifelong management of type 2 diabetes, so don't be put off.

- Review your routine and make adjustments in meal times, exercise, medication or wherever you feel tweaks need to be made.

- Set realistic goals (this is a big one) and be patient.

- Celebrate your small wins with something non-food related. This builds momentum and is good for mental health.

- Don't be afraid to seek support if you need it. Seek out peer groups, or try apps for tracking – this can reignite your motivation and help solve problems.

- Address underlying issues such as sleep problems, depression or any other health issues that could be affecting your blood glucose. If you're unwell, take time off to get on top of things, chat to your employer and be an open communicator.

Make sure you're having regular check-ins, creating achievable habits, seeking professional support and positive reinforcement. And guess what? You can get back on track and be living your best life.

MAINTAINING LONG-TERM REMISSION

Once you're in remission, your work has not stopped. You now need to maintain being in remission. Being in remission needs an ongoing commitment because there will always be the risk of relapsing. The condition will resurface when you start to gain weight again, or slowly slip back into those old habits that made you diabetic in the first place.

PRIORITISE MAINTAINING YOUR WEIGHT

Did you know that weight regain is the most common reason why people relapse with type 2 diabetes?

- Always make sure your focus is on fat loss while preserving muscle mass. This is the foundation of my weight-loss programs.

- Exercise is so important for muscle. Be sure you're doing your resistance training and exercise program. Even a walk counts. Make sure you are sticking to an exercise plan. Avoid long periods of inactivity.

- Dietary changes and physical activity are key.

KEEP EATING HEALTHY FOOD

- Stick to nutrient-dense, low-calorie foods. I don't mean food products here – rather, choosing non-starchy veggies over starchy ones.

- Be sure you have protein with every meal, good fats daily and some whole grains (always at the start of the day, never at dinner).

- Avoid all sugary snacks, watch your portions and avoid most processed foods.

GET SUPPORT AND STAY CONNECTED

- Seek support if you need it and always self-monitor. Remember to get regular check-ups and look for any early signs of blood sugar rising. Stay connected to your healthcare professionals. Long-term support gives you greater success to stay in remission.

- Understand that this journey will have ups and downs. Some days are easier than others and your motivation can fluctuate. Know that setbacks are just a bump in the road.

- Learning to recognise that setbacks are normal. I tell my patients that every day is a new day to start again. Also consider professional help if you're still struggling with stress, emotional eating or even transitions in life.

- There's no one-size-fits-all approach; tailor strategies to what is best for your needs and health. Continue your healthy habits as a way of life, because the risk of relapse is always going to be there.

Maintaining remission is a real accomplishment. Remember this: embrace the healthy lifestyle and diet and see it as a gift to yourself. Don't be disheartened by setbacks.

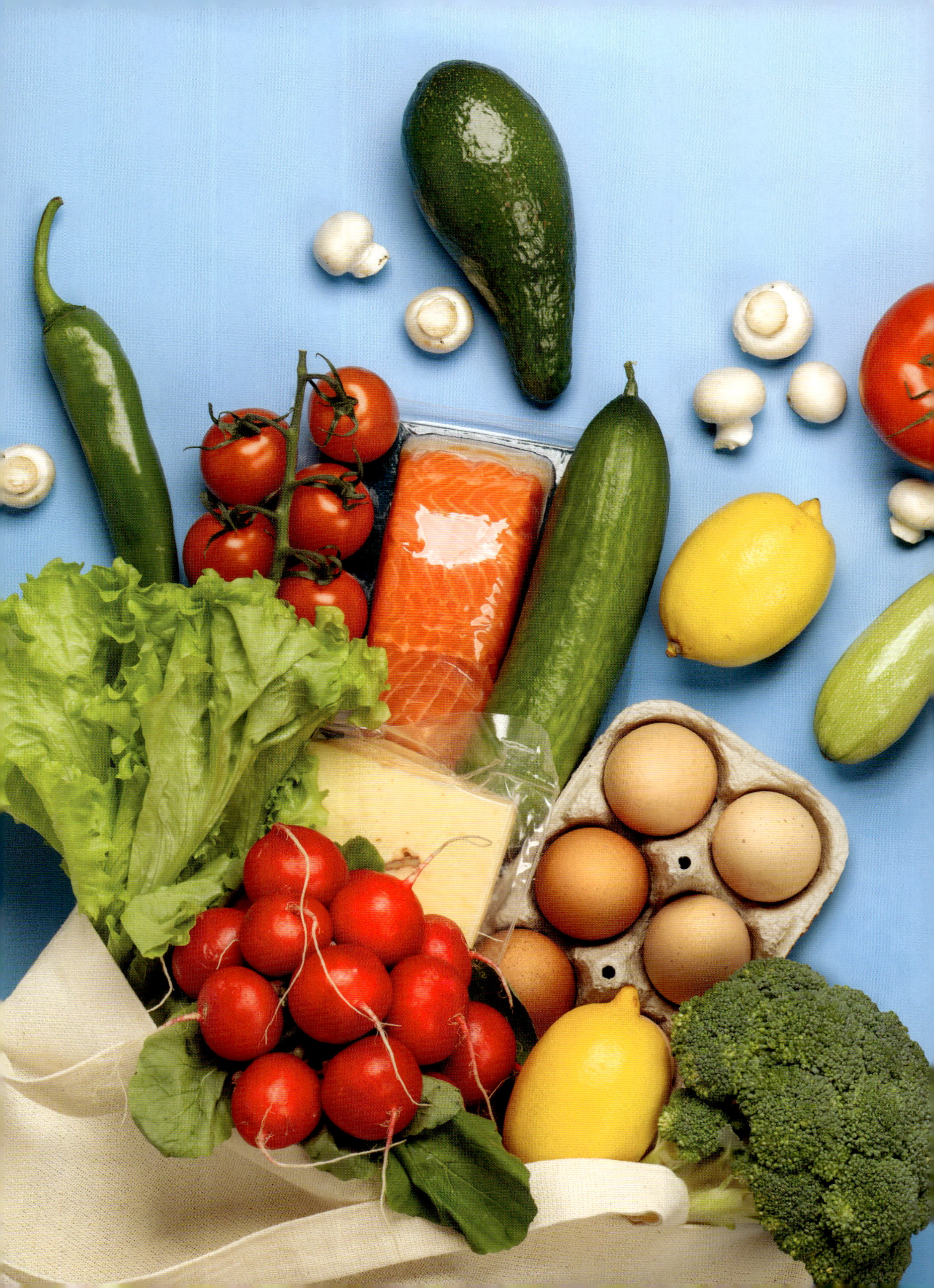

The 9-week program

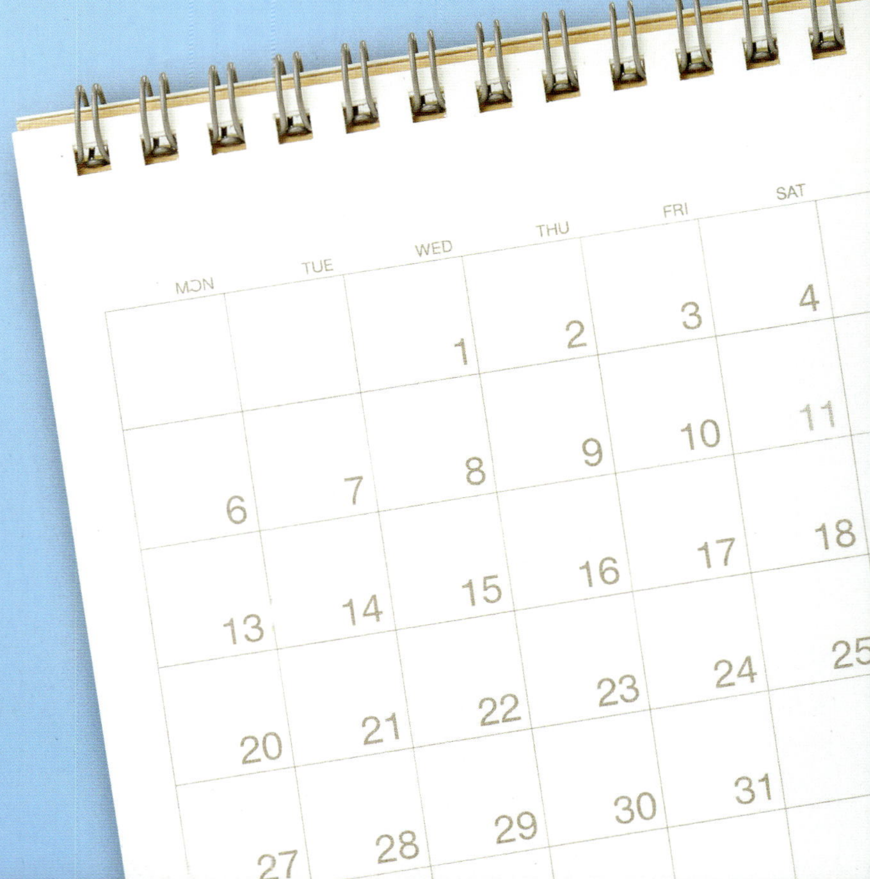

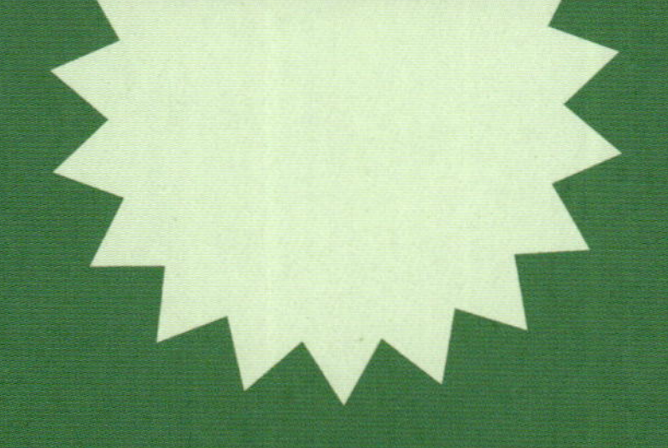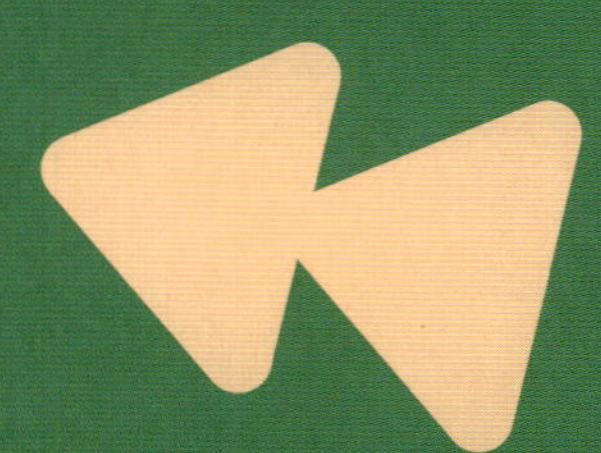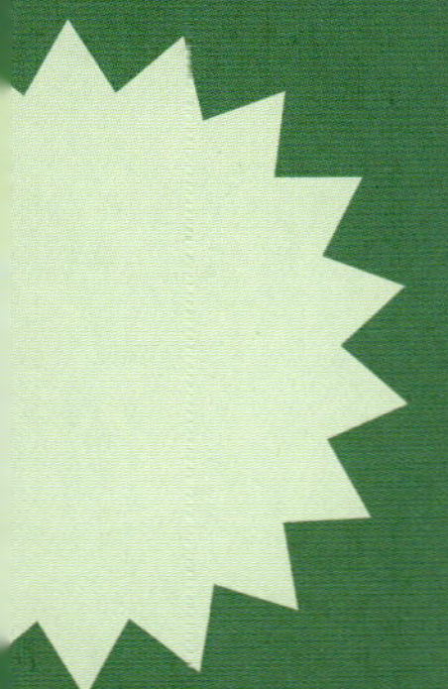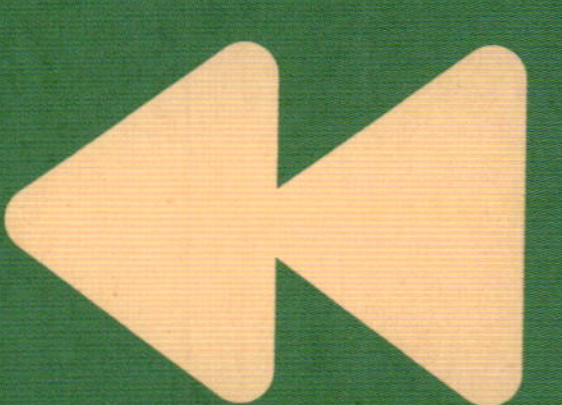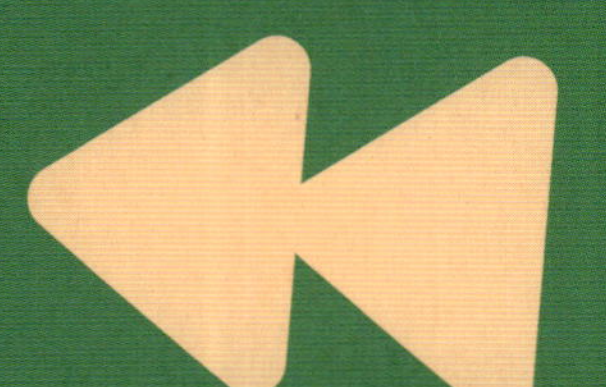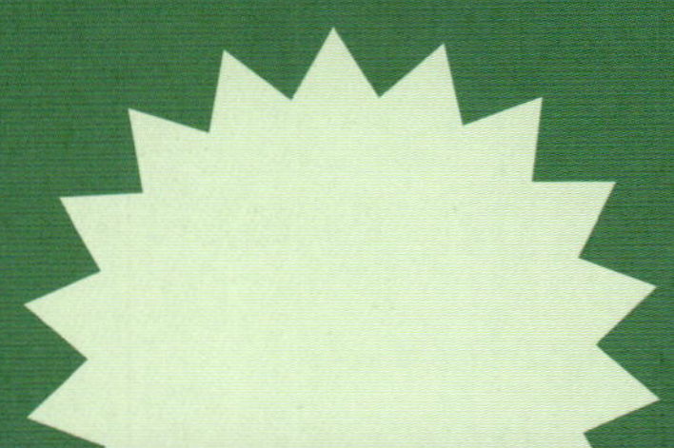

CHAPTER 12

Reversing diabetes

The 9-week program is a weight-loss program that I have specifically created for people with type 2 diabetes, but those with prediabetes, insulin resistance and obesity can do the program with success. About 80% of people with insulin resistance, prediabetes and type 2 diabetes are carrying too much weight. Remember, diabetes is a disease of the diet, and to treat disease you need to go to the cause – change your diet and get to a healthy weight.

My program is carefully put together to educate and arm you with all the information you need to help put type 2 diabetes into remission.

The program aims to reduce body fat and preserve that all-important muscle. It's designed for mild ketosis because I really believe in having a healthy, nutrient-dense diet rather than eating solely fats and protein. I see getting to a goal weight as something you need to do the healthy way, teaching you to embrace legumes, fruit and vegetables – but know which ones to choose: those that are high-fibre and low-carbohydrate.

As a practitioner, it is so important that this program is a fat-loss program.

The only effective way to lose fat is to be in a ketogenic state.

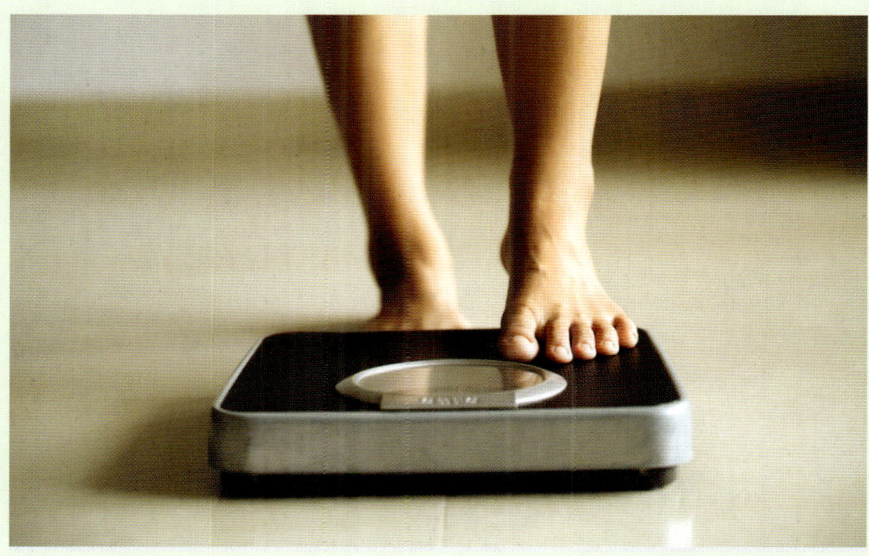

Fat loss in the pancreas and liver can restore the functions of these organs and glucose regulation; the greater the fat loss, the greater your chance of reversing type 2 diabetes and preventing all the long-term complications. Removal of fat is crucial because fat interferes with key functions required for glucose control. When the liver is fatty it drives insulin resistance, meaning the body needs more insulin to manage blood glucose and this is a foundational defect in type 2 diabetes. When you reduce liver fat, you'll improve insulin sensitivity and blood glucose control, and the results can be quick.

Fat in the pancreas, especially around the beta cells, impairs the ability of those cells to produce and release insulin. Lowering pancreatic fat lets the cells recover and function properly.

To get type 2 diabetes into remission, you need substantial weight loss to reduce excess fat in the liver and pancreas, allowing insulin production and insulin sensitivity to recover. The longer the diabetes persists, the harder it is to fully restore the pancreas and liver and achieve remission.

Excess fat is not a reservoir of energy as many think. It is inflammatory, releasing pro-inflammatory molecules and toxic metabolites that block insulin signalling and damage beta cell function. Removing fat is thus essential for normal blood glucose regulation. Basically, reducing fat in the liver and pancreas restores the machinery of glucose control at the root of T2D and is the foundation for remission.

The focus of my program is low-carbohydrate and non-starchy vegetables, low-carbohydrate fruit, healthy fats, and lean proteins. Half your plate should be non-starchy veggies at each meal.

Getting into ketosis is different for everyone.

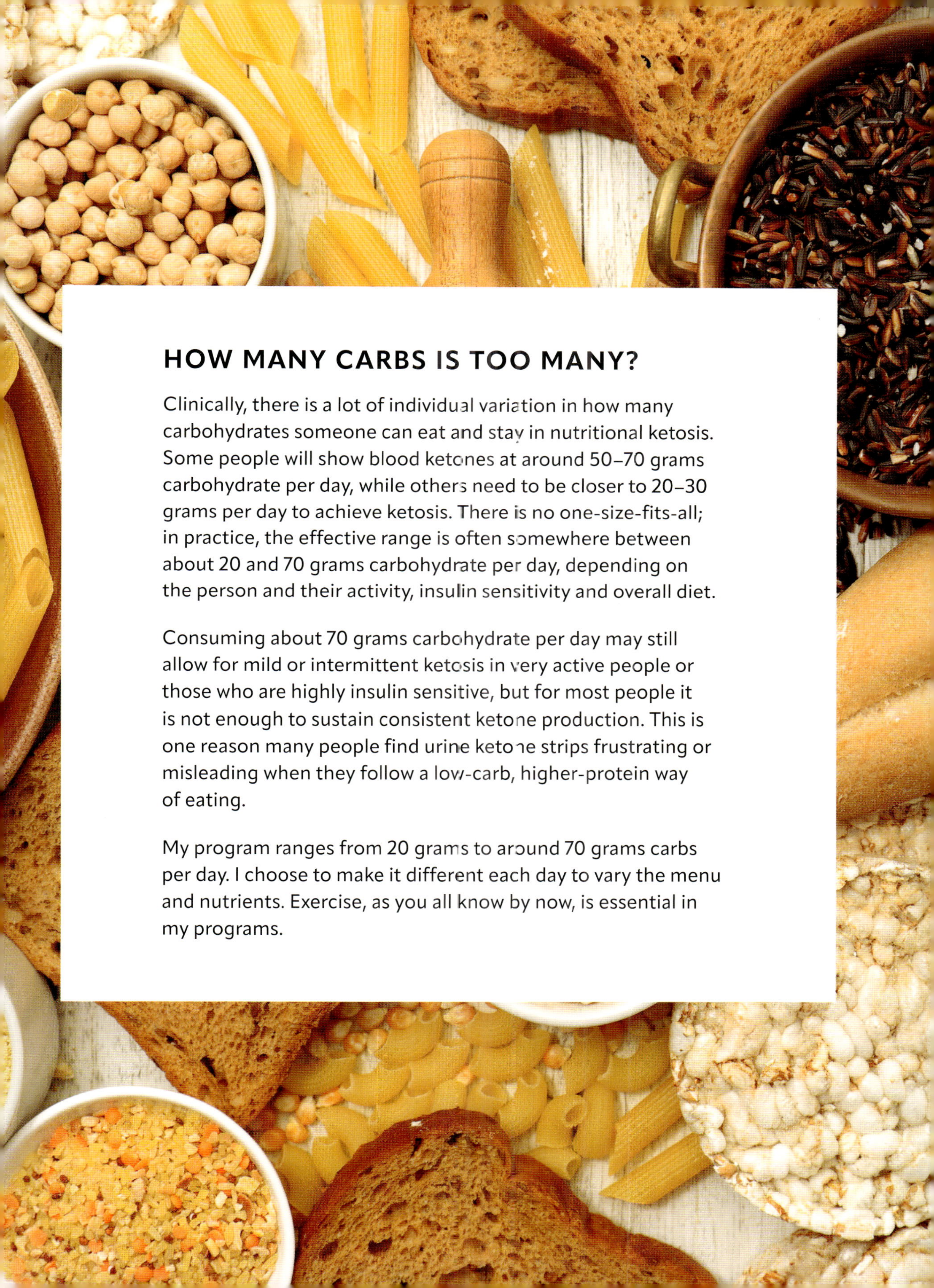

HOW MANY CARBS IS TOO MANY?

Clinically, there is a lot of individual variation in how many carbohydrates someone can eat and stay in nutritional ketosis. Some people will show blood ketones at around 50–70 grams carbohydrate per day, while others need to be closer to 20–30 grams per day to achieve ketosis. There is no one-size-fits-all; in practice, the effective range is often somewhere between about 20 and 70 grams carbohydrate per day, depending on the person and their activity, insulin sensitivity and overall diet.

Consuming about 70 grams carbohydrate per day may still allow for mild or intermittent ketosis in very active people or those who are highly insulin sensitive, but for most people it is not enough to sustain consistent ketone production. This is one reason many people find urine ketone strips frustrating or misleading when they follow a low-carb, higher-protein way of eating.

My program ranges from 20 grams to around 70 grams carbs per day. I choose to make it different each day to vary the menu and nutrients. Exercise, as you all know by now, is essential in my programs.

Physical signs of being in ketosis – what to look out for.

If you're not interested in using ketone strips, there are physical signs of being in ketosis. These signs can be quite noticeable, especially in the first few days or weeks of starting a keto diet. In my experience, some people get a few of the signs, others can get the full-on 'keto flu', some get a headache and others just feel low energy. Everyone is different.

Common signs:

- **Bad breath (fruity or acetone smell).** This is one of the most distinctive signs. It's caused by higher levels of acetone (a ketone) being exhaled. It does not smell bad like a bacterial smell, and you can taste it. Usually, a loved one will tell you.

- **Frequent urination.** Higher ketone and water loss lead to increased urination. I find this one really common; people really notice this.

- **Dry mouth and increased thirst.** As ketones are excreted and the body loses water, people often experience persistent thirst and a dry mouth. This is not so common in my experience.

- **Short-term fatigue (keto flu).** In the early transition phase, you may feel tired, sluggish or irritable; have headaches or muscle soreness; or feel dizzy as your body adapts from burning glucose to fat.

- **Appetite suppression.** Many people in ketosis notice less hunger and better satiety between meals. This is one of the best things about being in ketosis – it just makes the weight-loss journey so much easier.

- **Digestive changes.** You may experience constipation or diarrhoea as your digestion adjusts to the new macronutrient balance. This usually resolves within the first month.

- **Muscle cramps.** Because of increased fluid and electrolyte losses, you can get leg cramps or spasms. Often it can be good in the first few 3 weeks to take an electrolyte drink. Just make sure you choose a good-quality one – nothing with artificial sweeteners or flavours.

To lose fat, you need to burn fat!

- **Weight loss.** Both rapid initial water weight reduction and fat loss over time. I find the water loss is only in the first 2 weeks, then it appears to be a pure fat loss.

- **Improved concentration or 'mental clarity'.** After adapting, many people report more stable energy and better focus. This is amazing and why ketosis can be a wonderful place to be.

To talk you through the journey:

A 9-WEEK PLAN IN THREE PHASES

This program is designed as a weight-loss program, but each week has a different theme to address complications of type 2 diabetes and give you the best possible outcome. For those of you without T2D, you can see it as a holistic approach to your weight-loss and health journey.

PHASE 1	**WEEKS 1–3**	**GETTING INTO KETOSIS**
	WEEK 1	Getting into the swing of it
	WEEK 2	Lowering inflammation
	WEEK 3	Supporting gut health
PHASE 2	**WEEKS 4–6**	**ADAPTATION AND CHECK-UP**
	WEEK 4	Supporting our heart and vascular system
	WEEK 5	Protecting our nervous system
	WEEK 6	Supporting eye health
PHASE 3	**WEEKS 7–9**	**CONTINUED WEIGHT LOSS**
	WEEK 7	Supporting skin and preventing infections
	WEEK 8	Supporting mental health and cognition
	WEEK 9	Supporting our immune system

Complications such as MASLD (formerly known as non-alcoholic fatty liver disease) are addressed within the program through getting into ketosis (fat-burning), consuming antioxidants, lowering inflammation, eating a nutrient-dense diet and making healthy lifestyle choices.

GETTING STARTED

When you start this program, it's important to understand and recognise where your health is at and how serious your condition is. I have some reminders and strategies you need to put into place when you embark on this program.

- **Pick a time to start that works for you.** Sometimes the best time to start is not now because life does get in the way. Choose what works best for you. And commit to it.

- **Tell family and friends what you are doing, for support.** This helps you manage social situations better. Also talk to your GP or healthcare provider about what you are planning on doing.

PRE-PROGRAM BLOOD TESTS

Get a check-up and request the following blood tests:

- insulin
- fasting glucose
- vitamin D
- iron
- HbA1c
- liver function
- cholesterol
- C-reactive protein
- erythrocyte sedimentation rate
- full blood count.

Also, get your blood pressure checked.

- **Think about what exercise you want to do and how you are going to do it.** If you're not a regular exerciser, then I suggest starting with daily walking. Make it brisk and a minimum of 30 minutes to start. Once you have more of a routine and feel your fitness is building or weight is lost, then start to implement a program of HIIT training, resistance training and cardiovascular exercise.

- **Address any possible stressful situations.** Find ways to navigate these without elevating your cortisol levels as elevated cortisol promotes fat storage.

- **Focus on your sleep.** Lack of sleep leads to weight gain; it increases ghrelin, the hunger hormone, and decreases leptin, the hormone that tells when we are full. We make poorer food choices when tired, plus lack of sleep increases cortisol levels. Focus on good-quality sleep patterns, and work out what changes you can make to suit you.

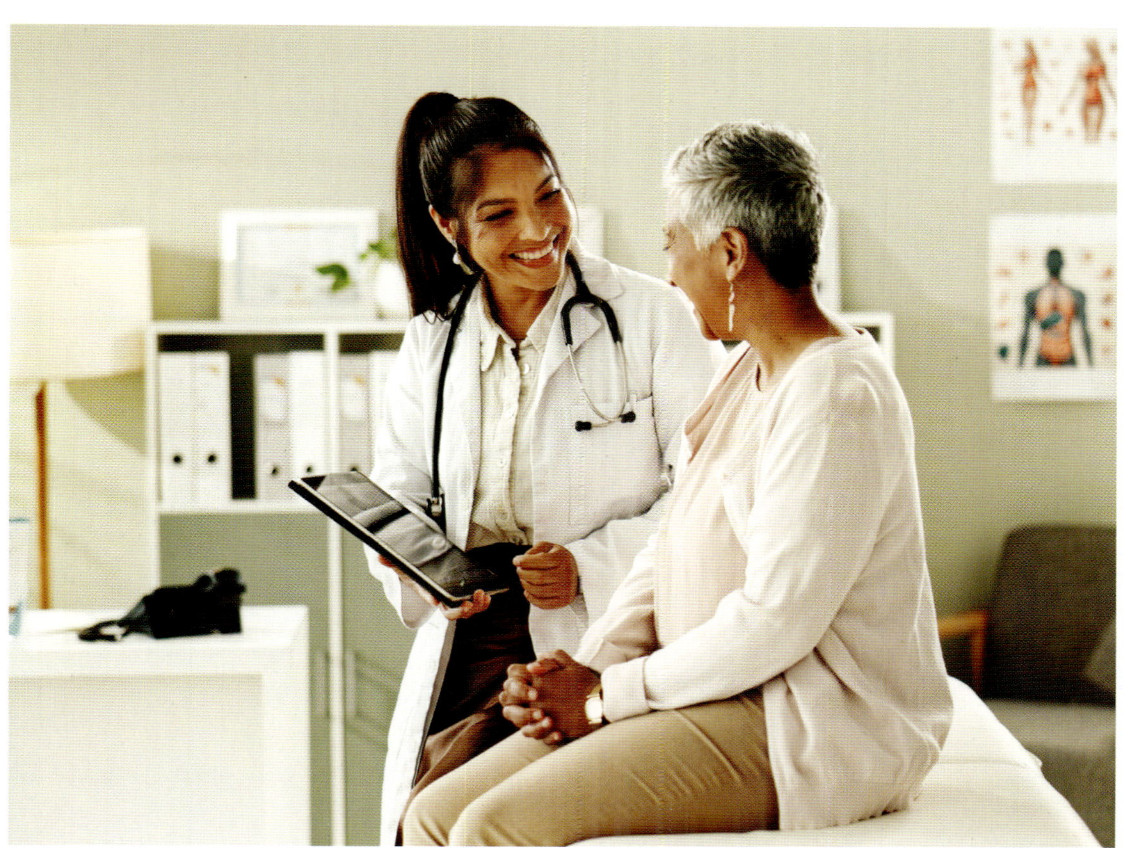

THE BEGINNING

Weeks 1 to 3 – Getting into the swing of it all, and ketosis

The first 3 weeks are really about getting into the swing of it all and into a ketogenic state. The focus of the program is as follows:

- Three meals a day – all low-carb with lean protein and non-starchy vegetables

- Very low carbohydrate – about 50 grams a day from non-starchy fibrous vegetables

- Protein – about 1.2 grams per kilogram of your body weight from healthy sources such as chicken, eggs, lean meat, tofu, turkey and fish

- Healthy fats – avocados, nuts, fatty fish and olive oil

- Hydration – water intake at 30 ml per kilogram of body weight

- Beverages – no more than 2 units of alcohol per week, but ideally remove altogether. Herbal teas, ideally black coffee and tea (a dash of milk is fine but not a big splash)

- Snacks – optional

- Fasting – 12 hours between dinner and breakfast

- Supplements – often in the beginning, you could take a multivitamin. An electrolyte supplement can help in early ketosis. I recommend one for the first 4 weeks of the program. Please email me for my recommendation contact@sarahdilorenzo.com

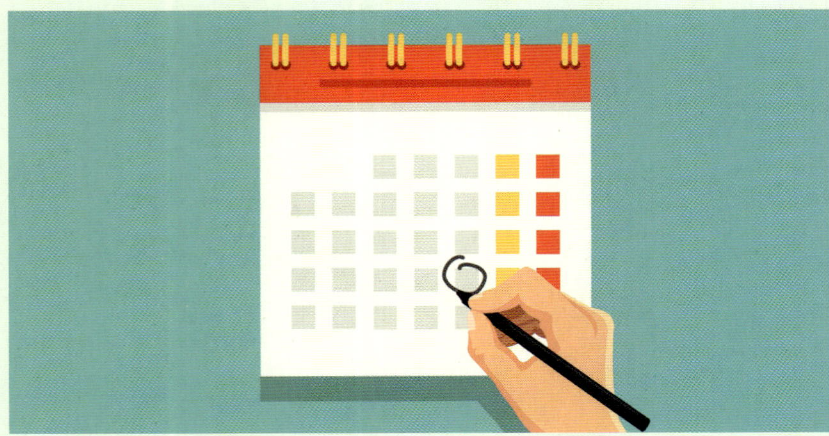

HYDRATION

Staying hydrated is essential when in ketosis. Here's why:

- Restricting carbs leads to rapid loss of water and salt.

- You have increased fluid needs for fat-burning.

- Electrolyte balance is crucial for energy, muscle and heart health.

- Water supports kidney filtration and reduces your risk of kidney stones.

- You'll help avoid dehydration-related side effects and keep your metabolism running smoothly.

You should drink at least 30 ml water per kilogram of your own body weight daily. Find ways to make sure you don't forget such as:

- having a water bottle

- setting a reminder on your phone every couple of hours

- having a special cup

- keeping track on an app.

HYPOGLYCAEMIA

Be prepared for the possibility of hypoglycaemia (hypos). In my experience, hypos don't affect everyone and are usually mild, but I do need to make people aware of this. If they do happen, it's only really at the beginning of the program.

As a practitioner, I always want people to be prepared, just in case. I have treated many people with type 2 diabetes who haven't experienced hypos in the start of their health journey with me, but some patients have. When picked up at the early stages, they can be well controlled. Education is key and knowledge is everything. I am overly cautious but feel a duty of care to do the best I can for my patients and all of you.

- **Monitor your blood glucose.** Consider wearing a continuous blood glucose monitor in the first 3 weeks of the program. You can easily get these from a chemist over the counter and they range between $100 and $300.

WATCH OUT FOR EARLY SIGNS OF HYPOGLYCAEMIA

Signs to be aware of:

- shakiness or trembling

- sweating, often for no obvious reason

- hunger or nausea

- light-headedness or dizziness, feeling faint or weak

- headache or 'brain fog'

- irritability, mood changes or confusion

- paleness, or feeling unwell or clammy

- rapid heartbeat

- sluggishness, tiredness or difficulty concentrating.

Be especially aware of these symptoms if you are taking insulin or sulfonylurea medication and haven't had the dosages adjusted. Please, if you have type 2 diabetes, consult with your doctor before starting the program.

It is important to know the difference between going into ketosis and hypos. The symptoms are generally different, so look out for being pale, sweating, nausea, a rapid heartbeat, confusion or a clammy feeling.

Know the difference between going into ketosis and hypoglycaemia.

I always feel relieved when my patients reach the 1-month mark because I know their chances of hypos are almost eradicated.

MANAGING A HYPO

I get my patients to have any of the following glucose sources on hand for the first month of the program. Many don't need this precaution, but it's best to be prepared.

ITEM	PORTION SIZE	CARBS (APPROX.)
BANANA	½ medium	15 grams
GRAPES	15	15 grams
RAISINS	2 tablespoons	14 grams
APPLE/ORANGE	1 small	15 grams
HONEY/MAPLE SYRUP	1 tablespoon	13–17 grams
APPLE SAUCE	½ cup	12–15 grams
MEDJOOL DATE	1 large	18 grams

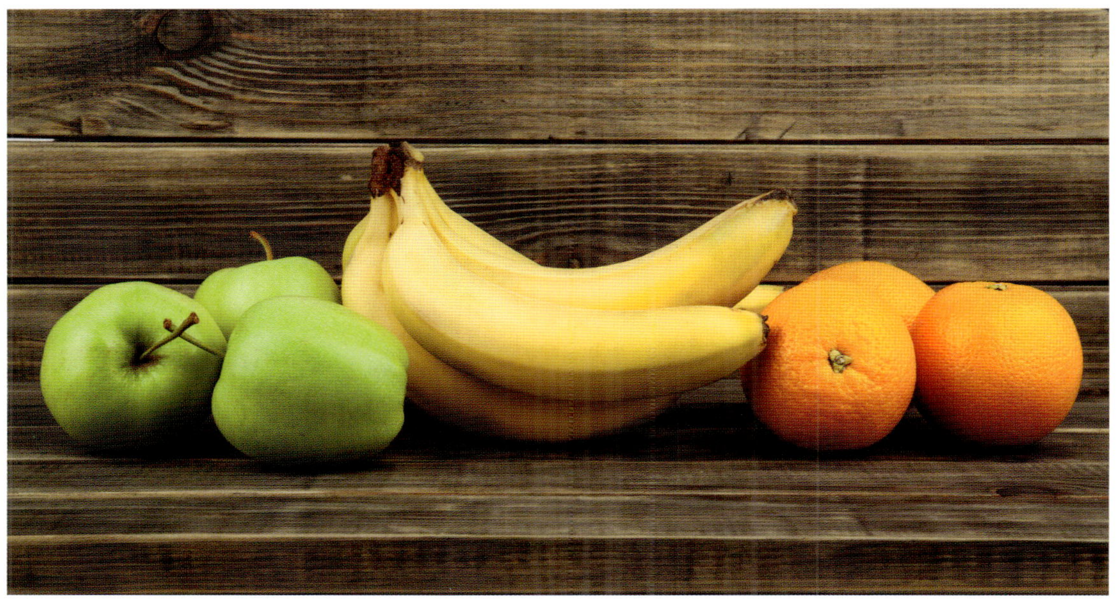

TRACKING YOUR SUCCESS

I really do love this part of the journey. It's so good to see all the non-scale victories along the way: reducing medications, wearing new clothes, having more energy, lowering disease risk, having better mood, sleeping better, libido returning and getting your life back the way it should be. Have T2D is like having another job, managing the condition and its complications. To move away from this disease means gaining an entirely new way of life. As a practitioner, seeing my patients get their life back is the most rewarding thing ever – the freedom, the happiness and the new lease on life. This is why I do what I do!

To start:

- Get a journal, either hardcopy or use an app or your phone.

- Take your measurements.

- Consider using a belt to measure yourself; it's so good to see the notches go down.

- Take pictures of yourself in swimwear or underwear.

- Weigh yourself.

- Think about setting a realistic goal weight.

- Set yourself a day of the week to weigh yourself. Weighing yourself is something quite individual; it helps some people feel success but may discourage others.

- Make an appointment with your doctor.

- Join my Facebook community – The Sarah Di Lorenzo Community – for extra support. You'll find a community full of like-minded people who are kind and all about lifting each other up.

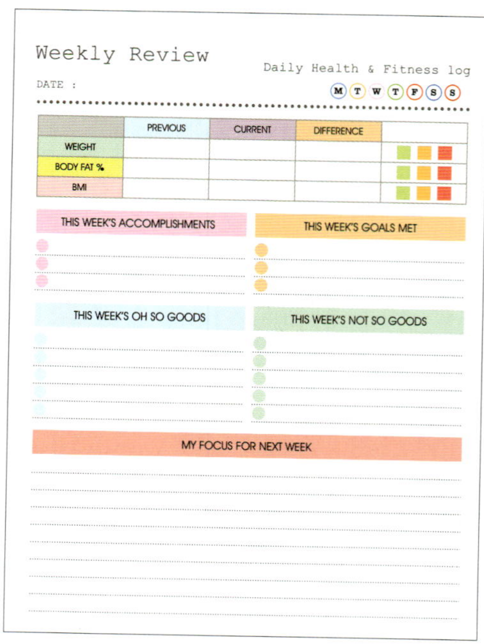

OTHER IMPORTANT THINGS

The key to success is preparation:

- Have a good look in your pantry. Clear out all the tempting treats, biscuits, white flour, white bread, white pasta, lollies, fried foods, fatty foods, etc. You can either give them away or dispose of them in the bin.

- Get your shopping done.

- Schedule in your exercise. Consider exercise like a visit to the doctor.

- Focus on going to bed at the right time and getting good-quality sleep. Lack of sleep = weight gain.

- Make sure you have stress management techniques in place.

- Keep drinking your water – find a way to track this that works for you.

- At the end of each week, reflect on your success and plan for the next week.

THE PROGRAM NITTY-GRITTY

Alcohol consumption – for best results, avoid alcohol all together. Otherwise, stick to 2 units per week. Water intake is essential. Aim for 30 ml per kilogram of your body weight.

Note: You can repeat meals and interchange your proteins of choice.

ORDER OF EATING FOODS

Remember the order of the eating pattern to help with glycaemic control. Eating fibre and protein before carbohydrates slows down stomach emptying and glucose absorption, reducing blood sugar spikes and demands for insulin. Glucose and insulin responses are flatter when eating carbs last, with a post-meal glucose level 30% lower than when eating carbs first.

1. **Non-starchy vegetables (fibre).** Begin the meal with salads, leafy greens, broccoli and any other non-starchy vegetables

2. **Protein and healthy fats.** Move to protein sources such as chicken, fish, tofu, eggs, lean meat and healthy fats such as avocado and nuts.

3. **Carbohydrates.** Finish with complex carbohydrates such as whole grains, legumes, starchy vegetables or fruit. This is for when you're maintaining a healthy weight.

SALT

I do season my recipes with salt and pepper. Many wonder why, given salt's bad reputation.

I know this is going to be controversial, but several studies and reviews have found that low-salt diets can lead to an increased fasting insulin, elevated glucose levels and worse markers of insulin resistance. This effect is thought to be related to activation of the renin–angiotensin–aldosterone system and sympathetic nervous system, which can interfere with glucose metabolism.

The evidence suggests that strict or short-term low-salt diets are associated with higher insulin resistance, while moderate salt reduction over longer periods may have neutral or beneficial effects for some populations.

While low-salt diets can be recommended for lowering blood pressure, excessive salt restriction may harm metabolic health and worsen insulin sensitivity.

So I'm not telling you all to go and eat lots of salt, but to have it in moderation, just lightly seasoning your meals. I have salt with every meal.

Help regulate your blood glucose after meals with calf raises or a 10-minute walk.

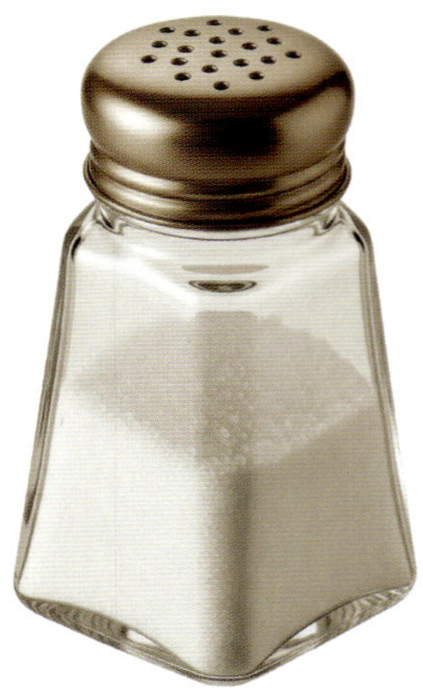

SLOW IT DOWN!

Think about how many times you are chewing your food.
I'd say most people chew around five times per mouthful.
Slowing down your chewing and eating pace can support
higher GLP-1 (glucagon-like peptide-1) levels. This really
helps with satiety and appetite regulation.

Multiple studies show that when people chew their food
thoroughly and slow down their pace of eating, they have
a greater and more sustained release of GLP-1, as well as
other 'fullness' hormones such as peptide YY (PYY).

PYY is a powerful gut–brain hormone that helps regulate
appetite by slowing digestion and sending fullness signals to
the brain. It rises after eating protein- and fibre-rich meals, and
is extremely important for maintaining energy balance and
preventing overeating.

Aim for 20 chews per mouthful.

Slow, mindful chewing prolongs the early phase of digestion,
giving the gut time to sense food and secrete hormones such as
GLP-1, which in turn slows gastric emptying, enhances fullness
and reduces later calorie intake.

ROAD BLOCKS TO WEIGHT LOSS

Weight loss is a journey. Always remember why you need to get to a healthy goal weight. Take the program day by day mentally, but have your food prepared for the week ahead.

Every morning is a new start.

Something I want you to think about is your relationship with food. How did you end up with type 2 diabetes? Was it how you were raised, emotional eating, boredom eating or stress eating? Could it be that you never really thought about what you were eating, and made it up as the day went on – what I call an ad lib eater?

To beat the disease, you need to face and truly understand how you got to where you are in the first place. This is what created the disease.

- Write down what you think it was and try to understand it, so you can make the changes you need. This is a reflection for you. What I want you to do is put a plan in place to get to the core of your issue with food and put steps in place so it never happens again.

- Write a list of six things you love that give you a dopamine hit and make you feel good that aren't food related. It could be:

  - swimming in the ocean

  - going to a gallery

  - having your hair done

  - getting a massage

  - going phone-free for a few hours

  - lying on a blanket in the sun

  - visiting someone you love

  - knitting

  - painting.

- Every time you feel that you want to reach for food – because of boredom, stress or emotion, for instance – do something from this list. Be kind to yourself, as if you were your own best friend. Treat yourself how you treat others. Self-care and self-love is so important in this journey.

I write a lot more about weight loss in The 10:10 Plan – my ten-week weight-loss program.

GO FOR 12/12 FASTING

For as long as I can remember, I've told all my patients to eat their dinner as early as possible, at least 3 hours before they go to bed. I have never really promoted it as a 'fast' but more of a way of life we all should live by. Sometimes when you label something, people may see it as a thing to do for a fixed amount of time rather than a way of life.

Ideally, your last meal would be around 6 p.m. and your first meal would be after 6 a.m. In between, you can have water, herbal tea, black coffee and mineral water.

When it comes to type 2 diabetes, there are many beneficial factors to fasting:

- **Insulin and blood glucose regulation.** Fasting for 12 hours allows insulin levels to decrease after meals, preventing constant insulin production and promoting increased insulin sensitivity.

- **Reduced glucose spikes.** By giving the body a break from constant eating, 12/12 fasting limits the period of post-meal glucose spikes, reducing your overall exposure to high blood glucose and supporting pancreatic recovery.

- **Alignment with circadian rhythms.** Eating during a consistent 12-hour window, especially earlier in the day, aligns your food intake with natural hormonal patterns, which can help optimise glucose metabolism, lower blood pressure and reduce inflammation.

- **Weight loss and fat mobilisation.** People tend to consume fewer calories during the eating window, promoting weight loss and visceral fat reduction, which as you know are essential for reversing T2D. Note: fat mobilisation is the release and use of stored body fat for energy, enabling your body to adapt to fasting, exercise and metabolic changes.

- **Improved insulin sensitivity.** Research shows that even moderate forms of fasting, such as 12/12, can improve markers of glycaemic control, including lower fasting glucose and HbA1c.

The evidence does support success in reversing diabetes with time-restricted eating such as 12/12 fasting. You'll support decreasing your weight and body fat, reducing insulin resistance, lowering fasting glucose, improving glucose tolerance, and having greater control over blood pressure and lipid levels. These are all so important for diabetes remission and metabolic health improvements, especially when paired with a balanced, healthy, gorgeous, nutrient-rich diet.

WHAT ABOUT SNACKING?

I have always been a believer in snacking. For starters, it can get you to the next meal without overeating, but it's also a great way to get more nutrients in your diet and include foods such as nuts and fruit daily.

High-fibre fruit and nuts are amazing for snacking.

In this program, my snacking options are generally foods such as cheese, non-starchy vegetable sticks and low-carb fruits. For best results in the program, however, avoid snacking.

Note: this isn't a calorie-counting program, but focuses on macronutrients, in particular carbohydrates, proteins and fats.

ELECTROLYTES AND KETOSIS

The electrolytes sodium, potassium and magnesium are important during the initial stages of ketosis. The shift to a low-carb diet changes how your body handles water and minerals, leading to increased water and electrolyte losses.

When you restrict carbs, your insulin levels can drop quickly. When insulin is lower, it triggers the kidneys to excrete more sodium and water, and the result is loss of electrolytes. We need electrolytes for energy production, hydration, and proper functioning of muscles, nerves and the heart. Deficiencies cause cramps, heart palpitations and fatigue.

The keto flu is a road bump you may experience at the beginning of the program – anything from a headache to fatigue, poor concentration and feeling dizzy. This is due to the loss of electrolytes.

Supplementing with electrolytes during early ketosis can help with energy and metabolism, and prevent keto flu. Plus, for every gram of glycogen, you lose about 3 grams water, this is why you urinate a lot in the early phases.

Other drinks:

- **Beverages.** These are listed at the bottom of each week as reminders. The only non-negotiable is having water daily. The remainder are optional.

- **Coffee and tea.** Both coffee and tea are welcome throughout the program. My recommendation is to choose black for best results, but if you do wish to add milk, make it a dash not a splash, and avoid all sweeteners, especially artificial sweeteners.

You can email contact@sarahdilorenzo.com for my recommendations for supplements, including electrolytes.

For my protein bars and products – sarahdilorenzo.com

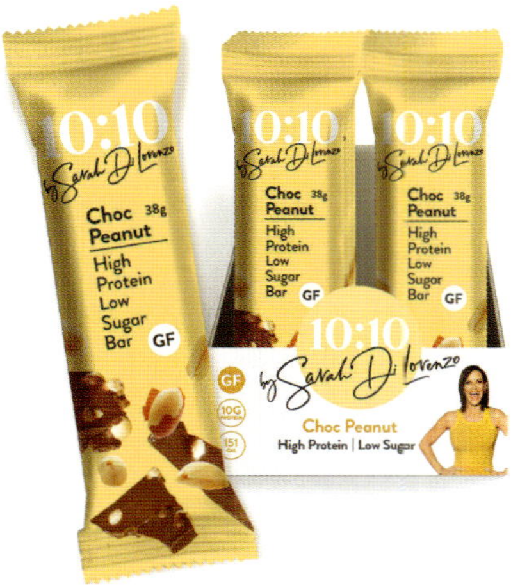

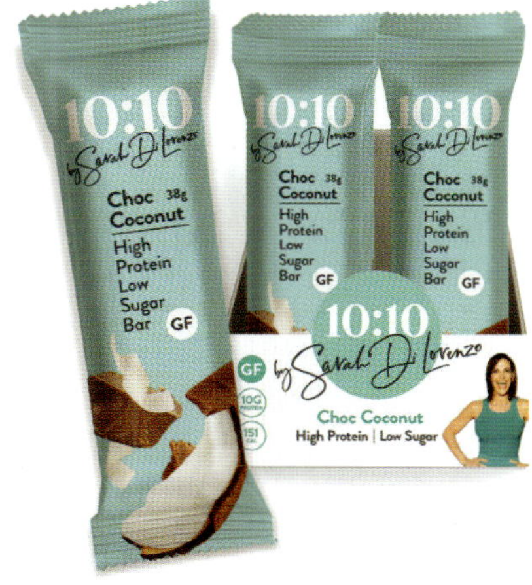

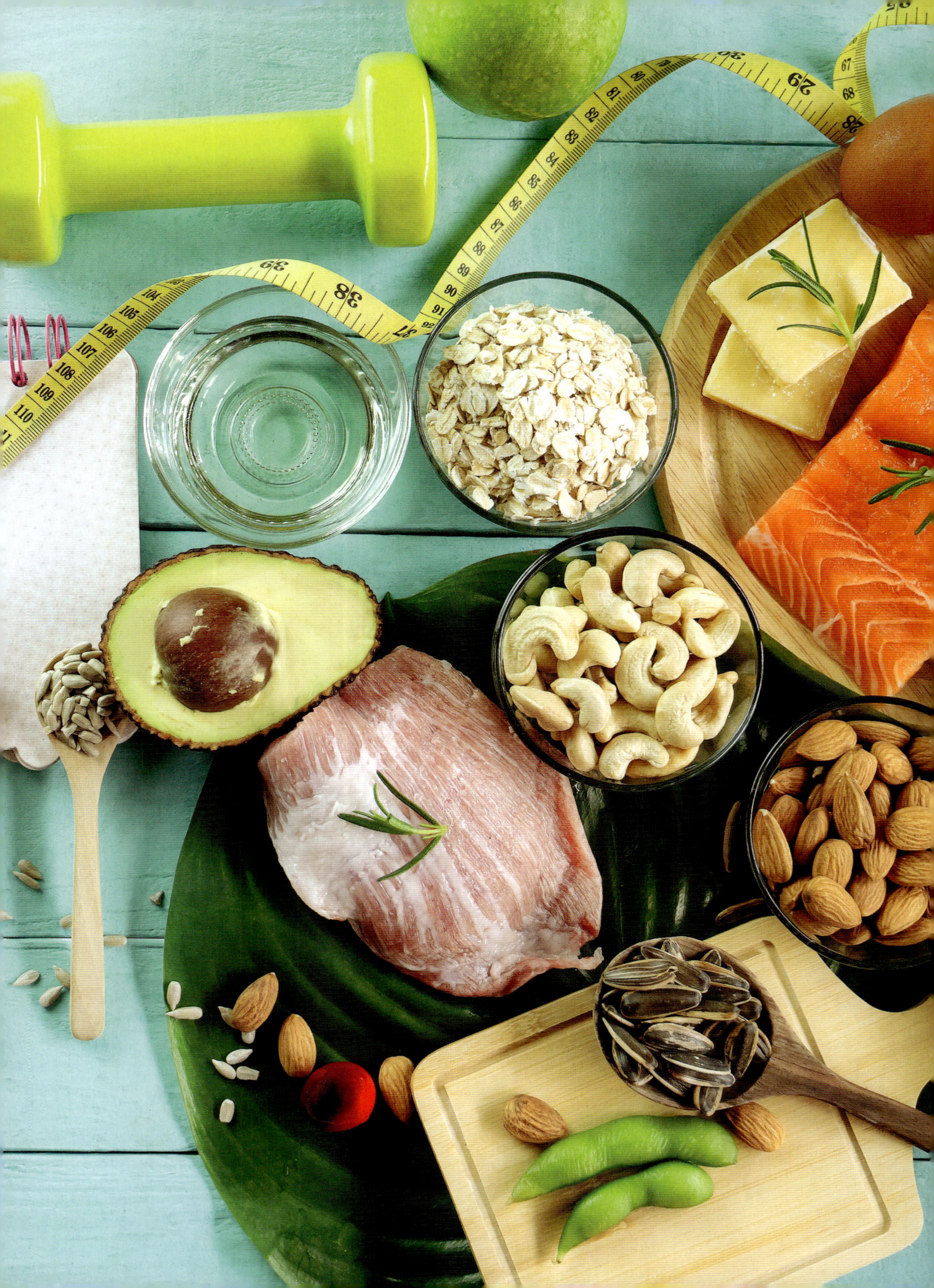

PHASE 1 (WEEKS 1–3):

Getting into ketosis

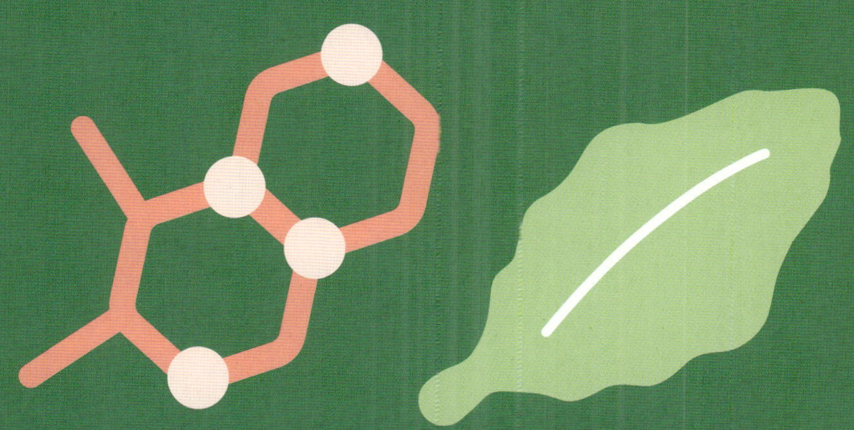

Getting into the swing of it

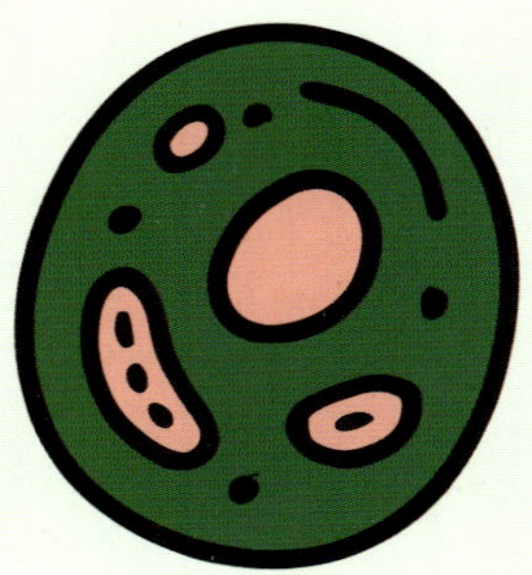

Focus: Gut health and lowering inflammation

Make sure you time your final meal to be 12 hours before your breakfast!

Reminders

- What is your exercise routine?

- Have you started tracking your measurements?

- Have you addressed sleep, socialising or any stress?

- Are you using a continuous blood glucose monitor or tracking your blood glucose? Do you need to check your blood pressure?

- Don't forget – walking after each meal, order of eating (good to keep in the habit) and doing 12/12 fasting.

	BREAKFAST	MID-MORNING	LUNCH	MID-AFTERNOON	DINNER
MONDAY	2 poached eggs with 1 cup spinach leaves and 1 tablespoon feta	5 pecans	120 grams grilled chicken breast with ¼ avocado and a green salad	½ cup strawberries	120 grams salmon with 1 cup steamed broccoli, ½ cup sliced zucchini and ½ carrot
TUESDAY	⅔ cup Greek yoghurt with 1 tablespoon chia seeds, ½ teaspoon cinnamon, 1 teaspoon honey and 5 strawberries	10 almonds	Tofu burger (page 273)	2 dates	Beef mince cups with coriander (page 274)
WEDNESDAY	Green diabetes-friendly smoothie (page 269)	10 pistachios	Sarah's garden salad (page 275) with a small tin of tuna and 2 tablespoons cottage cheese	Boiled egg	One-tray bake – 120 grams chicken, 1 sliced zucchini, 1 cup eggplant slices. Bake for 15 minutes. Garnish with oregano and 1 teaspoon olive oil
THURSDAY	Omelette with mushrooms, tomatoes and herbs (page 274)	Apple	Salmon health bowl (page 276)	10 almonds	Tofu stir-fry with cauliflower rice, bok choy, capsicum (page 278)
FRIDAY	Diabetes-friendly chia pudding (page 270)	Skip	Greek salad (page 275) with 100 grams tuna	1 tablespoon hummus with 1 carrot	120 grams poached chicken with ½ cup steamed broccoli, ½ cup steamed cauliflower, garnished with fresh herbs and a drizzle of olive oil and fresh cayenne chilli (optional)
SATURDAY	Sarah's favourite breakfast (page 268)	Skip	Cottage cheese wrap (page 268), with lettuce and ½ tomato sliced and some red onion	10 cashews	120 grams fish, 5 steamed asparagus spears, 1 cup steamed broccoli and cauliflower, garnish with fresh herbs, 1 teaspoon olive oil, chilli flakes
SUNDAY	2 Cottage cheese, egg and herb muffins (page 267)	5 walnuts	120 grams grilled chicken breast with ¼ avocado and a green salad	10:10 SDL protein bar or 10 cashews	Mackerel curry with ginger and vegetables (page 279)
BEVERAGES Water, plus optional coffee, tea, green tea, herbal tea, electrolytes					

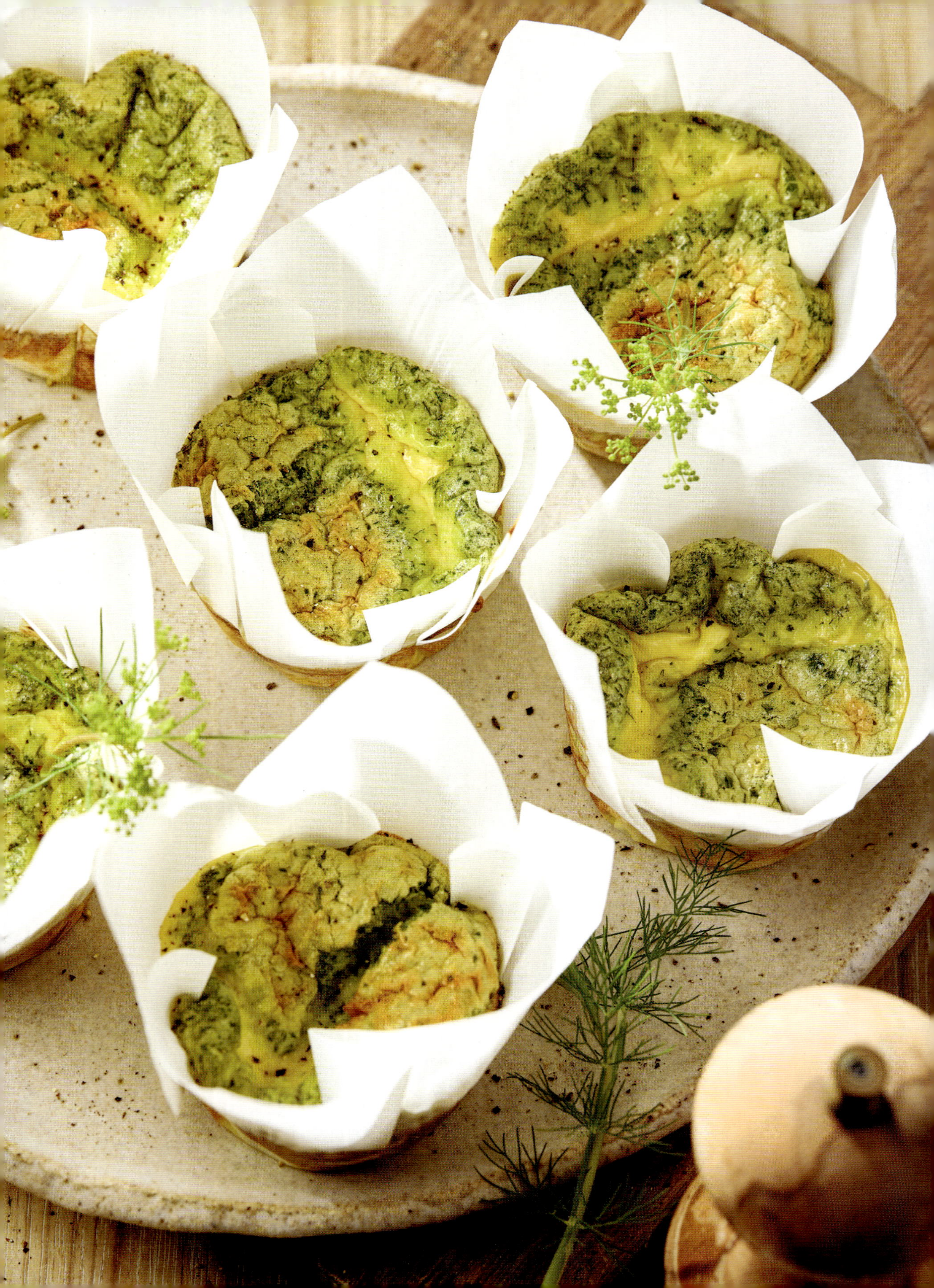

COTTAGE CHEESE, EGG AND HERB MUFFINS

MAKES 10 (2 PER SERVE) • CARBS PER SERVE: 2.6 GRAMS

8 eggs

1 cup cottage cheese

pinch of salt and pepper

¼ cup chopped fresh parsley

2 tablespoons chopped fresh dill

1. Preheat the oven to 170°C. Line the holes of a muffin tin with baking paper.

2. Blend all the ingredients together until smooth. Add evenly to the muffin tin and bake for about 20 minutes.

Tip: These are perfect for breakfast or lunch with a salad, and freeze well.

SARAH'S FAVOURITE BREAKFAST

SERVES 1 • CARBS PER SERVE: 21 GRAMS

1 diced kiwifruit
(skin on)

⅔ cup Greek yoghurt

¼ cup blueberries

1 tablespoon chia seeds

½ teaspoon ground
cinnamon

½ teaspoon ground
ginger

Add all the ingredients to a bowl. Mix together and enjoy.

Tip: If you want to sweeten, honey will add carbs (about 6 grams for 1 teaspoon). You could add granulated stevia to the yoghurt and mix in.

COTTAGE CHEESE WRAP

MAKES 2 WRAPS (1 WRAP PER SERVE)
CARBS PER SERVE: 3.5 GRAMS

extra-virgin olive
oil spray

240 grams cottage
cheese

2 eggs (or ¼ cup
egg whites)

salt and pepper

1. Preheat the oven to 180ºC. Line a baking tray with baking paper, then spray a bit of oil onto the baking paper.

2. Put the ingredients into a blender or food processor and process for 2 minutes to make a smooth batter.

3. Pour the batter into an even layer on the baking paper. Transfer to the oven and bake for about 35 minutes or until golden brown, or the wrap has set.

4. Remove from the oven and let cool for 10 minutes.

5. Fill with your favourite filling and enjoy!

GREEN DIABETES-FRIENDLY SMOOTHIE

SERVES 1 • CARBS PER SERVE: 12 GRAMS

1 cup baby spinach or kale

½ small avocado

½ cup frozen or fresh blueberries or raspberries

½ cup unsweetened almond milk

⅓ cup full-fat Greek yoghurt

½ scoop unflavoured whey protein isolate

1 tablespoon chia seeds

½ teaspoon ground cinnamon

stevia (optional)

Add all the ingredients to a blender. Blend until smooth and creamy. Pour into a glass and serve immediately.

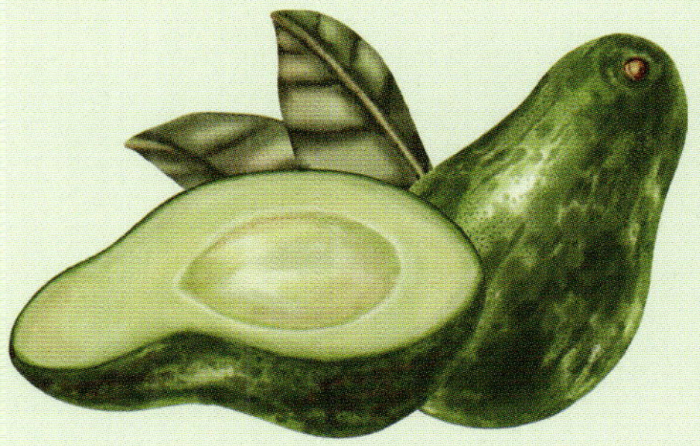

DIABETES-FRIENDLY CHIA PUDDING

SERVES 1 • CARBS PER SERVE: 8 GRAMS

3 tablespoons chia seeds

⅔ cup unsweetened almond milk

⅓ cup full-fat Greek yoghurt

½ teaspoon ground cinnamon

½ teaspoon ground ginger

granulated stevia (optional)

¼ cup fresh or frozen berries (blueberries, raspberries, strawberries)

1 tablespoon chopped walnuts

1. In a jar or bowl, combine the chia seeds, almond milk, Greek yoghurt, cinnamon, ginger and stevia (if using). Stir well, cover and refrigerate for at least 4 hours, or overnight, until thickened.

2. In the morning, stir again and top with berries and nuts. Enjoy chilled.

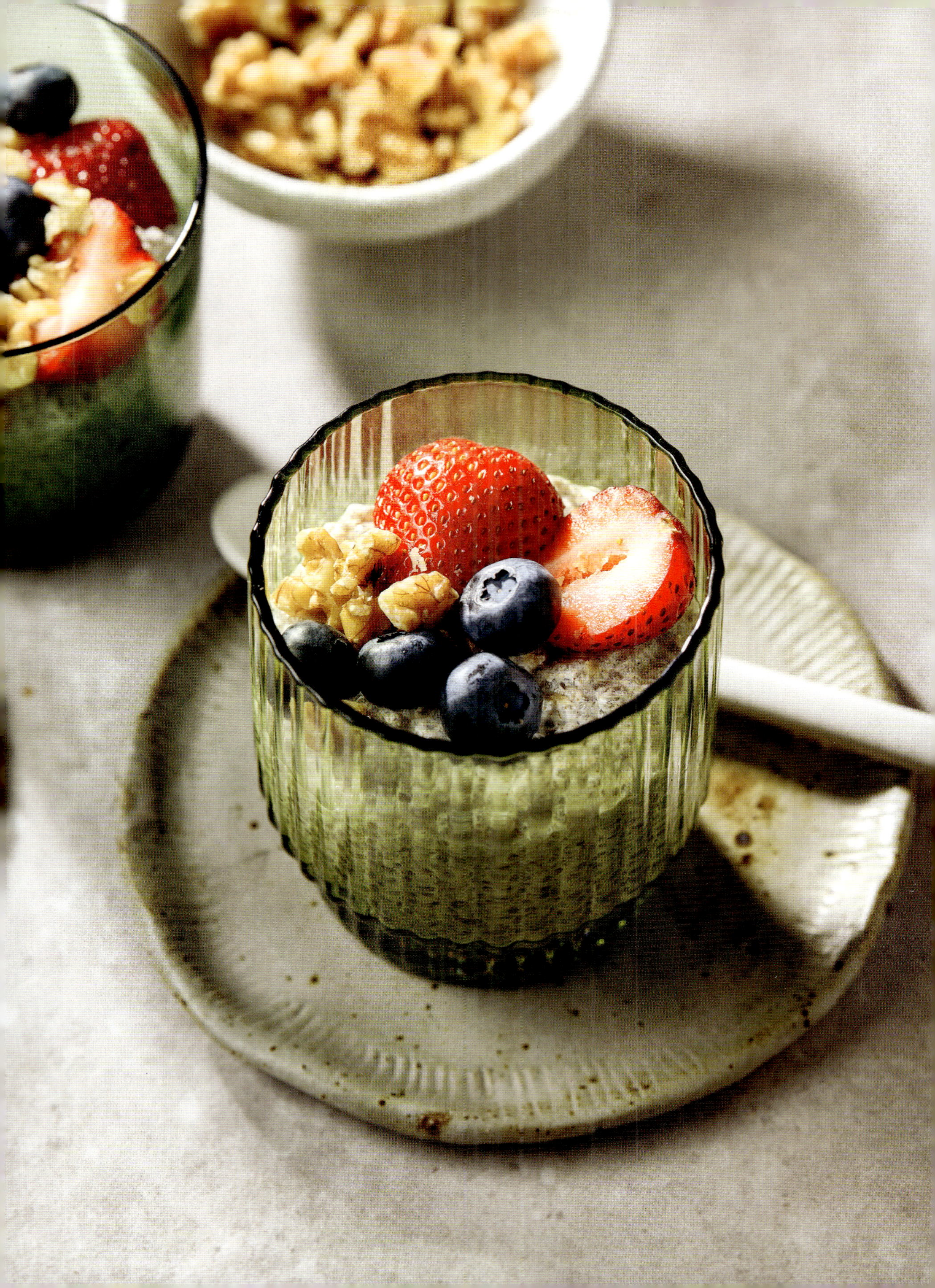

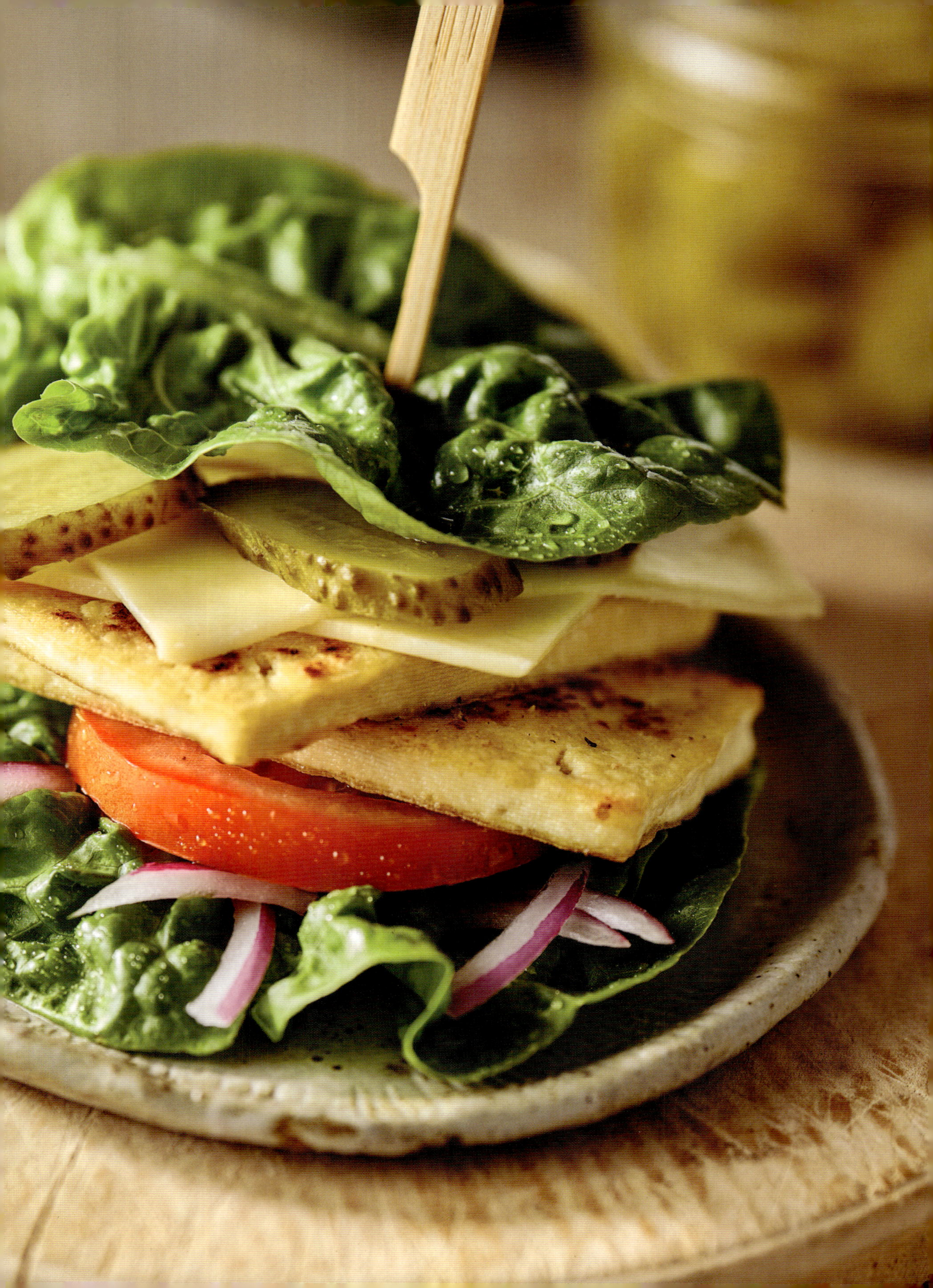

TOFU BURGER

SERVES 1 • CARBS PER SERVE: 4.9 GRAMS

---

100 grams firm tofu

½ teaspoon extra-virgin olive oil

salt and pepper

2 iceberg lettuce leaves

1 slice cheddar cheese

½ tomato, sliced

1 tablespoon sliced red onion

pickles (optional)

1. Cook the tofu in a pan in the oil until golden brown, then season with salt and pepper.

2. Assemble the ingredients as you would a burger with the lettuce leaves as the bun. Enjoy!

Tip: If you don't like tofu, then change to a lean protein you prefer.

BEEF MINCE CUPS WITH CORIANDER

SERVES 1 • CARBS PER SERVE: 10 GRAMS

---

120 grams beef mince

1 teaspoon extra-virgin olive oil

½ teaspoon ground cumin

½ teaspoon paprika

4 cos lettuce leaves

5 cherry tomatoes, diced

1 cucumber, chopped

1 tablespoon chopped fresh coriander

1. Cook the beef in a frying pan with the oil and spices.

2. Add the meat to the lettuce, top with the tomatoes and cucumber, then scatter the coriander over the top.

OMELETTE WITH MUSHROOMS, TOMATOES AND HERBS

SERVES 1 • CARBS PER SERVE: 3.6 GRAMS

---

extra-virgin olive oil, for frying

2 eggs

½ cup thinly sliced mushrooms

½ tomato, sliced

1 tablespoon chopped fresh dill

1 tablespoon chopped fresh parsley

Heat a frying pan and add a little bit of olive oil. Whisk the eggs and add them to the pan. Add mushrooms, tomato and herbs to one-half of the egg mixture. Cook and fold over. Serve.

GREEK SALAD

SERVES 2 • CARBS PER SERVE: 11 GRAMS

---

2 tomatoes, cut into wedges

2 cucumbers, chopped

½ small red onion, sliced

100 grams feta

50 grams pitted olives

1 tablespoon extra-virgin olive oil

juice of 1 lemon

Assemble your salad ingredients in a serving bowl. Drizzle the olive oil and lemon juice over the top and serve.

SARAH'S GARDEN SALAD

SERVES 1 • CARBS PER SERVE: 6 GRAMS

---

1 cup chopped iceberg lettuce

5 cherry tomatoes, halved

1 tablespoon chopped red onion

1 Lebanese cucumber, chopped

salt and pepper

extra-virgin olive oil, to serve

fresh lemon juice, to serve

Add all the ingredients to a bowl and toss. Season with salt and pepper, and serve with a drizzle of extra-virgin olive oil and squeeze of fresh lemon juice.

SALMON HEALTH BOWL

SERVES 1 • CARBS PER SERVE: 8.2 GRAMS

120 grams fresh salmon, cooked

1 cup baby spinach leaves

1 cucumber, chopped

½ cup grated carrot

¼ avocado, sliced

1 teaspoon pepitas, to garnish

Assemble all the ingredients in a bowl and serve.

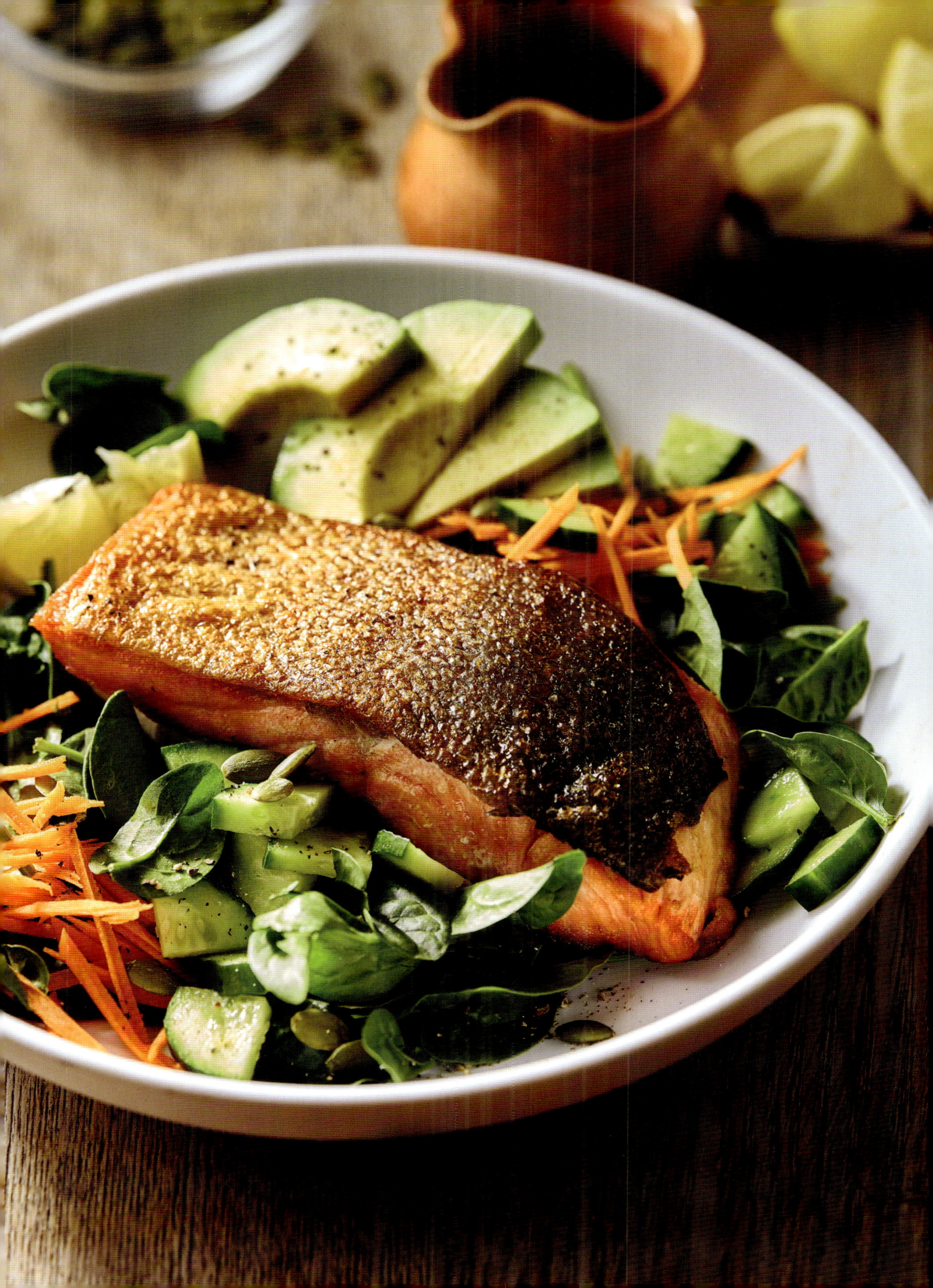

TOFU STIR-FRY WITH CAULIFLOWER RICE, BOK CHOY AND CAPSICUM

SERVES 1 • CARBS PER SERVE: 5 GRAMS

---

1 cup cauliflower florets

1 tablespoon extra-virgin olive oil

100 grams firm tofu, diced

1 bok choy, sliced

½ capsicum, sliced

1 teaspoon grated fresh ginger

1 clove garlic, minced

2 teaspoons tamari

spring onions, to garnish

fresh coriander, to garnish

1. To make the cauliflower rice, chop or pulse the cauliflower in a food processor. Add to a frying pan with 1 teaspoon olive oil, cook for 5 minutes, then season and set aside.

2. In a frying pan with the remaining olive oil, cook the tofu until brown on all sides. Add the veggies, ginger, garlic and tamari and cook for another few minutes.

3. Add the cauliflower rice to a bowl and top with the stir-fry. Garnish with the spring onions and fresh coriander.

Tip: If you don't like tofu, use another lean protein such as chicken.

MACKEREL CURRY WITH GINGER AND VEGETABLES

SERVES 2 • CARBS PER SERVE: 16 GRAMS

extra virgin olive oil (for cooking)

½ red onion, diced

2 mushrooms, sliced

1 zucchini, sliced

1 can diced tomatoes

½ cup Greek yoghurt

2 tablespoons tomato paste

1 tablespoon curry powder

1 tablespoon peanut butter

1½ teaspoons ground ginger

½ teaspoon ground coriander

½ teaspoon ground cumin

½ teaspoon ground turmeric

pinch of chilli power (optional)

1 broccoli head

125 grams canned mackerel

salt and pepper

Garnishes: fresh coriander leaves, sesame seeds, sesame oil

1. Cook the onion, mushrooms and zucchini in the pan. Add all the other ingredients except the fresh coriander, broccoli and mackerel.

2. Cook for about 5–7 minutes, add the mackerel and broccoli, season with salt and pepper, and cook for a couple of minutes only (you want to keep the broccoli firm).

3. Garnish with fresh coriander, sesame seeds and a small drizzle of sesame oil.

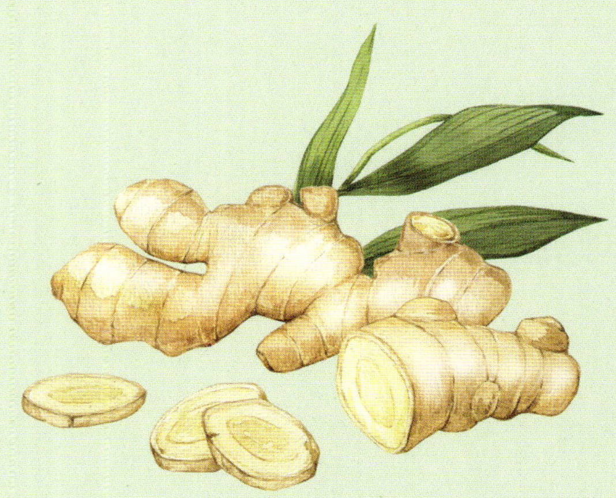

Lowering Inflammation

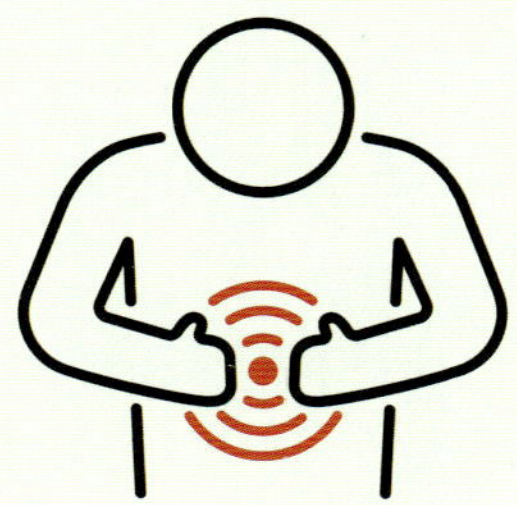

Focus: Settling into ketosis, losing weight and lowering chronic inflammation

Chronic inflammation drives chronic disease such as type 2 diabetes.

At the beginning of this week, most of you will be in a ketogenic state. In my experience, it can take anywhere from 2 to 10 days for people to get into ketosis. The younger you are, the easier it is. Aging does slow down metabolic adaptation, and for older people the delayed keto adaptation is because they have higher glycogen reserves, differences in hormones and much slower metabolic flexibility. Other factors that seem to affect people getting into ketosis include exercise, diet prior to starting and any intermittent fasting.

The first 10 days of the program are the hardest. But once you reach the 10-day mark, it all becomes a lot easier and, in my opinion, really enjoyable. When you are truly in a ketogenic state, you stop thinking about food. The food noise leaves your mind, you have clarity of thinking, loads of energy, sleep better and feel great.

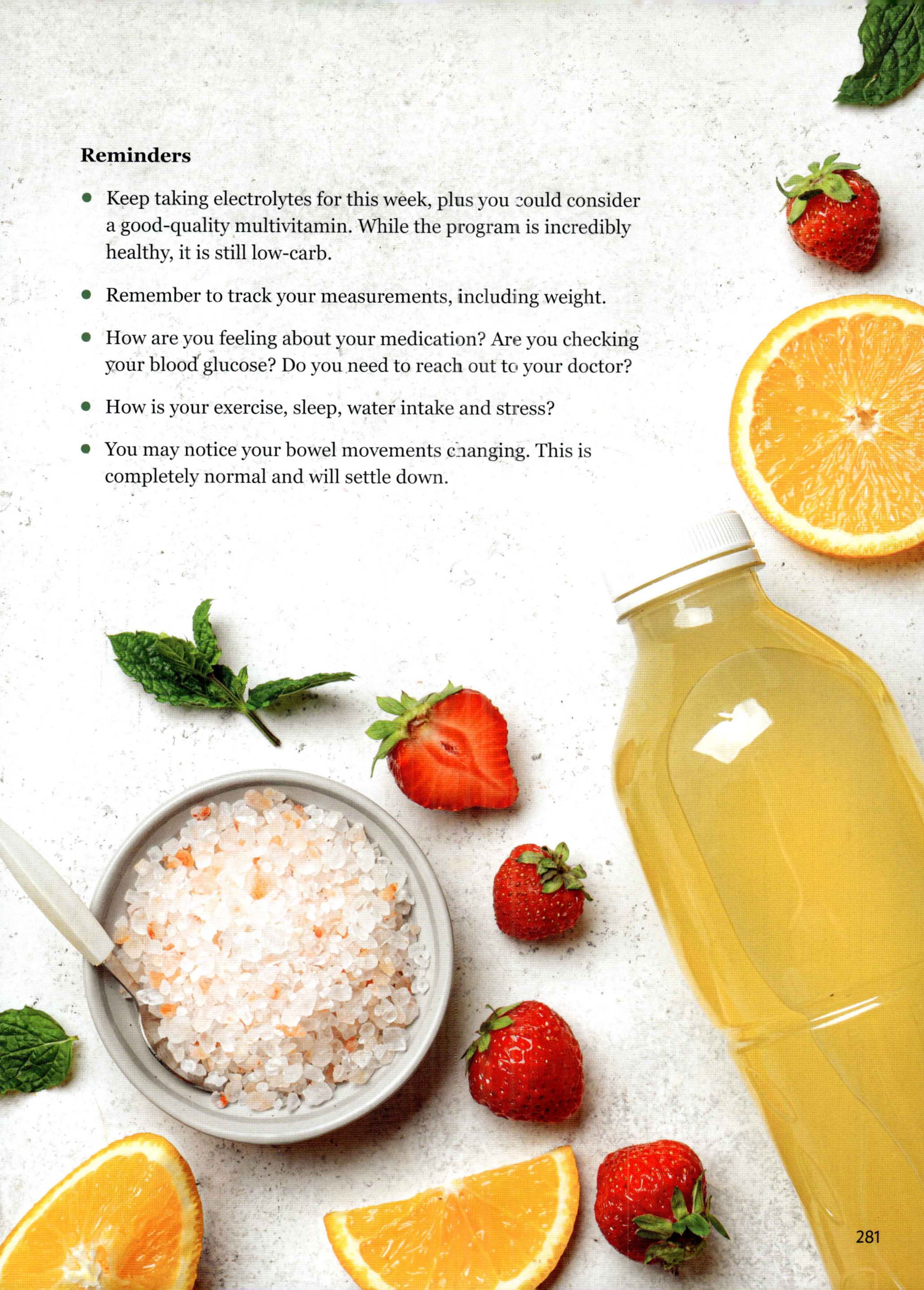

Reminders

- Keep taking electrolytes for this week, plus you could consider a good-quality multivitamin. While the program is incredibly healthy, it is still low-carb.

- Remember to track your measurements, including weight.

- How are you feeling about your medication? Are you checking your blood glucose? Do you need to reach out to your doctor?

- How is your exercise, sleep, water intake and stress?

- You may notice your bowel movements changing. This is completely normal and will settle down.

	BREAKFAST	MID-MORNING	LUNCH	MID-AFTERNOON	DINNER
MONDAY	Anti-inflammatory smoothie (page 283)	Skip	Avocado and salmon low-carb lunch bowl (page 289)	5 walnuts	Greek salad (page 275) with 100 grams poached chicken
TUESDAY	2 poached eggs with ¼ avocado, ½ cup cooked spinach and 2 cherry tomatoes	Apple	Cottage cheese wrap (page 268) with onion, tomato and lettuce	Turmeric latte (page 284)	Tofu burger (page 273)
WEDNESDAY	Anti-inflammatory smoothie (page 283)	Skip	Sardine salad (page 292)	10 cashews	Lean beef steak with grilled eggplant and steamed brussels sprouts (page 291)
THURSDAY	⅔ cup Greek yoghurt, ¼ cup raspberries, ½ teaspoon cinnamon	10 almonds	Sarah's garden salad (page 275) with 2 boiled eggs	10:10 SDL protein bar	Grilled chicken breast salad (page 292)
FRIDAY	High-protein, low-carb cinnamon pancakes with strawberries (page 286)	Turmeric latte (page 284)	Salmon health bowl (page 276)	1 tablespoon hummus with 1 celery stick	Simple cauliflower fried rice (page 288), served with 100 grams cooked shredded chicken
SATURDAY	Anti-inflammatory smoothie (page 283)	Skip	Cabbage pizza (page 293)	10:10 SDL protein bar	Spiced salmon and Mediterranean veggie tray bake (page 294)
SUNDAY	2 soft-boiled eggs with 1 zucchini, lightly steamed, cut into strips to dip into the egg	½ cup strawberries	Sarah's grated salad (page 285) with 100 grams tuna	10 almonds	Beef mince cups with coriander (page 274)

BEVERAGES Water, plus optional coffee, tea, green tea, herbal tea, electrolytes

ANTI-INFLAMMATORY SMOOTHIE

SERVES 1 • CARBS PER SERVE: 15 GRAMS

1 cup baby spinach

1 cup coconut or almond milk

½ cup frozen pineapple pieces

juice of 1 lemon

1 tablespoon grated fresh ginger

1 tablespoon chia seeds

1 teaspoon olive oil

½ teaspoon ground turmeric

pinch of black pepper

Blitz and enjoy!

STRAWBERRY DIABETES-FRIENDLY SMOOTHIE

SERVES 1 • CARBS PER SERVE: 21 GRAMS

1 cup strawberries

½ cup water

½ cup almond milk

1 serve protein powder

5 cashews

1 pitted medjool date

½ teaspoon ground cinnamon

4 ice cubes

Blend all the ingredients and enjoy.

TURMERIC LATTE

SERVES 1 • CARBS PER SERVE: 1.4 GRAMS (WITHOUT HONEY), 4.4 GRAMS (WITH HONEY)

½ cup water

½ cup almond milk

1 teaspoon ground turmeric

¼ teaspoon black pepper

½ teaspoon honey (optional)

Put all the ingredients in a saucepan. Bring to the boil and let simmer for a couple of minutes. Enjoy!

SARAH'S GRATED SALAD

SERVES 2 (MAIN) OR 4 (SIDE) • CARBS PER SERVE: 14 GRAMS (MAIN) OR 7 GRAMS (SIDE)

---

2 carrots, grated

1 beetroot, grated

1 cup chopped fresh coriander

1 cup chopped fresh parsley

1 red onion, chopped

2 tablespoons pepitas, to garnish

DRESSING

juice of 1 lemon

2 tablespoons extra-virgin olive oil

salt and pepper

1. To make the dressing, combine all the ingredients in a jar and shake well to combine.

2. To make the salad, add all the ingredients to a bowl and toss. Drizzle dressing over the top.

Tip: This is great to make up in a batch and enjoy over a couple of days with a different protein.

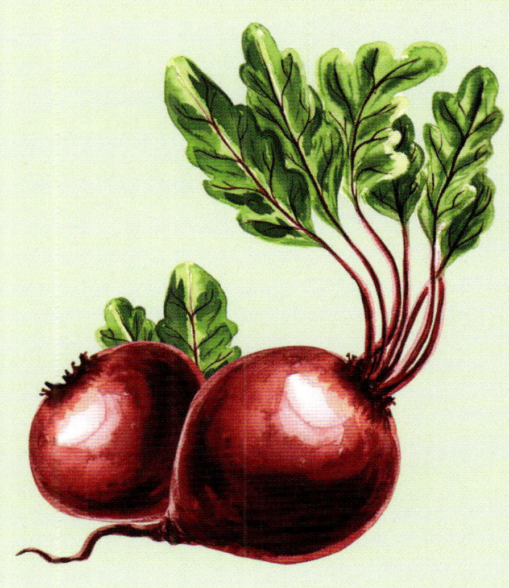

HIGH-PROTEIN, LOW-CARB CINNAMON PANCAKES WITH STRAWBERRIES

SERVES 1 • CARBS PER SERVE: 7.5 GRAMS

1 large egg

2 tablespoons full-fat Greek yoghurt, plus extra to serve

1 scoop (about 30 grams) vanilla or plain protein powder

1 tablespoon almond flour

½ teaspoon baking powder

½ teaspoon cinnamon

1–2 tablespoons milk of your choice (optional)

fresh strawberries, to serve

1. Whisk the egg, yoghurt and protein powder in a bowl until smooth.

2. Stir in the almond flour, baking powder and cinnamon, adding a little milk (only if batter is too thick)

3. Heat a non-stick frying pan over medium heat. Pour in batter to form 2–3 small pancakes. Cook for 1–2 minutes each side, until golden and set.

4. Serve warm with fresh strawberries and a dollop of Greek yoghurt.

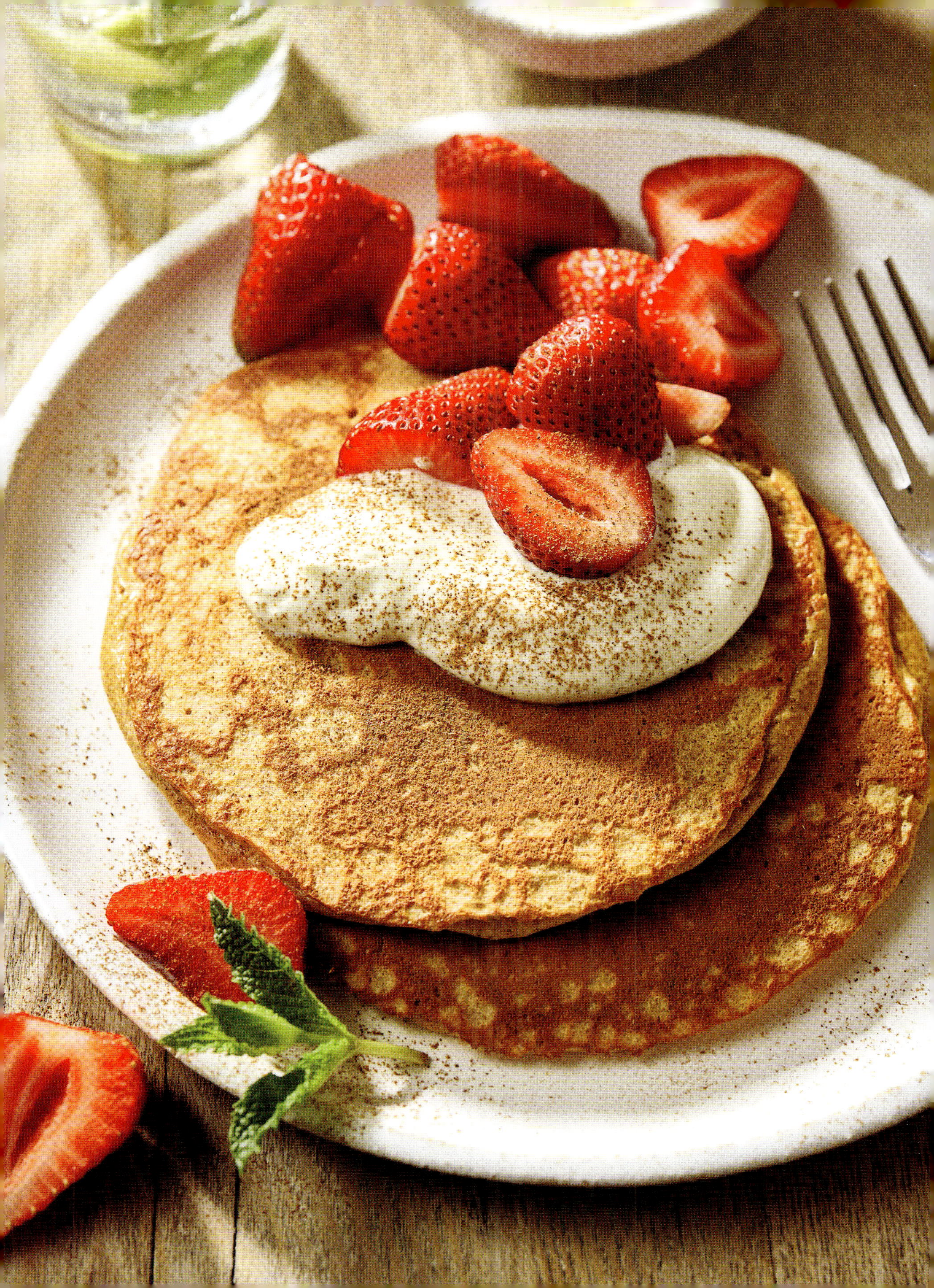

SIMPLE CAULIFLOWER FRIED RICE

SERVES 4 • CARBS PER SERVE: 10 GRAMS

---

1 small cauliflower head or 1 x 300-gram bag pre-riced cauliflower

3 tablespoons tamari

2 tablespoons mirin

1 teaspoon maple syrup

2 large eggs, beaten

2 tablespoons sesame oil

2 shallots, thinly sliced

1 medium carrot, cut into matchsticks

4 cloves garlic, crushed

½ cup frozen peas

salt and pepper

1 teaspoon sesame seeds, to garnish

2 spring onions, sliced, to garnish

¼ cup chopped parsley, to garnish

1. Prepare the cauliflower 'rice' by grating or pulsing in a food processor (skip if using pre-riced cauliflower).

2. Mix the tamari, mirin and maple syrup in a small bowl.

3. Add the eggs to a frying pan and scramble. Set aside.

4. Add 1 tablespoon sesame oil to the pan then sauté the shallots, carrot, garlic and peas for 1–2 minutes. Add the riced cauliflower and cook for another 2–3 minutes until softened.

5. Add the mirin mixture and the remaining sesame oil.

6. Return scrambled egg to the pan. Serve hot, garnished with sesame seeds, spring onions and parsley.

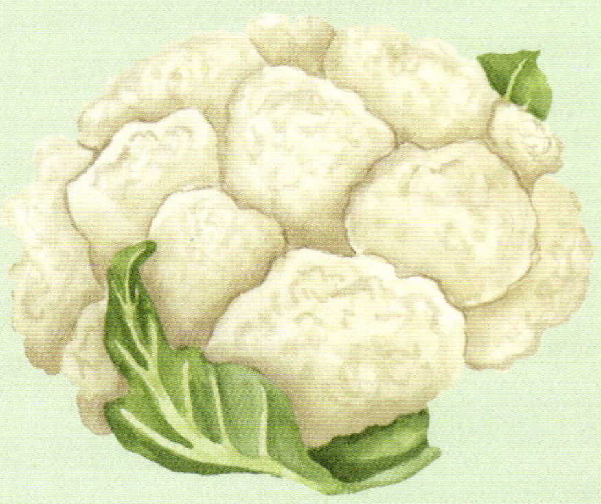

AVOCADO AND SALMON LOW-CARB LUNCH BOWL

SERVES 1 • CARBS PER SERVE: 5 GRAMS

1 cup baby spinach or mixed greens

½ medium avocado, sliced

120 grams cooked salmon fillet (steamed, grilled or poached)

½ cup chopped cucumber

½ cup halved cherry tomatoes (optional)

1 tablespoon extra-virgin olive oil

juice of ½ lemon

salt and pepper, to taste

1 tablespoon chopped fresh dill or parsley, to garnish

sprinkle of pepitas, to garnish

1. Place the greens in a wide bowl as your base. Top with slices of avocado and place the cooked salmon fillet on top. Add cucumber and cherry tomatoes (if using).

2. Drizzle with the olive oil and lemon juice, and season with salt and pepper. Garnish with fresh herbs and pepitas.

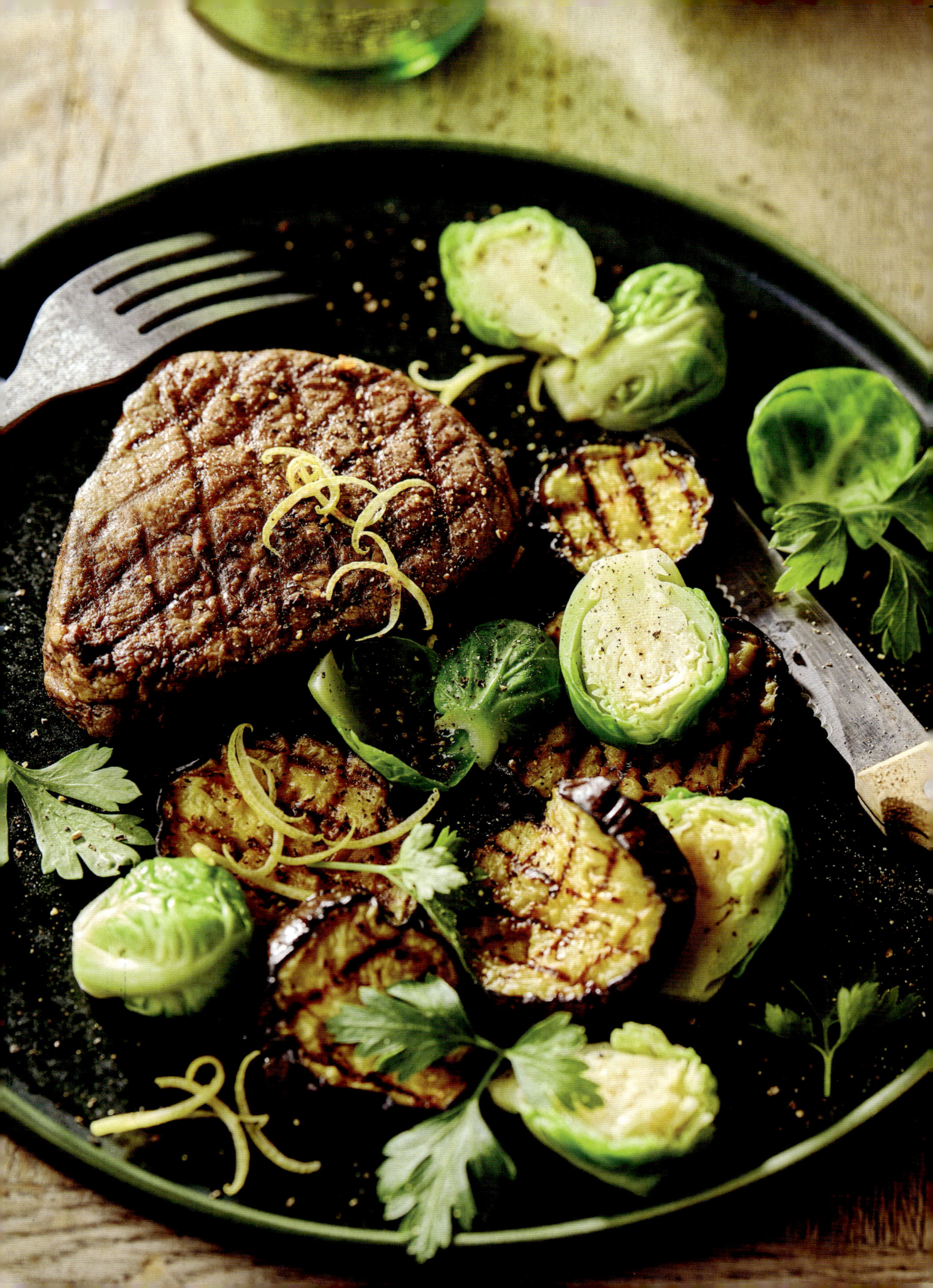

LEAN BEEF STEAK WITH GRILLED EGGPLANT AND STEAMED BRUSSELS SPROUTS

SERVES 1 • CARBS PER SERVE: 12 GRAMS

1 cup sliced eggplant (approx. 82 grams)

1 teaspoon extra-virgin olive oil

salt and pepper

1 cup brussels sprouts

120 grams lean beef steak

sprinkle of fresh parsley, to garnish

lemon zest, to garnish

1. Preheat the grill or a grill pan. (I use a grill pan.) Brush the eggplant slices with olive oil, season with salt and pepper, and grill for 4–5 minutes each side, until tender and slightly charred.

2. Steam the brussels sprouts for 5 minutes.

3. Season the beef steak with salt and pepper. Grill on high for 2–3 minutes each side for medium-rare, or longer to your liking. Rest briefly, then slice.

4. Serve the steak alongside the grilled eggplant and steamed brussels sprouts. Garnish with parsley and lemon zest.

GRILLED CHICKEN BREAST SALAD

SERVES 1 • CARBS PER SERVE: 3.5 GRAMS

---

120 grams chicken breast, boneless and skinless

salt and pepper

1 cup mixed leafy greens (spinach, rocket, cos lettuce)

¼ avocado, sliced

½ medium cucumber, chopped

1 tablespoon extra-virgin olive oil

juice of ½ lemon

1. Preheat a grill or grill pan to medium-high heat. Season the chicken breast with salt and pepper.

2. Grill chicken for 3–5 minutes each side or until cooked through and the juices run clear. Remove and slice into strips.

3. Place the mixed greens in a serving bowl. Arrange the avocado and cucumber over the greens. Top with grilled chicken slices.

4. Drizzle the olive oil and lemon juice over the salad. Season to taste with salt and pepper. Toss gently and serve immediately.

SARDINE SALAD

SERVES 1 • CARBS PER SERVE: 7.5 GRAMS

---

1 cup mixed green leaves

120 grams canned sardines (oil drained)

30 grams olives, sliced

½ capsicum, chopped

1 tablespoon chopped red onion

½ cup chopped cherry tomatoes

¼ cup chopped fresh parsley, plus extra to garnish

extra-virgin olive oil, to garnish

apple cider vinegar, to garnish

Assemble the salad in a bowl and enjoy.

CABBAGE PIZZA

SERVES 6 • CARBS PER SERVE: 18 GRAMS

1 green cabbage

4 tablespoons extra-virgin olive oil

¼ cup grated parmesan cheese

½ teaspoon onion powder

½ teaspoon garlic powder

½ teaspoon dried oregano

½ teaspoon chilli powder

salt and pepper

SUGGESTED TOPPINGS

¾ cup no-added-sugar pasta sauce

1 cup grated mozzarella

chilli flakes

1 capsicum, chopped

feta

dried oregano

spinach leaves

1. Preheat the oven to 220ºC and line a baking tray with baking paper.

2. Slice the cabbage into 2 cm-thick slices.

3. In a small bowl, mix the olive oil, parmesan, spices and salt and pepper. Brush the mixture onto the cabbage slices on one side then bake in the oven for 15 minutes.

4. Remove from the oven. Turn the cabbage slices over, brush the other side with the mixture and bake for a further 15 minutes.

5. Top with the toppings as you would a pizza, starting with your sauce (or you could even use pesto). Then add the mozzarella and other desired toppings. Return to the oven and cook until your cheese melts.

SPICED SALMON AND MEDITERRANEAN VEGGIE TRAY BAKE

SERVES 1 • CARBS PER SERVE: 6 GRAMS

½ medium zucchini, sliced

¼ medium eggplant, cubed

½ red capsicum, sliced

¼ small red onion, sliced

5 cherry tomatoes, halved

1 tablespoon extra-virgin olive oil

½ teaspoon smoked paprika

¼ teaspoon ground cumin

½ teaspoon dried oregano

salt and pepper

120 grams salmon fillet

handful of fresh parsley or basil, chopped, to serve

lemon wedge, to serve

1. Preheat the oven to 200°C. Line a baking tray with baking paper.

2. In a bowl, toss the zucchini, eggplant, capsicum, onion and tomatoes with olive oil, half the herbs and spices, plus salt and pepper to taste.

3. Spread the vegetables over half the tray. Place the salmon fillet on the other half. Sprinkle over the remaining paprika, cumin and oregano, plus salt and pepper to taste.

4. Roast in the oven for 12–15 minutes, or until salmon is just cooked through and vegetables are tender.

5. Serve with a handful of fresh herbs and lemon wedge.

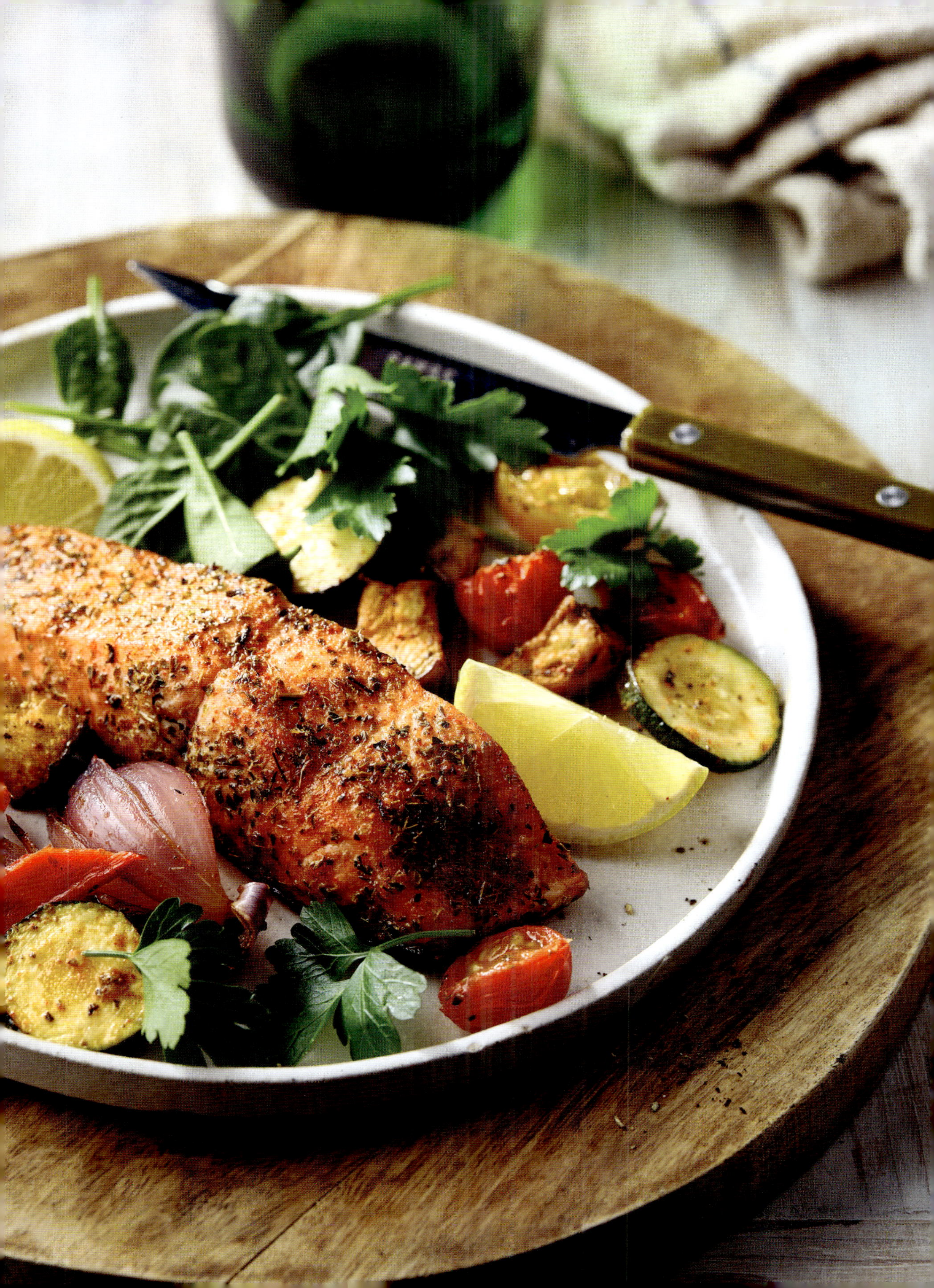

Supporting Gut Health

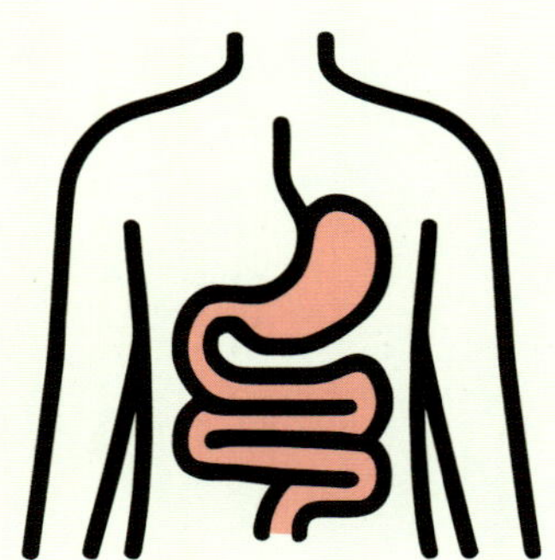

**Focus: Supporting your gut health
– the core of good health**

**Taking care of our gut is so important for overall
health and wellness – we really want to support
good health outcomes.**

This week, you may experience some constipation because of the
dietary changes, and because you're eating less. This does resolve.
A good probiotic can be amazing! Email me for my recommendation:
contact@sarahdilorenzo.com

When we have good gut health, we have improved insulin sensitivity
because a healthy gut microbiome full of good bacteria can produce
short-chain fatty acids *and* gut hormones such as GLP-1 that reduce
inflammation and can really enhance how the body responds to insulin.
Good gut health means lower inflammation, which keeps the gut barrier
strong, improves glucose control and reduces complications.

The program, of course, is still very much a weight-loss program. I just
see things holistically.

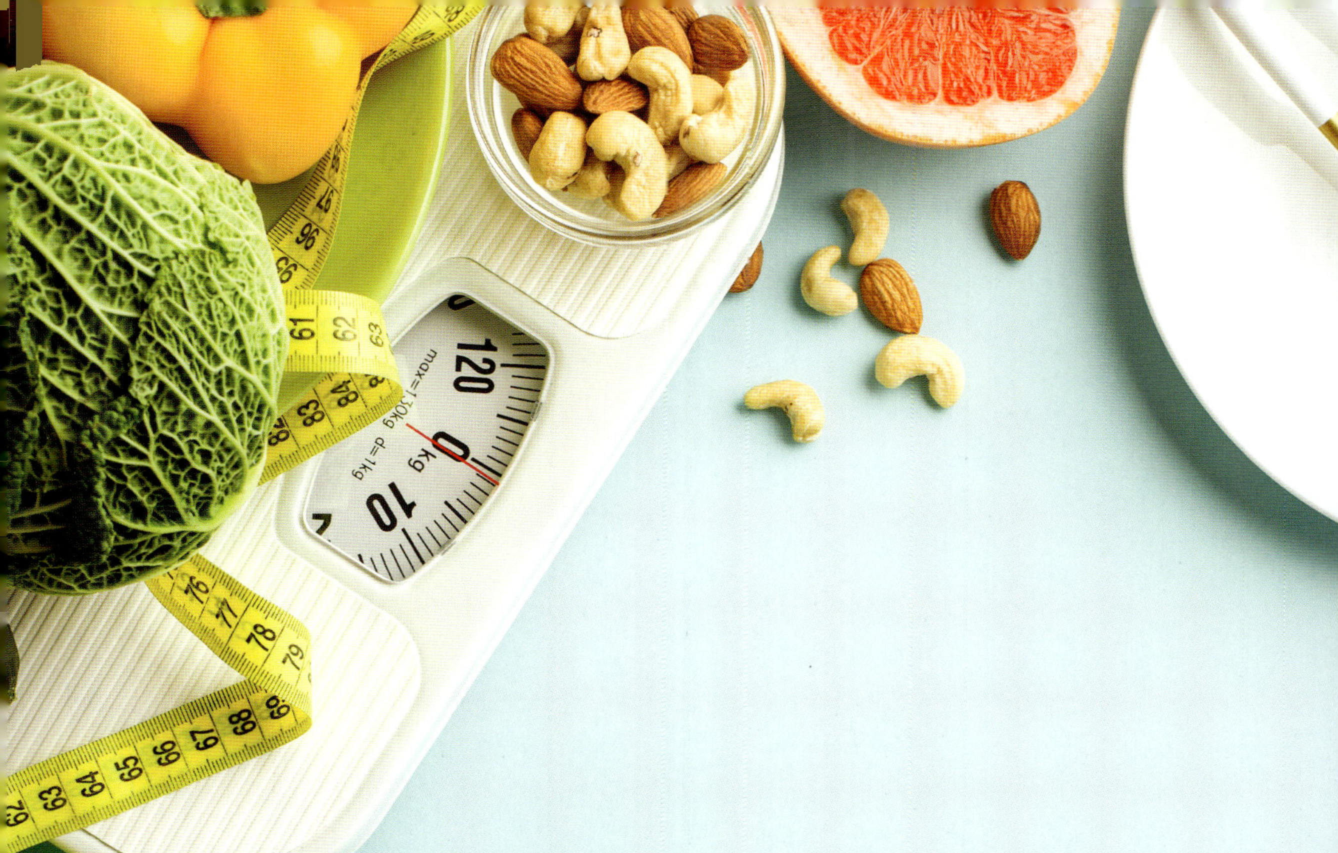

Reminders

- Don't forget to weigh in.

- Take your measurements.

- Do you need to get your medications checked?

- How is your exercise regime?

- Are you sleeping well?

- Are you making sure that dinner and breakfast are 12 hours apart?

- Are you keeping well hydrated?

	BREAKFAST	**MID-MORNING**	**LUNCH**	**MID-AFTERNOON**	**DINNER**
MONDAY	Gut-healthy green probiotic smoothie (page 299)	Skip	Black bean patties (page 308) served with Sarah's garden salad (page 275)	3 pickles and 25 grams cheese	Low-carb miso-glazed eggplant (page 306), served with 100 grams grilled fish
TUESDAY	2 cottage cheese egg and herb muffins (page 267)	½ cup raspberries	Salmon and sauerkraut salad (page 302)	15 pistachios	Gut-friendly zucchini boats (page 305)
WEDNESDAY	Sarah's favourite breakfast (page 268)	10 cashews	Sarah's garden salad (page 275) with 2 cottage cheese, egg and herb muffins (page 267) Serve with 1 tablespoon sauerkraut on the side.	1 tablespoon hummus with 2 celery stalks	Gut-friendly green soup (page 303) served with 100 grams shredded cooked chicken
THURSDAY	Gut-healthy green probiotic smoothie (page 299)	Skip	Gut-friendly green soup (page 303), served with 2 boiled eggs	¼ cup Greek yoghurt with ½ teaspoon cinnamon	Tofu burger (page 273)
FRIDAY	Greek yoghurt, berry and mint breakfast bowl (page 300)	Skip	Greek salad (page 275) with 125 grams canned sardines and ¼ cup sauerkraut	25 grams cheddar and 3 pickles	Black bean patties (page 308) with 1.5 cups of steamed broccoli, cauliflower and zucchini. Garnish with fresh parsley.
SATURDAY	2 soft-boiled eggs with 1 zucchini, lightly steamed, cut into strips to dip into the egg	10 almonds	Grilled chicken breast salad (page 292)	Apple	Gut-friendly green soup (page 303), served with 120 grams grilled fish
SUNDAY	Gut-healthy green probiotic smoothie (page 299)	Skip	Salmon and sauerkraut salad (page 302)	30 grams mixed nuts	Healthy mince bake (page 307)

BEVERAGES Water, plus optional coffee, tea, green tea, herbal tea, electrolytes

GUT-HEALTHY GREEN PROBIOTIC SMOOTHIE

SERVES 1 • CARBS PER SERVE: 7 GRAMS

¾ cup unsweetened almond milk or coconut milk

½ cup baby spinach

⅓ cup chopped cucumber

¼ cup full-fat Greek yoghurt

¼ small avocado

2 tablespoons chia seeds or linseeds (flaxseeds)

2 tablespoons frozen raspberries

½ teaspoon grated fresh ginger

½ teaspoon ground cinnamon

juice of ½ lemon

pinch of sea salt

stevia to sweeten (optional)

Put all the ingredients in a blender. Blend until smooth and creamy. Taste and adjust acidity or sweetness with a few extra raspberries or lemon juice. Pour and enjoy fresh.

GREEK YOGHURT, BERRY AND MINT BREAKFAST BOWL

SERVES 1 • CARBS PER SERVE: 18 GRAMS

⅔ cup Greek yoghurt

½ cup mixed fresh or frozen berries (blueberries, raspberries, strawberries)

1 tablespoon chia seeds or ground linseed (flaxseed)

8 walnuts or almonds, chopped

2 teaspoons pepitas

½ teaspoon ground cinnamon

½ teaspoon ground ginger

a few fresh mint leaves

1. Spoon the yoghurt into a bowl. Scatter berries evenly over the top. Sprinkle with chia seeds. Add chopped walnuts and pepitas.

2. Dust with cinnamon and ginger, and garnish with mint.

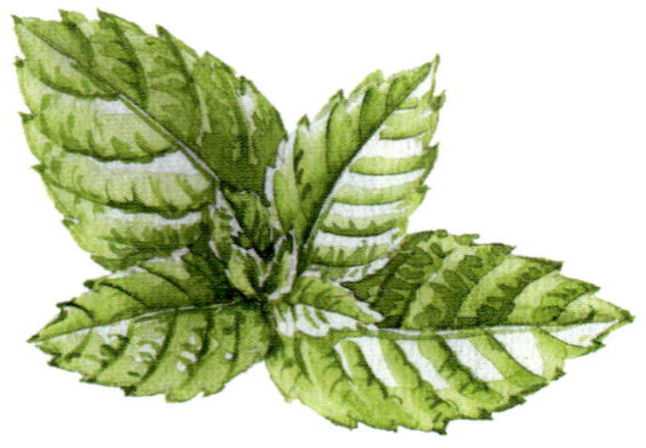

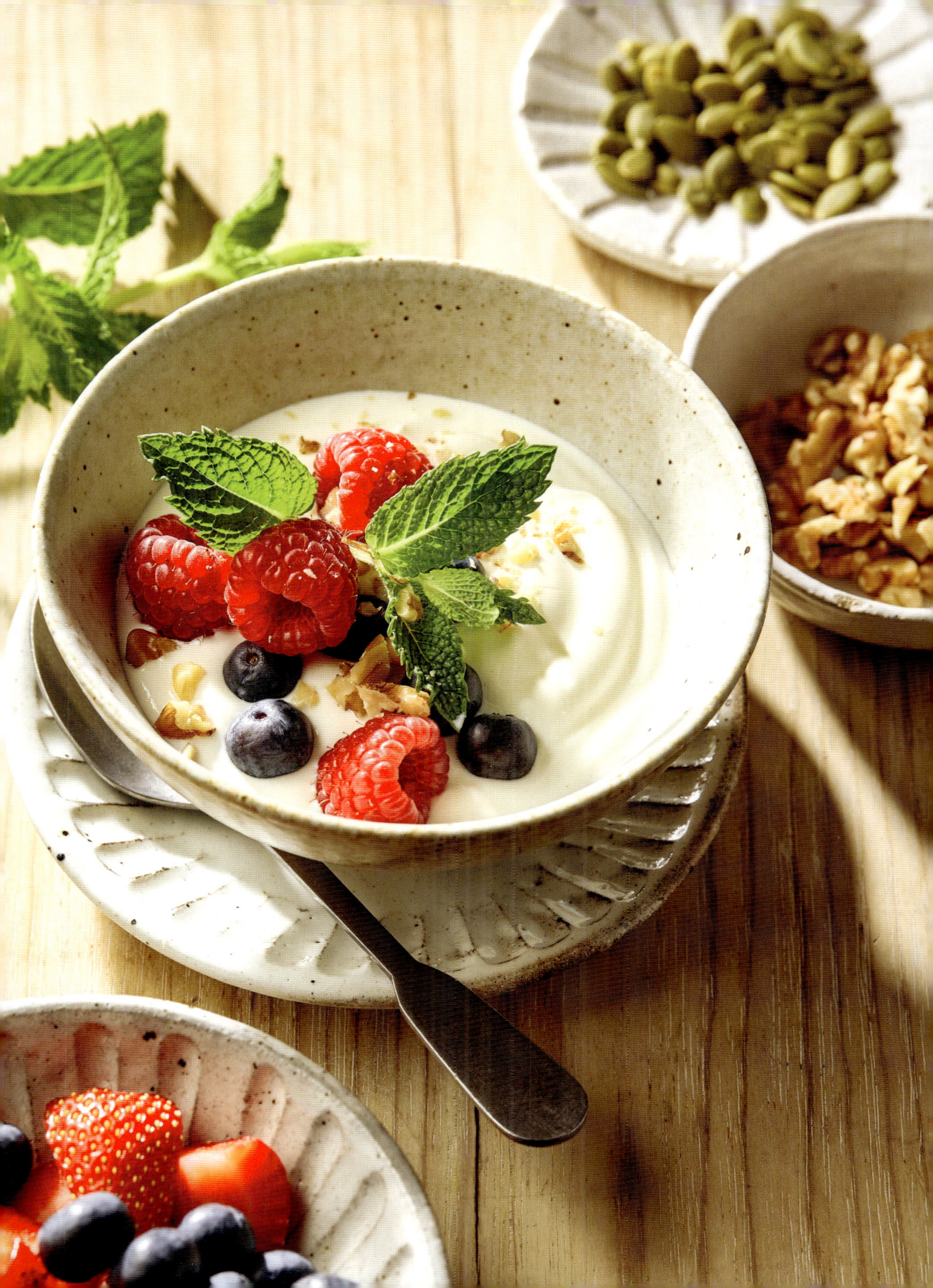

SALMON AND SAUERKRAUT SALAD

SERVES 1 • CARBS PER SERVE: 6 GRAMS

---

120 grams cooked salmon (or canned)

1 cup mixed leafy greens

½ cup chopped cucumber

¼ avocado, sliced

2 tablespoons sauerkraut (fermented for probiotic boost)

1 tablespoon extra-virgin olive oil

squeeze of lemon juice

salt and pepper

Assemble the salad and enjoy.

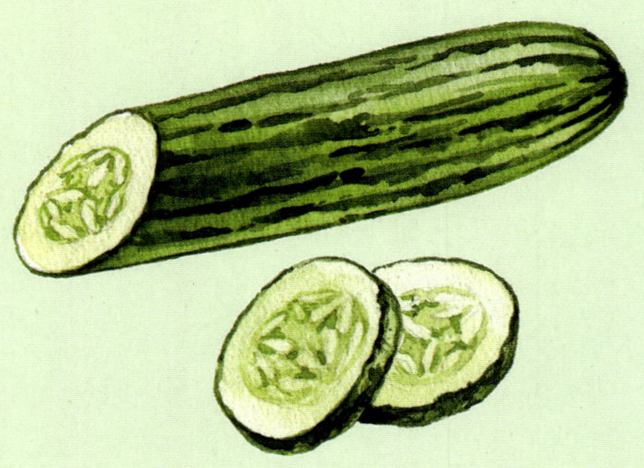

GUT-FRIENDLY GREEN SOUP

SERVES 2 • CARBS PER SERVE: 5 GRAMS

1 tablespoon extra-virgin olive oil

1 spring onion (or ½ leek, white part only), sliced

1 stalk celery, chopped

4 cloves garlic, minced

1 small zucchini, chopped

1 cup kale or silverbeet, chopped (stalks removed)

2 cups baby spinach

2 cups chicken bone broth

¼ cup chopped fresh parsley

2 tablespoons chopped fresh dill or basil

1 tablespoon fresh lemon juice

salt and pepper

2 tablespoons Greek yoghurt, to serve

1. Heat the olive oil in a saucepan over medium heat. Add spring onion, celery and garlic. Sauté for 2–3 minutes.

2. Add the zucchini, kale and spinach. Stir for 1–2 minutes until the greens wilt. Pour in broth. Bring to a gentle simmer, cover, and cook for 10 minutes.

3. Stir in the parsley, dill and lemon juice. Allow to cool slightly. Blend the soup with a hand-held or regular blender until very smooth.

4. Return to the pot, heat gently and season with salt and pepper. Serve hot, topped with a swirl of Greek yoghurt.

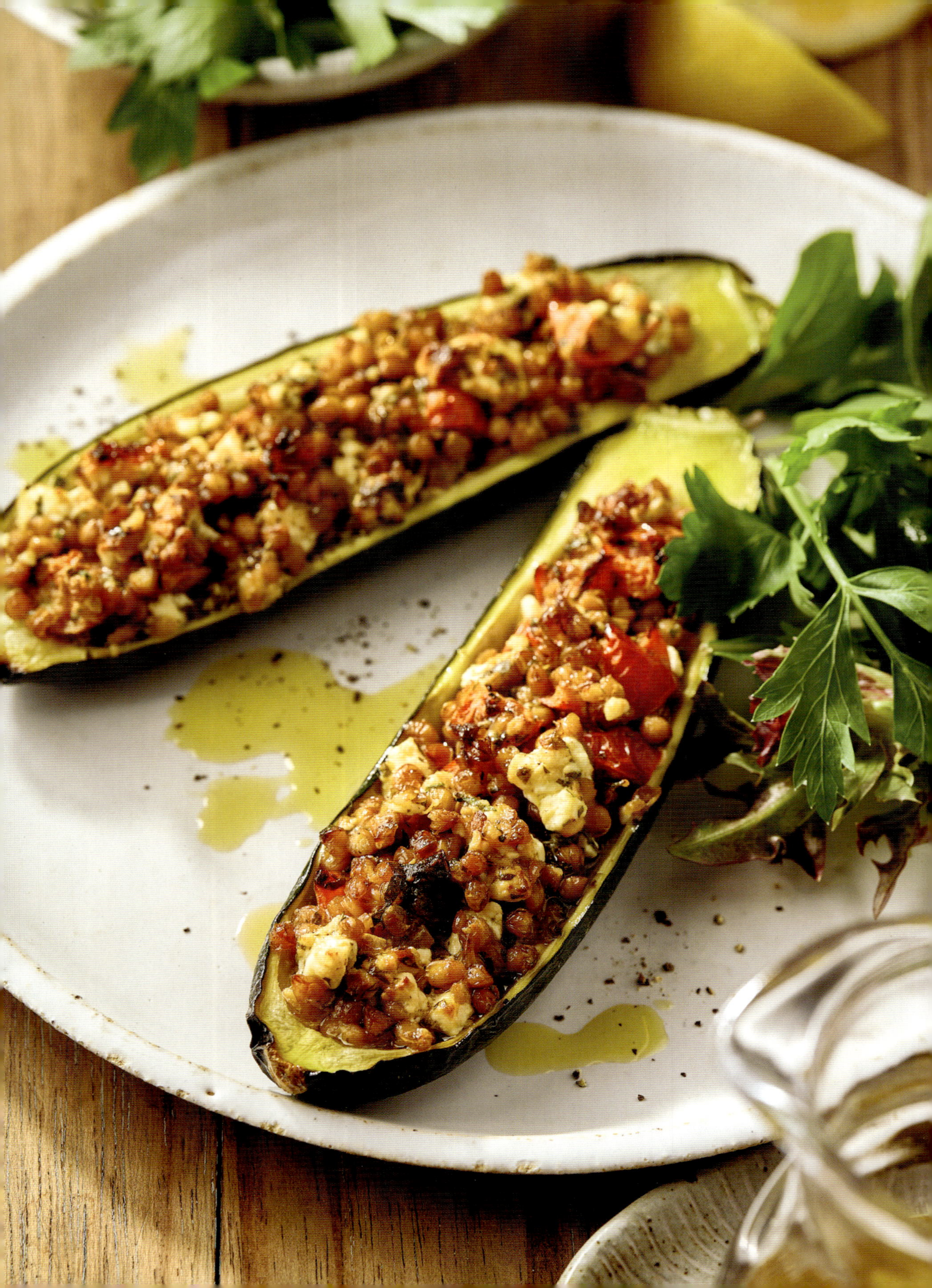

GUT-FRIENDLY ZUCCHINI BOATS

SERVES 1 • CARBS PER SERVE: 8 GRAMS

1 medium zucchini

2 teaspoons extra-virgin olive oil

¼ cup cooked lentils (brown or green, canned, drained and well-rinsed is fine)

3 cherry tomatoes, diced

2 tablespoons feta, crumbled

1 tablespoon chopped fresh parsley, plus extra to serve

salt and pepper

1 cup mixed leafy greens, to serve

1. Preheat the oven to 200°C.

2. Slice the zucchini in half lengthwise and scoop out the centre, leaving a cavity. Drizzle the zucchini halves with a little olive oil and season with salt and pepper. Place on a baking tray, cut side up.

3. In a bowl, combine the lentils, tomatoes, feta, parsley, 1 teaspoon olive oil, and a little salt and pepper.

4. Spoon the mixture evenly into the hollowed zucchini halves. Roast in the oven for 20 minutes or until the zucchini is tender and the filling is slightly golden.

5. Serve warm with a side of fresh leafy greens, dressed with the remaining olive oil and extra fresh parsley.

LOW-CARB MISO-GLAZED EGGPLANT

SERVES 1 • CARBS PER SERVE: 6 GRAMS

---

1 small eggplant

1 tablespoon miso paste

1 teaspoon apple cider vinegar

1 teaspoon tamari

½ teaspoon grated ginger

½ teaspoon sesame oil

pinch of chilli flakes

1 teaspoon extra-virgin olive oil

sprinkle of fresh coriander, to serve

sesame seeds (optional), to serve

1. Preheat the oven to 200°C.

2. Slice the eggplant in half lengthwise. Score the flesh with a criss-cross pattern.

3. In a bowl, mix the miso, vinegar, tamari, ginger, sesame oil and chilli flakes until smooth.

4. Brush each eggplant half with olive oil. Place skin-side down on a non-stick frying pan or lined baking tray. Roast for 12 minutes, turning once, until soft and golden.

5. Brush the cooked eggplant with all the miso glaze. Return to the oven or grill for 3 minutes more until caramelised and glossy.

6. Serve hot, topped with coriander and sesame seeds (if using).

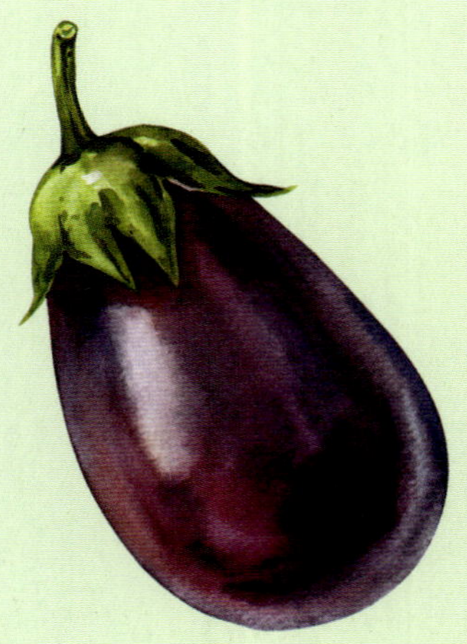

HEALTHY MINCE BAKE

SERVES 2 • CARBS PER SERVE: 10 GRAMS

1 medium zucchini, thinly sliced lengthways

1 small eggplant, thinly sliced

1 tablespoon extra-virgin olive oil

¼ onion, finely chopped

4 cloves garlic, minced

200 grams chicken mince

salt and pepper, to taste

1 tomato, finely sliced

1 teaspoon dried oregano

1 cup fresh baby spinach

¼ cup grated cheese

chopped fresh basil and parsley

1. Preheat the oven to 200°C. Line a baking tray with baking paper.

2. Arrange the zucchini and eggplant slices on the tray. Brush with half the olive oil and roast in the oven for 10 minutes, until softened.

3. In a frying pan, sauté the onion and garlic in the remaining olive oil for 2 minutes. Add the mince, season with salt and pepper, then add the tomato and oregano. Cook for a few minutes.

4. In a small dish, place the eggplant in a layer, then add layers with half the mince, zucchini, baby spinach, remaining mince and tomato slices. Sprinkle the cheese over the top. Bake uncovered for 15 minutes or until the cheese is browned.

5. Serve warm, garnished with fresh parsley.

BLACK BEAN PATTIES

SERVES 1 (1 LARGE OR 2 SMALL PATTIES)
CARBS PER SERVE: 6 GRAMS

¼ cup canned black beans, drained and rinsed

1 zucchini, grated

1 egg

1 tablespoon chopped fresh coriander or parsley

½ tablespoon finely diced red onion

¼ teaspoon ground cumin

¼ teaspoon smoked paprika

salt and pepper

1 teaspoon extra-virgin olive oil

freshly squeezed lime juice, to serve

1 tablespoon Greek yoghurt, to serve

Sarah's garden salad (page 275), to serve

1. Mash the beans in a bowl with a fork until mostly broken up.

2. Give the zucchini a squeeze to let out some of the excess water.

3. In a bowl, stir the egg, zucchini, herbs, onion, cumin, paprika, and salt and pepper to taste until well combined. Shape mixture into one large or two small patties.

4. Heat the olive oil in a non-stick pan over medium heat. Add the black bean patties and cook for 2–3 minutes each side, until golden and set.

5. Serve hot with a squeeze of lime or a spoonful of plain Greek yoghurt and my garden salad.

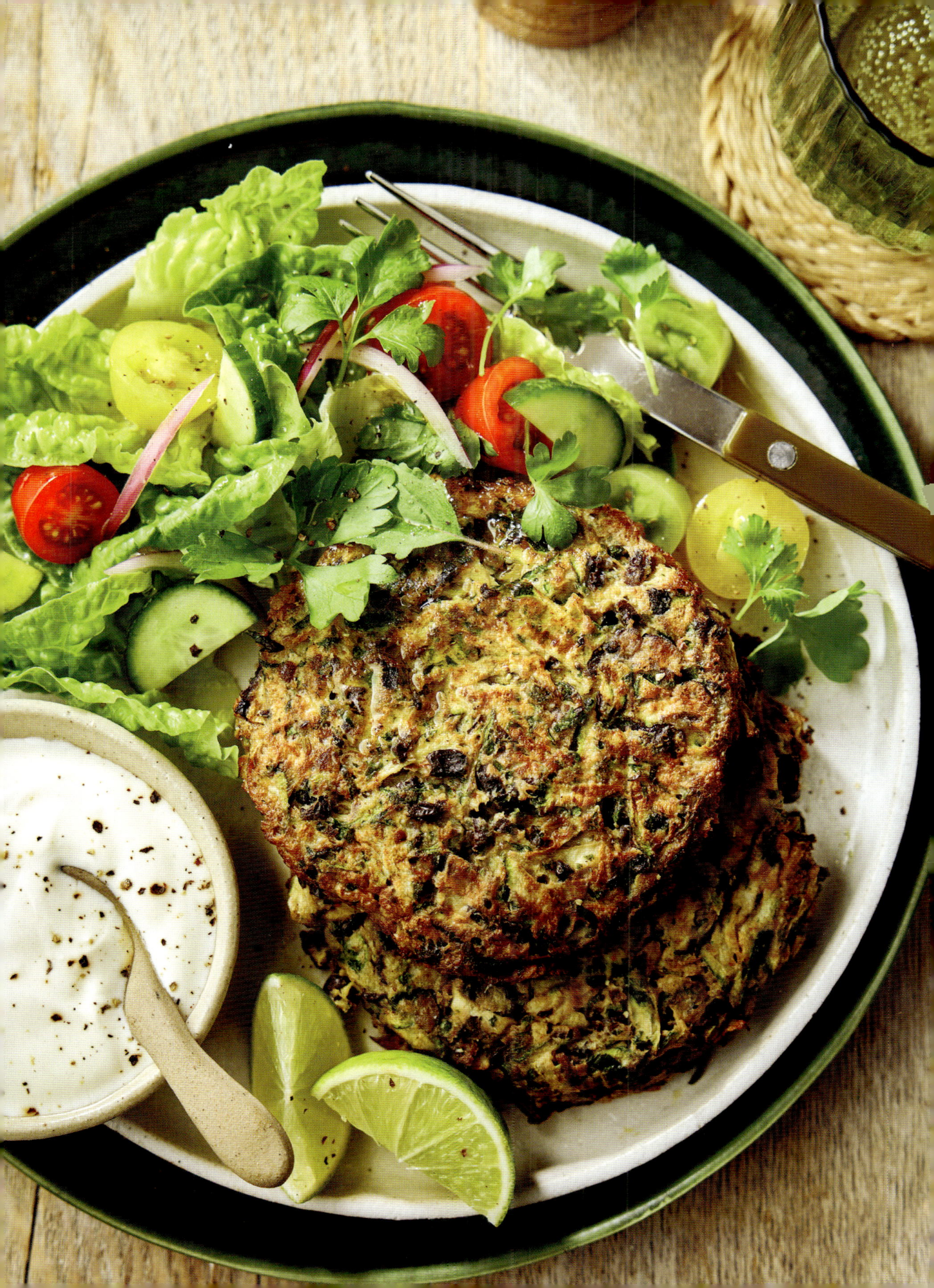

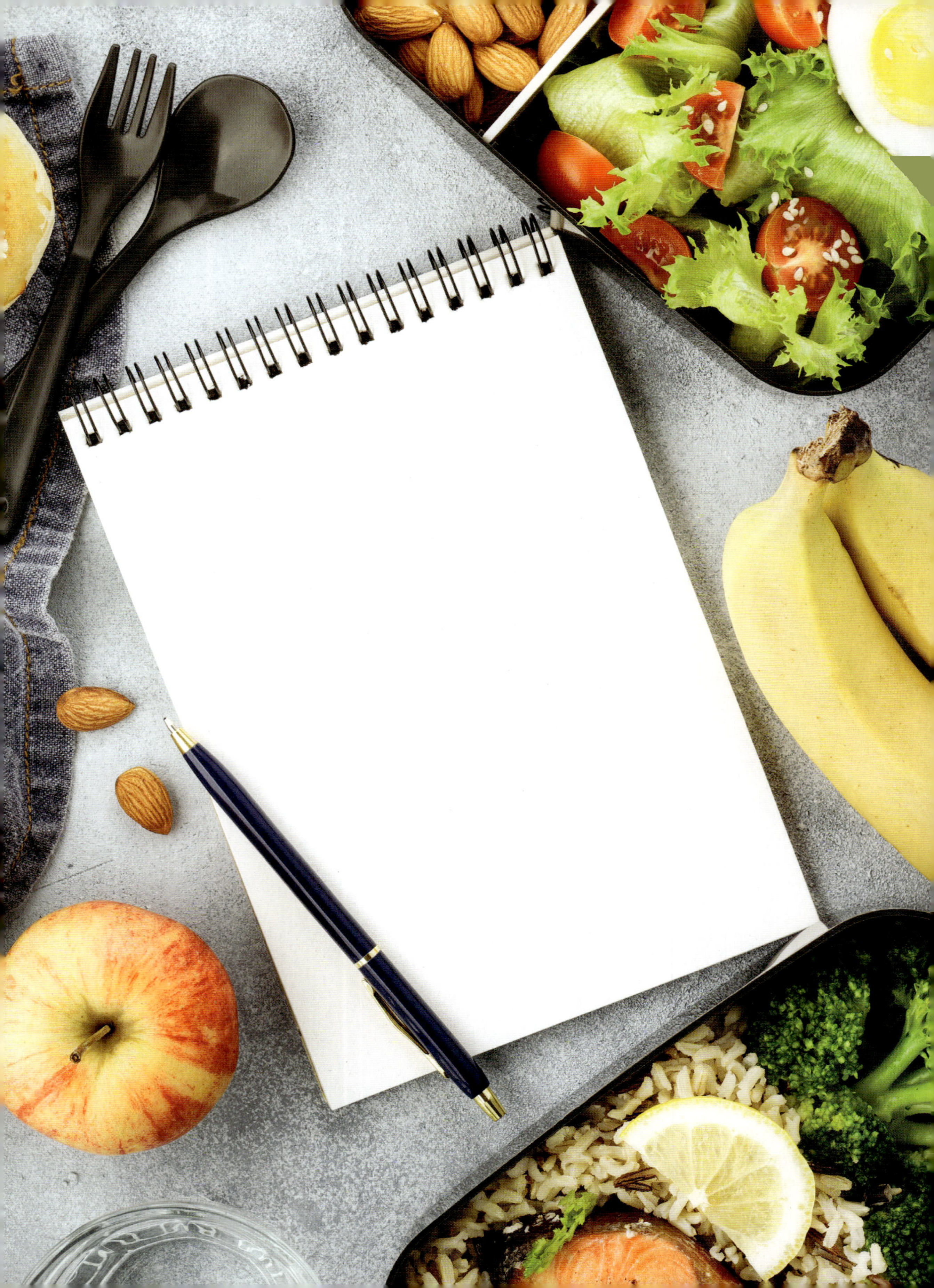

Adaptation and check-up

Supporting our heart and vascular system

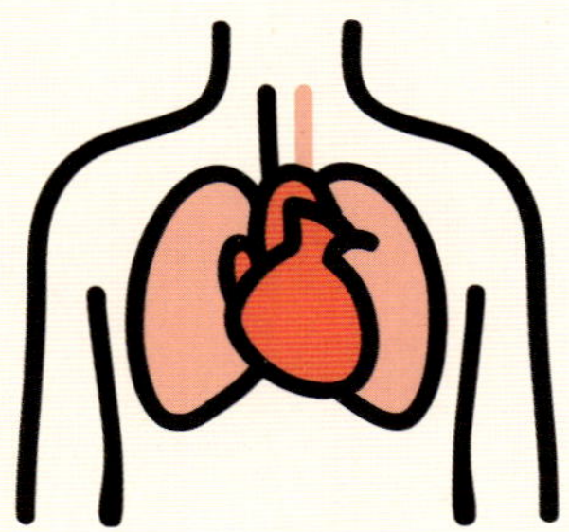

Focus: Lowering your risk of heart disease

By now, you should feel amazing and settled in the program.

This phase is where we can really start to see the possibility of fat loss in the liver and pancreas. In my clinical experience, this is where I see significant weight loss.

At this stage, you no longer need electrolytes. But make sure you're still staying well hydrated.

MEDICATION CHECK-UP

For those of you on blood pressure medication, you may want to check in with your GP.

- Do you still need to wear a continuous glucose monitor?

- Do a full medication review with your doctor as blood glucose levels may normalise.

This week is all about your heart and cardiovascular health.

The risk of heart disease with type 2 diabetes is so incredibly strong. Diabetes drives chronic inflammation, which promotes cholesterol build-up in blood vessels, impairs blood vessel relaxation and increases abnormal blood clotting. Together with insulin resistance and weight gain, these changes raise the risk of high blood pressure, cardiovascular disease and obesity-related complications.

People with T2D are four times more likely to develop heart disease, heart attacks, strokes and peripheral artery disease.

The best foods for our heart and vascular health are vegetables, fruits, whole grains and healthy fats. Leafy greens, such as spinach and broccoli, are rich in nitrates and vitamins that help protect arteries and reduce blood pressure. Fruits, such as berries, contain antioxidants that help lower LDL ('bad' cholesterol) and reduce inflammation. Whole grains and legumes, such as oats, brown rice and chickpeas, provide fibre and protein that help manage cholesterol. Fatty fish, such as salmon and tuna, provide high levels of omega-3 fatty acids, which improve blood pressure and lower triglycerides. Extra-virgin olive oil and avocadoes provide monounsaturated fats that protect heart health. And nuts and seeds, such as walnuts, almonds and flaxseed, are excellent for improving cholesterol levels and reducing heart disease risk.

Reminders

- Keep up your water intake.
- Are you getting good-quality sleep?
- Are you reducing your stress?
- Track your success – check your measurements and weight.
- Don't forget to follow the order of eating.
- Get regular exercise – walking after each meal or calf raises (if not walking).
- Are you having your last meal around 6 p.m. and your first meal 12 hours later?

	BREAKFAST	MID-MORNING	LUNCH	MID-AFTERNOON	DINNER
MONDAY	Strawberry diabetes-friendly smoothie (page 283)	Skip	Herb, egg and spinach slice (page 316), served with a green salad	25 grams cheese	Chicken and vegetable stew (page 322)
TUESDAY	2 poached eggs with ¼ avocado and 1 cup spinach, garnished with chopped fresh chives	5 walnuts	Chicken and celery salad (page 318)	½ cup berries	120 grams grilled white fish fillet, served with ½ cup steamed broccoli, ½ cup steamed cauliflower and ½ cup chopped zucchini Garnish with fresh parsley and a squeeze of lemon
WEDNESDAY	Green berry and fibre smoothie (page 315)	Skip	Avocado and salmon low-carb lunch bowl (page 289)	2 celery stalks with 2 teaspoons almond butter	Chicken and vegetable stew (page 322)
THURSDAY	Low-carb oat breakfast bowl (page 318)	Skip	Herb, egg and spinach slice (page 316) with Greek salad (page 275)	10:10 SDL protein bar	Mackerel patties (page 319) with 1½ cups mixed steamed green vegetables (broccoli, zucchini, brussels sprouts)
FRIDAY	Greek yoghurt, berry and mint breakfast bowl (page 300)	Skip	Grilled chicken breast salad (page 292)	1 gold kiwifruit with skin on (wash well)	Prawn and bok choy broth (page 325)
SATURDAY	2 poached or boiled eggs with 3 cherry tomatoes, ¼ avocado and ½ cup baby spinach leaves, garnished with chilli and fresh chives	5 walnuts	Salmon health bowl (page 276)	½ cup blueberries	Beef mince cups and coriander (page 274)
SUNDAY	Green berry and fibre smoothie (page 315)	Skip	Low-carb green goddess salad with chicken (page 321)	Skip	Spiced salmon and Mediterranean veg tray bake (page 294)
BEVERAGES Water, plus optional coffee, tea, green tea, herbal tea, electrolytes					

GREEN BERRY AND FIBRE SMOOTHIE

SERVES 1 • CARBS PER SERVE: 12 GRAMS

½ cup almond milk

½ cup water

½ cup Greek yoghurt

½ cup frozen mixed berries

½ cup baby spinach or kale

½ small avocado

6 walnuts

1 tablespoon ground linseed (flaxseed) or chia seed

½ teaspoon ground cinnamon

squeeze of lemon juice

ice cubes or water, to thin (optional)

Put all the ingredients in a blender and blend until completely smooth. Add ice or a splash of water for a thinner texture. Taste and adjust with more lemon or cinnamon as desired.

HERB, EGG AND SPINACH SLICE

SERVES 8 • CARBS PER SERVE: 4 GRAMS

2 tablespoons extra-virgin olive oil, plus extra for greasing

4 leeks, chopped

2 bunches silverbeet, trimmed and sliced

180 grams Danish feta

150 grams parmesan cheese, finely grated

1½ cups almond flour

8 large eggs

½ cup almond milk

½ cup chopped fresh parsley

¼ cup chopped fresh chives

¼ cup chopped fresh dill

¼ cup chopped fresh mint

salt and pepper

extra fresh herbs, to garnish

1. Preheat the oven to 200°C. Grease a baking dish with a little olive oil and line with baking paper.

2. Heat olive oil in a frying pan. Cook the leeks over medium heat for 5 minutes, until softened.

3. Add the silverbeet; cook until wilted and tender. Remove from heat and let cool slightly.

4. Stir the feta, parmesan and almond flour into the vegetable mixture.

5. In a separate bowl, whisk eggs and milk until well combined. Add the herbs and salt and pepper to taste, then combine with the vegetable mixture.

6. Pour everything into the prepared baking dish and smooth the top. Bake in the oven for 30 minutes until golden and just set in the centre.

7. Cool slightly, slice and serve garnished with extra fresh herbs.

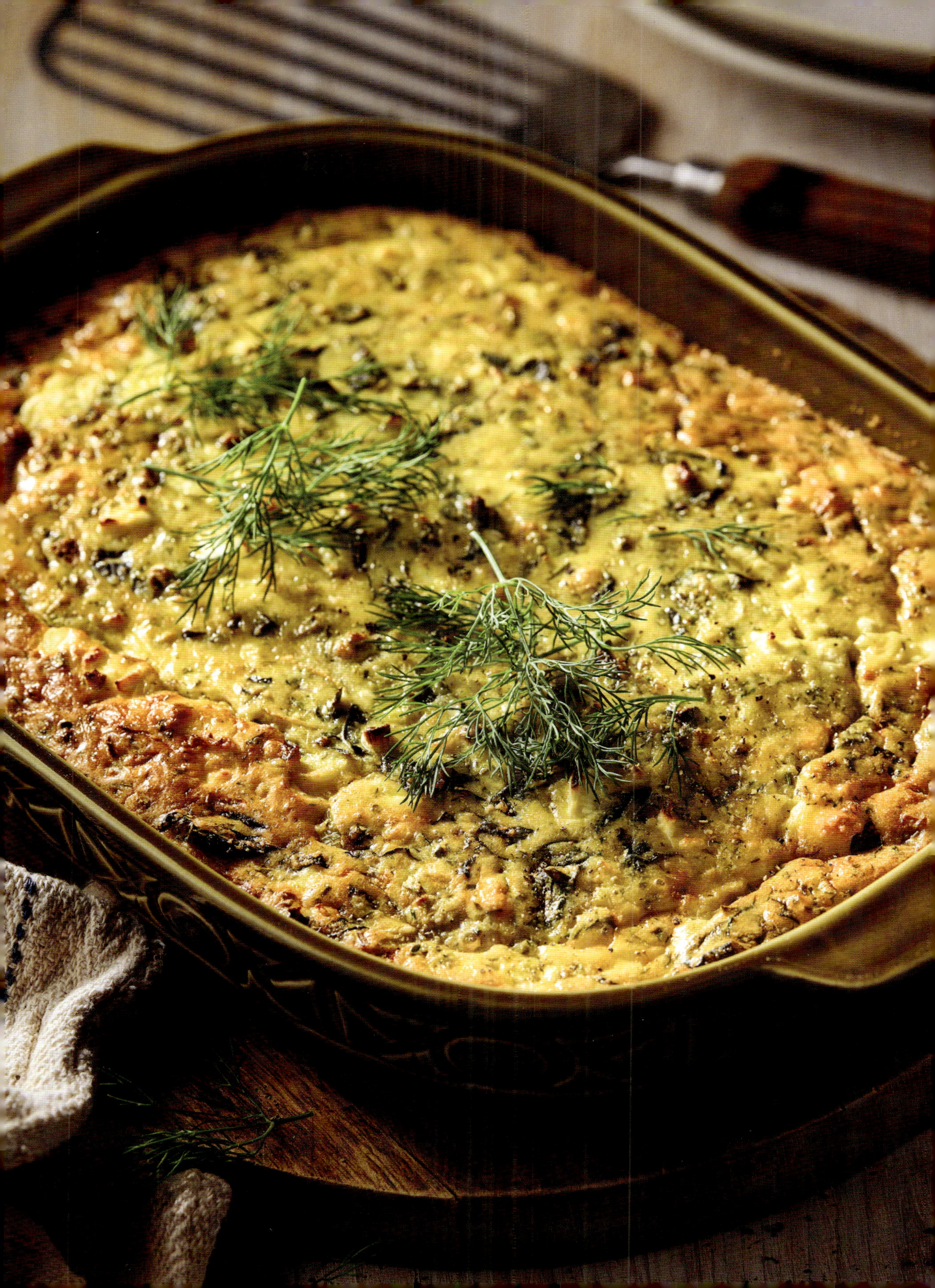

LOW-CARB OAT BREAKFAST BOWL

SERVES 1 • CARBS PER SERVE: 14 GRAMS

---

2 tablespoons steel-cut oats

2 tablespoons crushed walnuts

1 tablespoon chia seeds

1 tablespoon ground linseed (flaxseed)

1 serve whey protein isolate

½ teaspoon ground ginger

pinch of salt

½ cup unsweetened almond milk

2 tablespoons full-fat Greek yoghurt

¼ cup fresh raspberries

½ teaspoon ground cinnamon

1. Combine the oats, walnuts, chia seeds, linseeds, protein powder, ginger, salt and almond milk in a jar or bowl. Mix well and soak overnight in the fridge.

2. In the morning, stir in the Greek yoghurt, berries and cinnamon. Add a splash more milk or yoghurt if needed.

CHICKEN AND CELERY SALAD

SERVES 1 • CARBS PER SERVE: 19 GRAMS

---

200 grams shredded cooked chicken breast (rotisserie is an easy option)

1 cup cottage cheese

1 cup chopped celery

1 apple, chopped

¼ red onion, chopped

¼ cup crushed roasted cashews

2 tablespoons Greek yoghurt

1 tablespoon extra-virgin olive oil

1 teaspoon Dijon mustard

salt and pepper

lettuce leaf, to serve

Mix all the ingredients together in a bowl and serve in a lettuce leaf.

MACKEREL PATTIES

MAKES 6 PATTIES (2 PER SERVE)
CARBS PER PATTY: 1.5 GRAMS

---

400 grams canned mackerel, drained and flaked

2 large eggs

½ cup almond flour

¼ cup grated parmesan cheese

4 cloves garlic, minced

2 tablespoons chopped fresh parsley

½ teaspoon onion powder

1 tablespoon Dijon mustard

1 tablespoon lemon juice

salt and pepper

2 tablespoons extra-virgin olive oil for cooking

lemon wedges, to serve

salad or steamed greens, to serve

1. Combine the mackerel, eggs, almond flour, parmesan, garlic, parsley, onion powder, mustard, lemon juice, and salt and pepper in a large bowl. Mix until well combined.

2. Shape the mixture into six equal-sized patties.

3. Heat the olive oil in a large frying pan over medium heat. Cook the patties for 3–4 minutes each side, until cooked through and golden.

4. Serve immediately with lemon wedges and salad or steamed greens alongside.

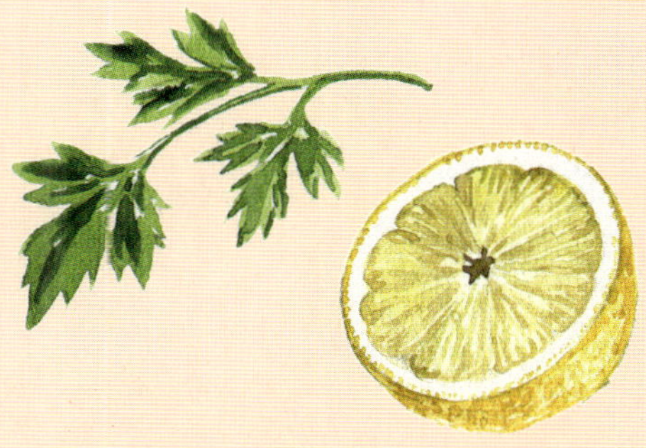

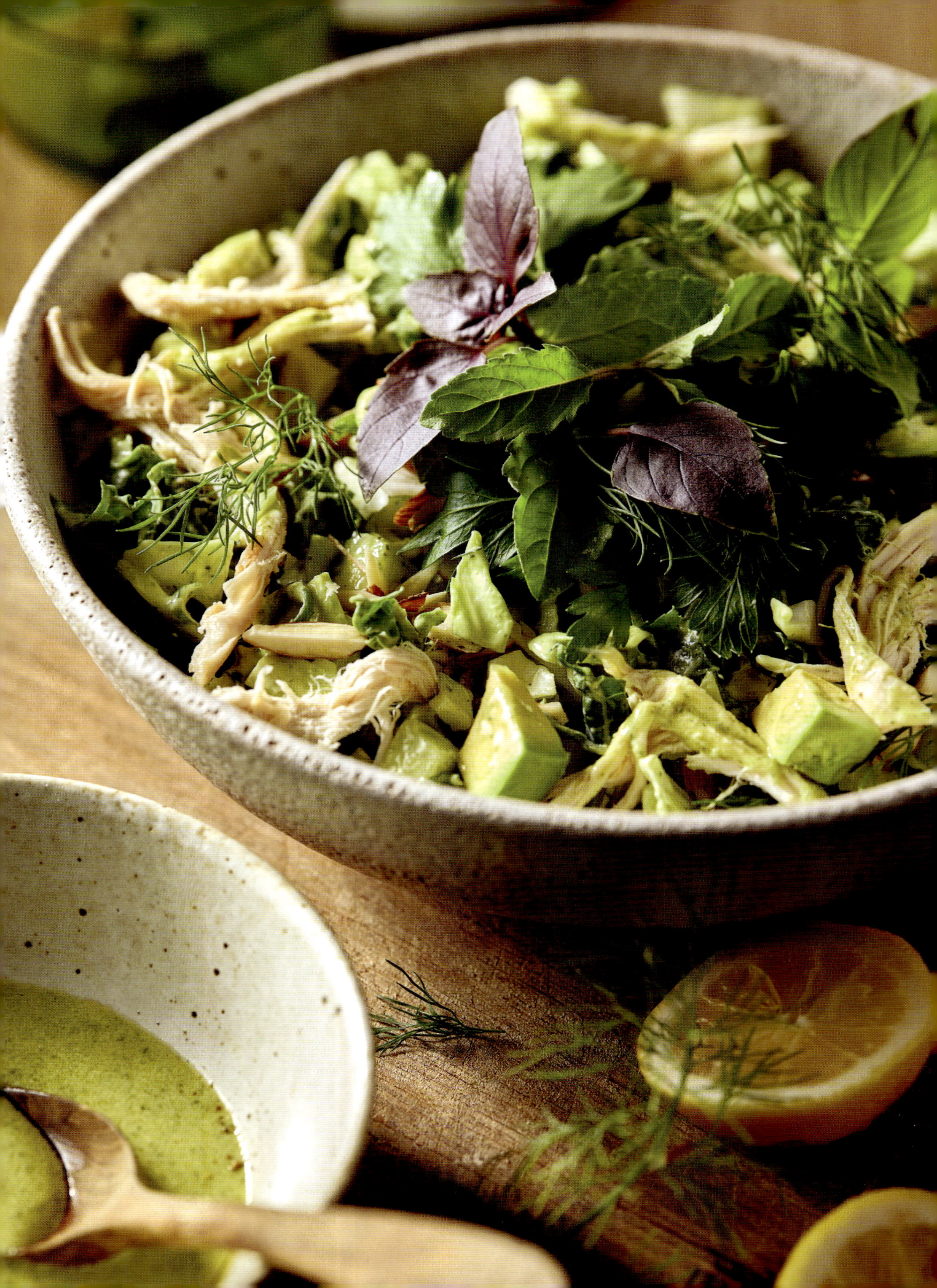

LOW-CARB GREEN GODDESS SALAD WITH CHICKEN

SERVES 1 • CARBS PER SERVE: 8 GRAMS

---

1 cup chopped cabbage (green or red)

1 cup baby spinach or chopped kale

½ cup cucumber, diced

½ avocado, cubed

1 spring onion, sliced

2 tablespoons fresh parsley, dill and chives (mixed)

120 grams cooked chicken breast, shredded

1 tablespoon slivered almonds

GREEN GODDESS DRESSING

juice of ½ lemon

¼ avocado

1 tablespoon extra-virgin olive oil

1 tablespoon Greek yoghurt

1 tablespoon fresh herbs (parsley, chives, dill)

2 teaspoons Dijon mustard

1 small clove garlic, minced

salt and pepper, to taste

1. Combine the cabbage, spinach, cucumber, avocado, spring onion and fresh herbs in a large bowl. Add the shredded chicken breast and almonds.

2. To make the dressing, blend all the ingredients until creamy and smooth. Adjust seasoning.

3. Toss salad with the dressing and serve immediately.

CHICKEN AND VEGETABLE STEW

SERVES 4 • CARBS PER SERVE: 8 GRAMS

1 tablespoon extra-virgin olive oil

1 medium onion, chopped

6 cloves garlic, minced

2 skinless chicken breasts

2 carrots, sliced

1 capsicum chopped

1 zucchini, diced

1 x 400-gram can diced tomatoes

2 cups chicken stock

1 teaspoon dried thyme

1 teaspoon dried oregano

black pepper

2 cups baby spinach

juice of ½ lemon, to serve

2 tablespoons chopped fresh parsley and dill, to serve

1. Heat the olive oil in a large pot over medium heat. Add the onion and garlic and cook for a few minutes.

2. Cut the chicken into bite-sized pieces and cook until browned.

3. Stir through the carrots, capsicum and zucchini and cook for another 2–3 minutes.

4. Add the tomatoes, stock, thyme, oregano and pepper. Bring to the boil, then reduce heat and simmer for 20 minutes.

5. Stir in spinach for 5 minutes, until wilted.

6. Serve with fresh lemon juice, parsley and dill on top.

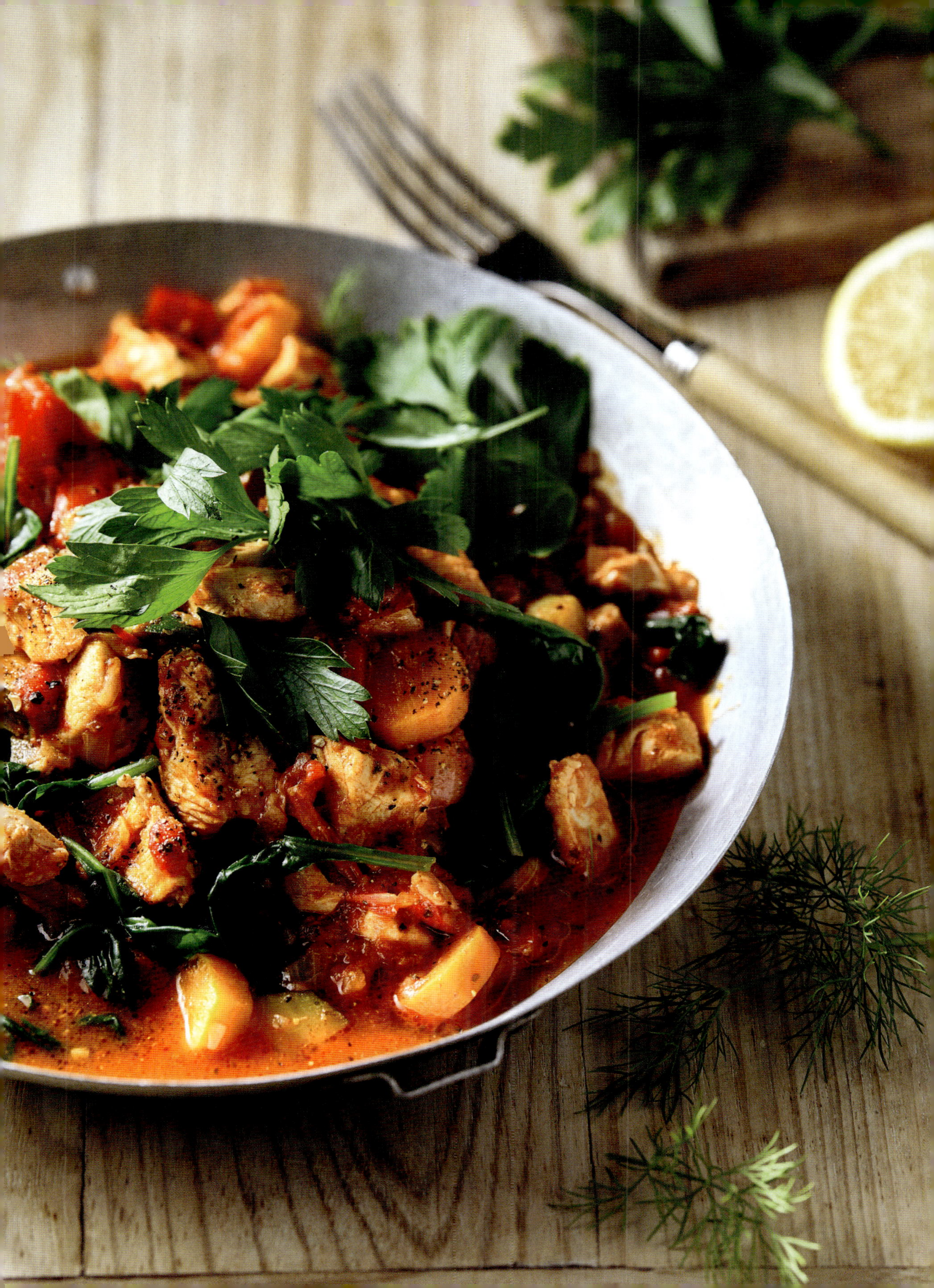

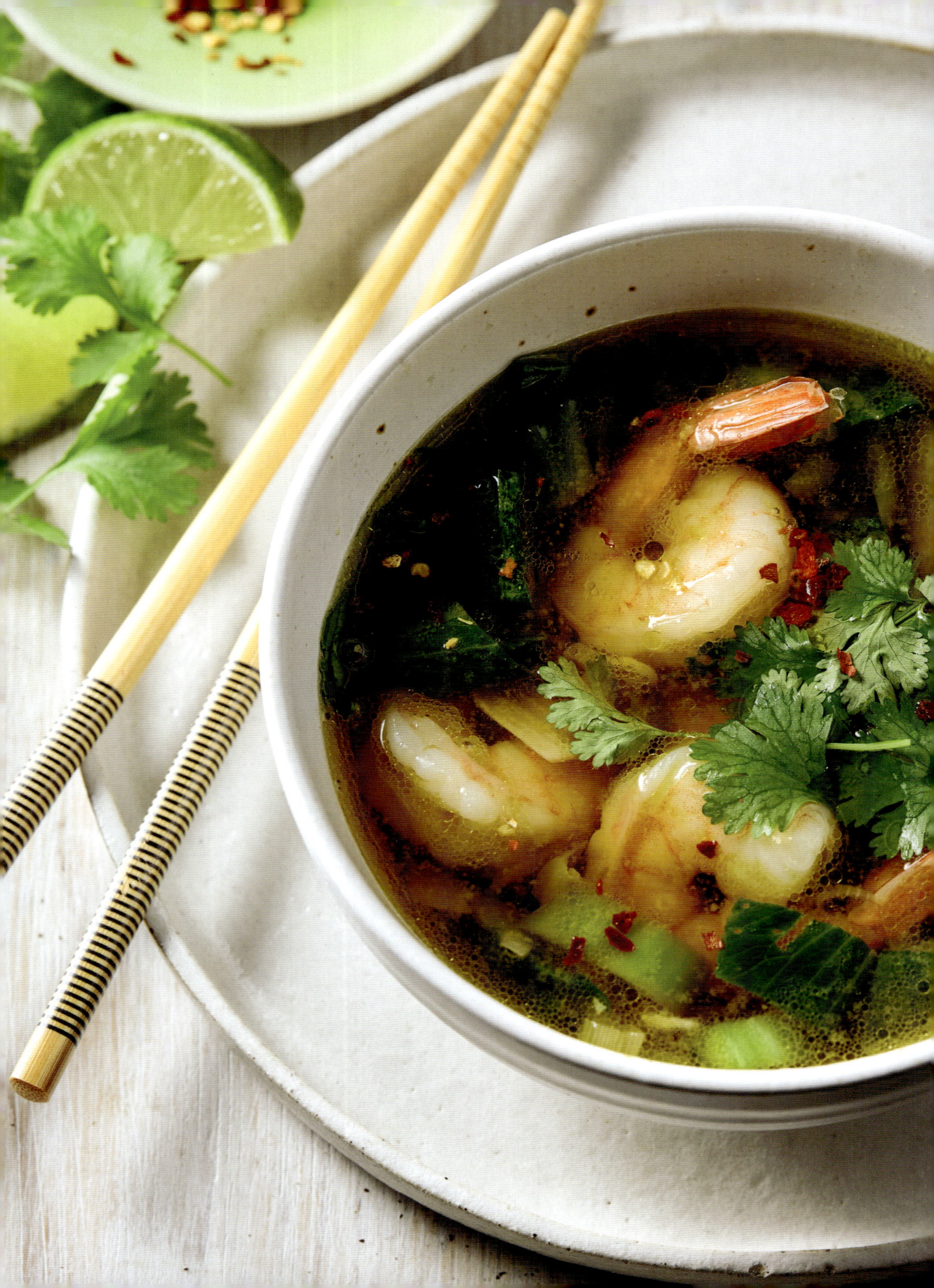

PRAWN AND BOK CHOY BROTH

SERVES 1 • CARBS PER SERVE: 3 GRAMS

2 teaspoons extra-virgin olive oil

2 cloves garlic, sliced

2 teaspoons sliced fresh ginger

1 spring onion, sliced (white part only)

2 cups chicken stock

2 teaspoons tamari

150 grams raw prawns, peeled and deveined

1 small bok choy (about 100 grams), sliced

juice of ¼ lime

salt and pepper

chilli flakes, to garnish

fresh coriander, to garnish

1. Heat the olive oil in a saucepan. Add the garlic, ginger and spring onion, and sauté for 1 minute.

2. Add the stock and tamari. Simmer for 5 minutes.

3. Add the prawns and bok choy. Simmer for 3 minutes until prawns are opaque and bok choy is wilted. Season with lime juice, salt and pepper. Garnish with chilli flakes and fresh coriander.

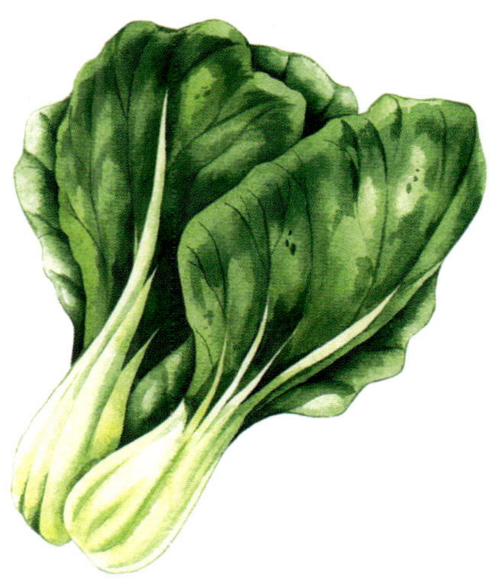

Protecting our nervous system

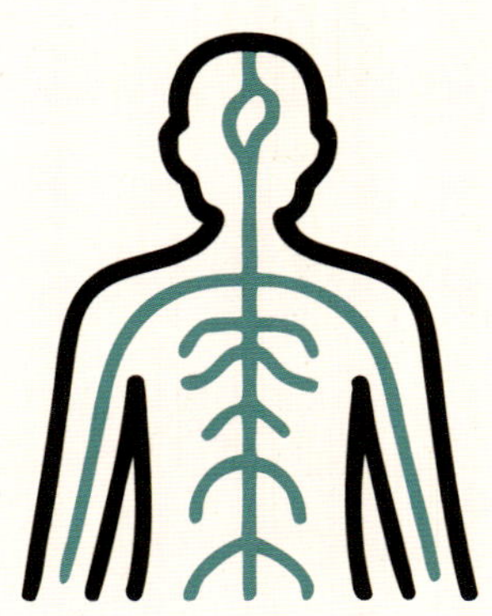

Focus: Continued weight loss while nurturing your nervous system

It's so important to protect your nervous system when you have type 2 diabetes. Our nervous system controls all muscle movements and organ function. High blood glucose can damage the central and peripheral nerves. The consequences include complications such as neuropathy, nerve pain, balance issues, memory changes, impaired movement, digestive problems, circulatory problems and possible cognitive decline.

High blood glucose can injure the small blood vessels supplying nerves, drive inflammation and oxidative stress, and disrupt the function of nerve cells. All this makes everything so much harder, as well as driving diabetes to progress.

Supporting and protecting our nervous system is central for improving quality of life and preventing complications.

THE BEST FOODS FOR OUR NERVOUS SYSTEM

- Omega-3 rich foods reduce inflammation and support nerve cell repair.

- Leafy greens and colourful vegetables protect nerve cells from sugar-induced damage.

- Nuts and seeds help support nerve signalling, antioxidant defence and myelin sheath maintenance.

- Eggs, fish, dairy and lean meats are high in vitamin B12, essential for preventing and helping heal nerve injury.

- Low-GI fruit delivers vitamin C, antioxidants and fibre that protects both blood vessels and nerves.

- Whole grains and legumes contain B vitamins for nerve health, fibre for glucose stability, and magnesium.

- Magnesium and vitamin D sources (e.g. almonds, eggs, oily fish) help prevent deficiencies which are linked to neuropathy risk and slowing nerve repair.

- We need to protect our nerves for our brain to function, and for our mobility, independence with aging and overall quality of life. Food is medicine; it can help repair and protect in conjunction with a healthy diet and lifestyle.

Reminder

While continuing with the program as you know it, think about your current exercise regime. Is it time to increase your resistance training? I do recommend this. Muscle is *so* important to help regulate blood sugar levels and for mobility, sleep, healthy aging and maintaining a healthy weight.

	BREAKFAST	MID-MORNING	LUNCH	MID-AFTERNOON	DINNER
MONDAY	Smoked salmon and veggie scramble (page 335)	5 walnuts	Turkey and mixed veg lunch bowl (page 339)	½ cup strawberries	Baked chicken and brussels sprouts (page 336)
TUESDAY	Nerve health green smoothie (page 332)	Skip	Baked chicken and brussels sprouts (page 336)	1 orange	Tofu burger (page 273)
WEDNESDAY	Chia bread (page 329) with sautéed mushrooms, spinach and garlic	10 almonds	Nerve-loving frittata (page 330) with Sarah's garden salad (page 275)	10:10 SDL protein bar	120 grams lean red meat cooked to your liking, with Greek salad (page 275)
THURSDAY	2 soft-boiled eggs (cooked for 4 minutes) with 5 asparagus spears to dip in	½ cup blueberries	2 slices of chia bread (page 329) with 2 boiled eggs, ¼ avo, 2 lettuce leaves, ½ tomato sliced, 1 teaspoon chopped red onion	30 grams pepitas and sunflower seeds	Nerve-loving frittata (page 330) with 1½ cups steamed mixed green veggies
FRIDAY	Nerve health green smoothie (page 332)	Skip	Chicken and celery salad (page 318)	25 grams cheese	Miso mushroom seafood soup (page 337)
SATURDAY	Sarah's favourite breakfast (page 268)	Skip	Turkey and mixed veg bowl (page 339)	10:10 SDL protein bar	Lean beef steak with grilled eggplant and steamed brussels sprouts (page 291)
SUNDAY	Omelette with mushrooms, tomatoes and herbs (page 274)	5 pecans	Sarah's grated salad (page 285) with 100 grams sardines	1 cup strawberries	Eggplant pizza (page 333) with a leafy green salad

BEVERAGES Water, plus optional coffee, tea, green tea, herbal tea, electrolytes

CHIA BREAD

MAKES 6 SLICES • CARBS PER SLICE: 1 GRAM

1¼ cups (200 grams) chia flour (or chia seeds)

1½ teaspoons baking powder

¼ teaspoon salt (optional)

1 cup water

1. Preheat the oven to 200°C. Line a baking sheet with baking paper.

2. If you don't have chia flour, grind chia seeds in a blender.

3. In a large bowl, whisk the chia flour, baking powder and salt. Stir in the water; the mixture will quickly become thick. Let it rest for 1–2 minutes.

4. Shape the mixture into a small loaf or divide into three mini-baguette shapes. Use a sharp knife to slash the tops for expansion. Bake in the oven for 55 minutes or until firm and dry.

5. Cool fully before slicing.

TOPPING SUGGESTIONS

- mashed avocado with lemon and herbs (2 grams carbs per ¼ avocado)
- cottage cheese and smoked salmon (<1 grams carbs per tablespoon)
- sliced hard-boiled or poached eggs (nearly 0 carbs)
- smoked salmon, sardines or tuna (0 carbs, high in omega-3s)
- thin layer of nut butter or tahini (1–2 grams carbs per tablespoon)
- sliced olives (minimal carbs, rich in healthy fats)
- sautéed mushrooms and spinach with garlic (about 2–3 grams carbs per serve).

NERVE-LOVING FRITTATA

SERVES 4 • CARBS PER SERVE: 2.5 GRAMS

---

1 tablespoon extra-virgin olive oil

½ cup sliced mushrooms

¼ cup diced red capsicum

1 cup baby spinach, chopped

6 eggs

¼ cup unsweetened almond milk

salt and pepper

½ cup grated cheddar or goat's cheese

green salad, to serve

1. Preheat the oven to 180°C.

2. Heat the olive oil in an ovenproof pan over medium heat. Add mushrooms and capsicum and sauté 2–3 minutes. Add the spinach and cook until wilted.

3. In a bowl, whisk the eggs, milk, and salt and pepper to taste. Stir in the cheese. Pour the egg mixture over the cooked vegetables and stir gently. Cook on the stovetop for 2–3 minutes until the edges start to set.

4. Transfer pan to the oven and bake for 12 minutes, or until it sets and is lightly golden.

5. Slice and serve the frittata with a green salad.

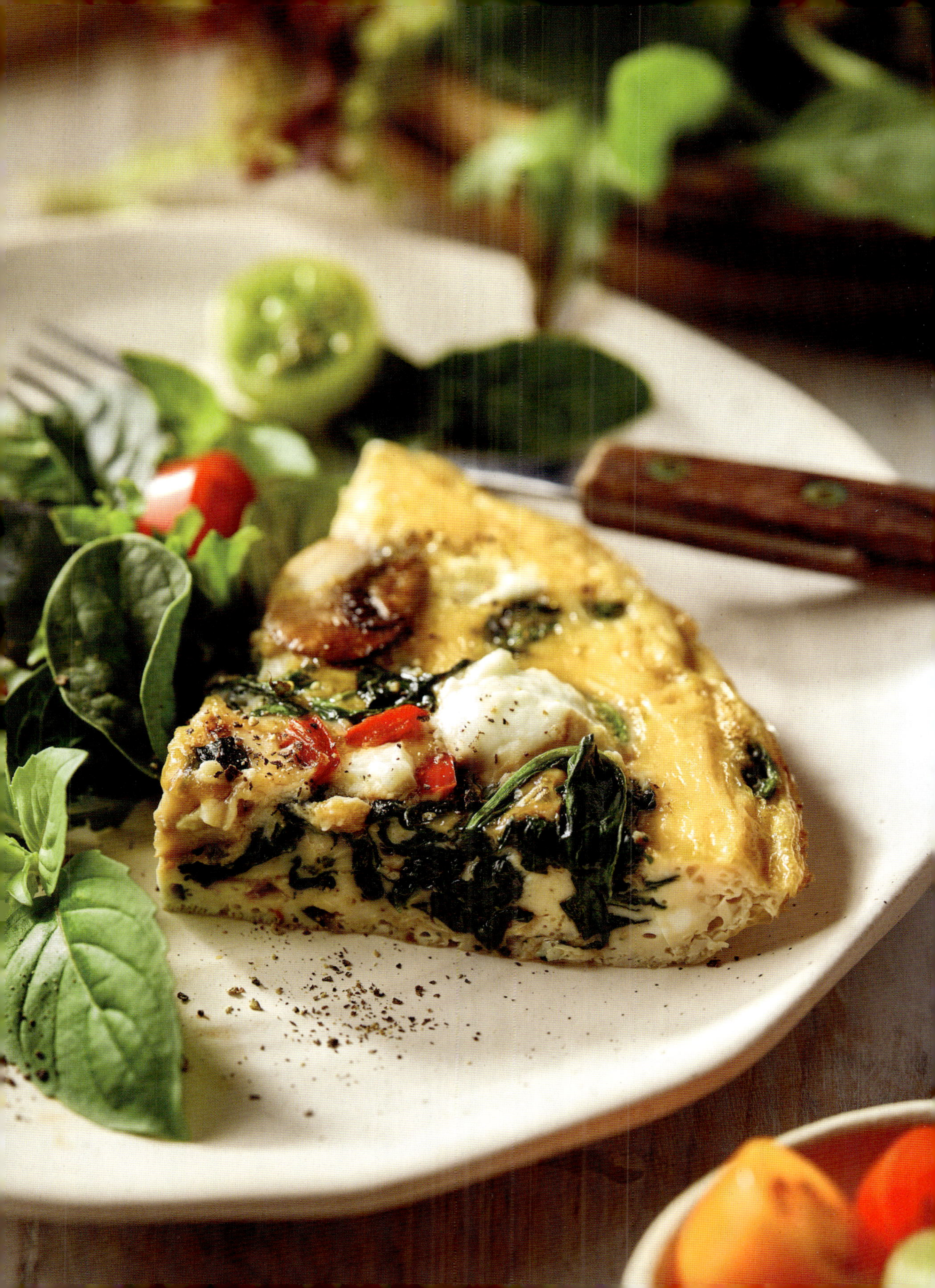

NERVE-HEALTH GREEN SMOOTHIE

SERVES 1 • CARBS PER SERVE: 10 GRAMS

---

1 cup unsweetened almond milk

1 cup baby spinach

½ small avocado or ⅓ larger avocado

¼ cup frozen raspberries

1 serve unflavoured protein powder

1 tablespoon chia seeds

1 tablespoon walnut pieces

½ teaspoon ground cinnamon

2 drops vanilla extract

ice cubes

Put all the ingredients in a blender, starting with the milk and spinach. Blend on high until very smooth and creamy. Pour into a glass and serve immediately.

EGGPLANT PIZZA

MAKES 6 PATTIES (2 PER SERVE) • CARBS PER SERVE: 13 GRAMS

¼ medium eggplant

2 teaspoons extra-virgin olive oil

salt and pepper

2 cloves garlic, minced

a few slices of onion

2 tablespoons no-sugar-added pasta or pizza sauce

¼ cup baby spinach

3 tablespoons grated mozzarella

1 tablespoon chopped fresh oregano

1. Preheat the oven to 200°C. Line a baking tray with baking paper.

2. Slice the eggplant into about 5-mm-thick pieces. Brush lightly with olive oil and season with salt and pepper. Place on the lined tray and roast for 7–10 minutes until beginning to soften.

3. Meanwhile, sauté the garlic and onion in a small frying pan with a little olive oil, until soft (about 3–4 minutes).

4. Add the pasta sauce and baby spinach. Cook for 1–2 minutes until the spinach wilts.

5. Remove eggplant from the oven and spread the sauce mixture evenly over the slices. Sprinkle the mozzarella and oregano on top. Return to the oven and bake for another 5 minutes or until the cheese is melted and bubbly.

6. Serve immediately.

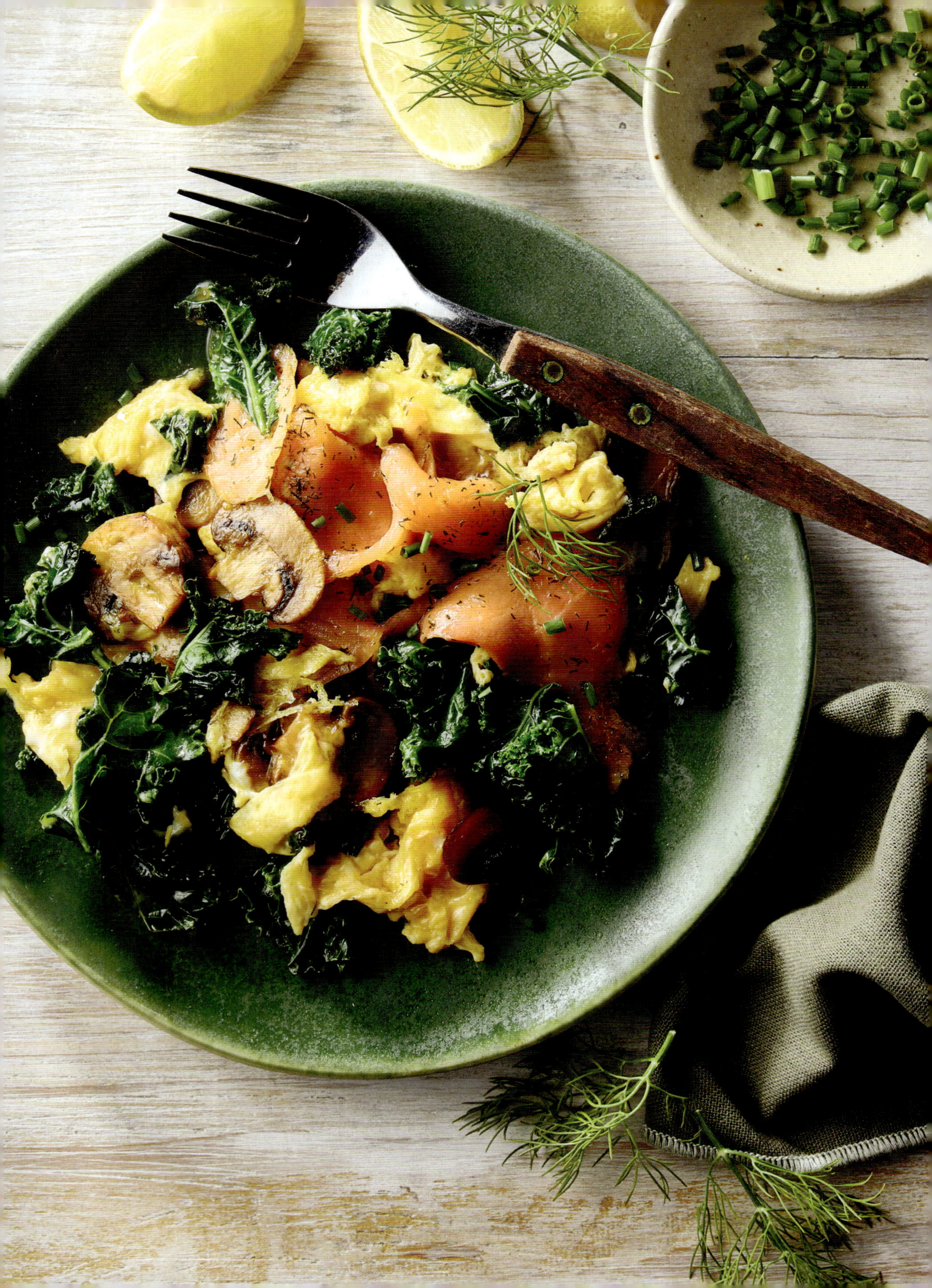

SMOKED SALMON AND VEGGIE SCRAMBLE

SERVES 1 • CARBS PER SERVE: 3 GRAMS

---

1 teaspoon extra-virgin olive oil

½ cup mushrooms, sliced

½ cup chopped fresh spinach or kale

2 eggs, beaten

50 grams smoked salmon, sliced

salt and pepper

fresh chives or dill, to garnish

1. Heat the olive oil in a non-stick frying pan over medium heat. Add the sliced mushrooms and sauté for 2–3 minutes until they begin to soften.

2. Add the leafy greens and cook, stirring, until just wilted (they really only need 1 minute).

3. Pour the eggs over the vegetables in the pan. Allow eggs to set slightly, then gently stir and fold to scramble them with the vegetables

4. When the eggs are nearly cooked through, fold in the smoked salmon and allow to warm (about 45 seconds).

5. Remove from the heat, season with salt and pepper to taste, and garnish with the fresh herbs. Serve immediately and enjoy!

BAKED CHICKEN AND BRUSSELS SPROUTS

SERVES 1 • CARBS PER SERVE: 9 GRAMS

---

100 grams brussels
sprouts, halved

35 grams broccoli
florets

⅓ small zucchini, sliced

2 garlic cloves, minced

1 teaspoon extra-virgin
olive oil

zest and juice of
⅓ lemon

salt and pepper

120 grams skinless
chicken breast

¼ teaspoon paprika

¼ teaspoon dried
thyme

½ cup baby spinach

¼ cup chopped fresh
parsley and basil

1. Preheat the oven to 200°C. Line a small baking
    tray with baking paper.

2. Toss the brussels sprouts, broccoli, zucchini and
    garlic with half the oil, half the lemon zest, and salt
    and pepper to taste. Arrange on the tray.

3. Rub the chicken with the remaining olive oil and
    lemon zest, and all the paprika, thyme and lemon
    juice. Season lightly. Place chicken among the
    vegetables on the tray.

4. Bake for 25 minutes, turning the chicken and
    tossing the veggies at the halfway point, until the
    chicken is cooked through and the vegetables are
    golden. In the final 3–4 minutes, scatter spinach
    over the veggies to wilt.

5. Remove the tray from the oven, finish with fresh
    herbs and serve immediately.

MISO MUSHROOM SEAFOOD SOUP

SERVES 1 • CARBS PER SERVE: 6 GRAMS

---

100 grams mushrooms, sliced

1 clove garlic, sliced

2 teaspoons tamari

1 teaspoon sesame oil

1 cup raw bok choy, chopped

1 teaspoon fresh ginger, grated

1½ cups chicken stock

100 grams seafood (prawns, scallops or white-fleshed fish)

1 tablespoon white miso paste

½ small red chilli, sliced, to garnish

½ spring onion, sliced, to garnish

chopped fresh chives and coriander, to garnish

1. Simmer mushrooms, garlic, tamari, sesame oil, bok choy and ginger in stock for 3–4 minutes.

2. Add the seafood and cook until just firm.

3. Remove from heat. Dissolve the miso paste in a little hot broth then return to the soup and stir through.

4. Garnish with the chilli, spring onion and fresh herbs to serve.

5. Serve immediately.

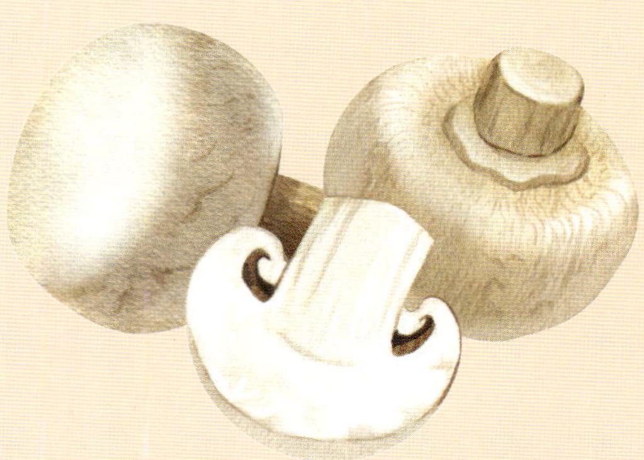

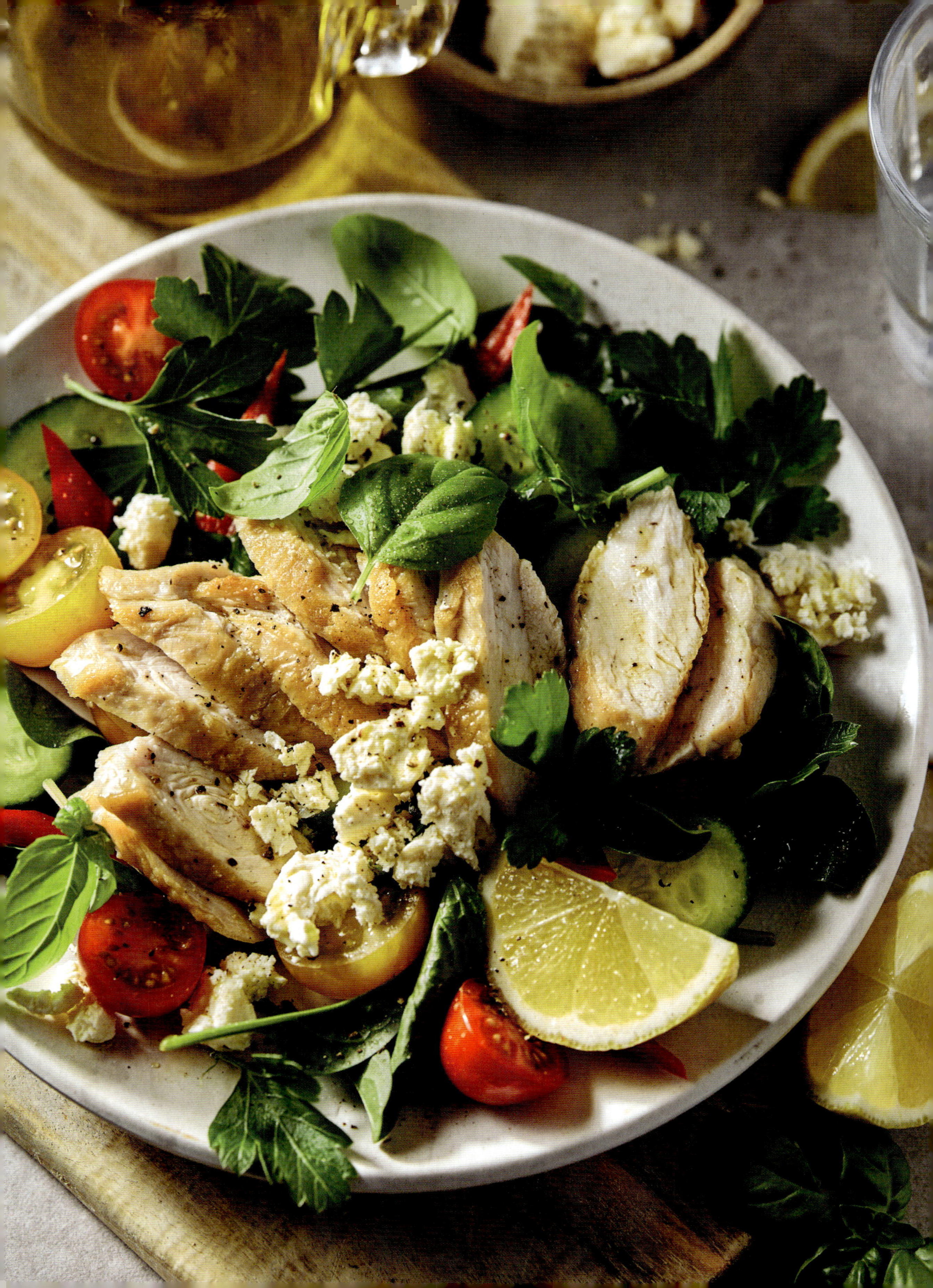

TURKEY AND MIXED VEG BOWL

SERVES 1 • CARBS PER SERVE: 8 GRAMS

120 grams turkey breast (raw, or precooked slices)

salt and pepper

juice of ½ lemon

1 teaspoon extra-virgin olive oil

1 cup baby spinach or mixed greens

½ cup halved cherry tomatoes

½ small cucumber, sliced

¼ red capsicum, sliced

2 tablespoons crumbled feta

1 tablespoon extra-virgin olive oil

chopped fresh parsley and basil, to serve

1. If raw, season turkey breast with a little salt, pepper and lemon juice. Pan-fry in olive oil for 8–10 minutes over medium heat, until cooked through. Remove from the heat, then slice.

2. Pile the greens in a serving bowl. Top with the veggies and turkey slices. Crumble the feta over, drizzle with olive oil and lemon juice, then sprinkle with fresh herbs.

3. Toss gently, taste, then season with extra salt, pepper or lemon if needed.

Supporting eye health

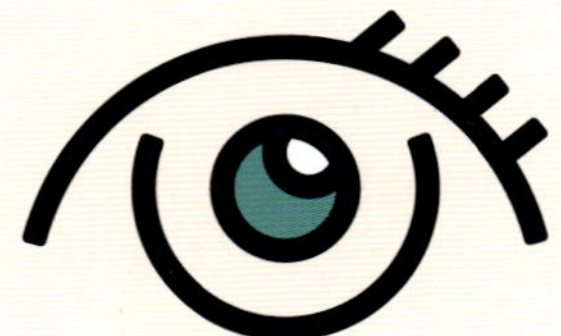

**Focus: Continued weight loss
and taking care of eye health**

Taking care of your eye health is critical with type 2 diabetes, because high blood glucose can damage the tiny delicate blood vessels in your eyes, leading to serious problems with vision and blindness. You have a higher risk for cataracts, glaucoma, macular oedema and diabetic retinopathy with T2D. These complications can be silent, and sadly you can't them reverse after the damage is done.

This is the last week of phase 2 – the adaptation phase.

For those of you who have 10 or more kilograms to lose, your weight loss should be quite significant, and can range from 4 kilograms for some up to 10 kilograms for others. Obviously, this is so individual for all.

Take time to see how far you have come. Around the 6-week mark is where I often see people relax a little bit once they've seen all the success so far – or they could see the dreaded weight-loss plateau. Don't be deterred by the weight-loss plateau. Like all things in life, it will pass. Stay strong and remember it is worth it.

By now, you have a real feel for non-starchy vegetables, what lean proteins to have and how to eat as someone with T2D, prediabetes or insulin resistance.

BEST FOODS FOR EYE HEALTH

Consuming foods rich in antioxidants, vitamins and minerals that support vision can help reduce the risk of eye complications. These include the following:

- **leafy greens** including spinach, kale, and collard greens
- **oily fish** including salmon, sardines, and mackerel
- **orange/yellow vegetables** such as carrots, sweet potatoes, and pumpkin
- **eggs**
- **citrus fruits** such as oranges, lemons and grapefruit
- **nuts and seeds** including almonds, walnuts and sunflower seeds
- **legumes** such as beans and lentils.

Including these foods in a balanced diet, a ongside tight blood glucose control and regular eye exams, is key to supporting eye health for those with type 2 diabetes.

Reminders

- What are your measurements?
- What non-scale victories have you had, such as dropping clothes sizes, feeling more confident, coming off medication, sleeping better, no longer snoring, doing more exercise? I really do love all of these wins!

Daily habits

- regular exercise
- managing medications
- sleeping well
- walking after meals
- managing stress
- calf raises.

	BREAKFAST	MID-MORNING	LUNCH	MID-AFTERNOON	DINNER
MONDAY	Eye-health smoothie (page 343)	Skip	Cottage cheese wrap (page 268)	½ cup blueberries	Turkey lentil soup (page 345)
TUESDAY	2 cottage cheese, egg and herb muffins (page 267)	10 cashews	Herb, egg and spinach slice (page 316)	Kiwifruit (skin on)	Pumpkin chicken curry (page 349)
WEDNESDAY	Diabetes-friendly chia pudding (page 270)	Skip	Spinach, orange, feta and tuna salad (page 346)	10:10 SDL protein bar	Herb, egg and spinach slice (page 316)
THURSDAY	Eye-health smoothie (page 343)	Skip	Turkey and mixed veg bowl (page 339)	2 celery stalks and 2 teaspoons almond butter	Pumpkin chicken curry (page 349)
FRIDAY	Egg and sardine breakfast (page 344)	Skip	Low-carb green goddess salad with chicken (page 321)	1 orange	Turkey lentil soup (page 345)
SATURDAY	Greek yoghurt, berry and mint breakfast bowl (page 300)	5 walnuts	Spinach, orange, feta and tuna salad (page 346)	10:10 SDL protein bar	Spiced salmon and Mediterranean veggie tray bake (page 294)
SUNDAY	Eye-health smoothie (page 343)	Skip	Salmon health bowl (page 276)	15 pistachios	Healthy mince bake (page 307)

BEVERAGES Water, plus optional coffee, tea, green tea, herbal tea, electrolytes

EYE-HEALTH SMOOTHIE

SERVES 1 • CARBS PER SERVE: 13 GRAMS

½ cup unsweetened almond milk

¼ cup Greek yoghurt

1 cup baby spinach

½ cup chopped kale

1 medium carrot, peeled and chopped

¼ avocado, peeled

1 tablespoon ground linseed (flaxseed)

1 scoop whey protein isolate

½ teaspoon vanilla extract

½ teaspoon ground cinnamon

squeeze of lemon or lime juice

ice cubes (for a creamy texture)

1. Put all the ingredients in a high-speed blender, starting with the almond milk and yoghurt. Then add the greens, carrot, avocado, ground linseed, protein powder, vanilla and cinnamon. Finally, squeeze in some lemon juice and add some ice cubes. Blend until smooth and creamy. Adjust consistency with extra almond milk, if needed.

2. Taste and adjust the sweetness or spice. If desired, add a pinch of stevia powder for extra sweetness. Pour into a glass and serve immediately.

EGG AND SARDINE BREAKFAST

SERVES 1 • CARBS PER SERVE: 5 GRAMS

---

1 teaspoon extra-virgin olive oil

¼ small onion, finely diced

2 cloves garlic, minced

90 grams canned sardines

1 small tomato, chopped

2 large eggs

salt and pepper

fresh parsley or chives, to serve

squeeze of lemon, to serve

1. Heat the olive oil in a small frying pan over medium heat. Sauté the onion and garlic, until soft.

2. Add the sardines, breaking them up gently. Stir in the chopped tomato. Cook for 2–3 minutes.

3. Make two small wells and crack in the eggs. Lower heat, cover and cook for 3–4 minutes, until the eggs are set.

4. Season with salt and pepper to taste, and serve warm with the fresh herbs and a squeeze of lemon.

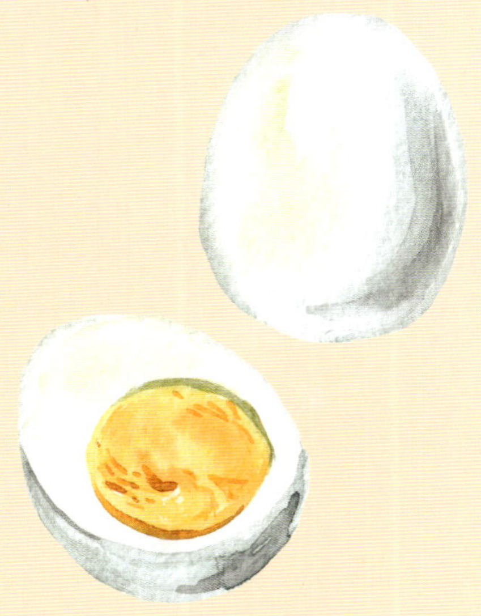

TURKEY LENTIL SOUP

SERVES 2 • CARBS PER SERVE: 12 GRAMS

1½ tablespoons extra-virgin olive oil

¼ medium onion, finely chopped

1 small carrot, sliced

1 celery stalk, sliced

225 grams turkey mince

½ teaspoon ground cumin

½ teaspoon ground coriander

½ teaspoon paprika

½ teaspoon ground turmeric

½ teaspoon ground ginger or 1–2 cm fresh ginger, grated

½ teaspoon salt (adjust to taste)

¼ teaspoon pepper

720 ml chicken stock

¾ cup grams canned diced tomatoes

½ cup shredded kale or spinach

2 bay leaves

½ cup canned lentils, drained and rinsed

juice of 1 lemon (optional)

fresh parsley leaves, to garnish

shaved parmesan, to garnish

1. Heat the olive oil in a large pot over medium heat. Add the chopped onion, carrot and celery. Sauté for about 5 minutes until the vegetables soften slightly.

2. Add the turkey mince to the pot and stir to combine. Cook for 3 minutes to brown the mince.

3. Stir in the cumin, coriander, paprika, turmeric, ginger, salt and pepper. Cook for another 2 minutes.

4. Add the stock, tomatoes, kale and bay leaves. Stir well. Bring soup to a simmer, cover partially and cook for 15–20 minutes until the vegetables are tender.

5. Stir in the lentils and simmer uncovered for another 10 minutes.

6. Remove from heat, stir in fresh lemon juice (if using) and adjust seasoning. Serve hot, garnished with fresh parsley and shaved parmesan.

SPINACH, ORANGE, FETA AND TUNA SALAD

SERVES 1 • CARBS PER SERVE: 10 GRAMS

2 cups baby spinach leaves

½ orange, cut into segments

30 grams feta, crumbled

70 grams canned flaked tuna

1 tablespoon chopped toasted walnuts or almonds, to serve

DRESSING

1 tablespoon extra-virgin olive oil

1 teaspoon apple cider vinegar

1 tablespoon chopped fresh mint and parsley

salt and pepper

1. Place the spinach in a serving bowl. Top with the orange segments, crumbled feta and flaked tuna.

2. To make the dressing, whisk the ingredients together in a small bowl.

3. Drizzle the dressing over salad, tossing gently to combine. Sprinkle with nuts to serve.

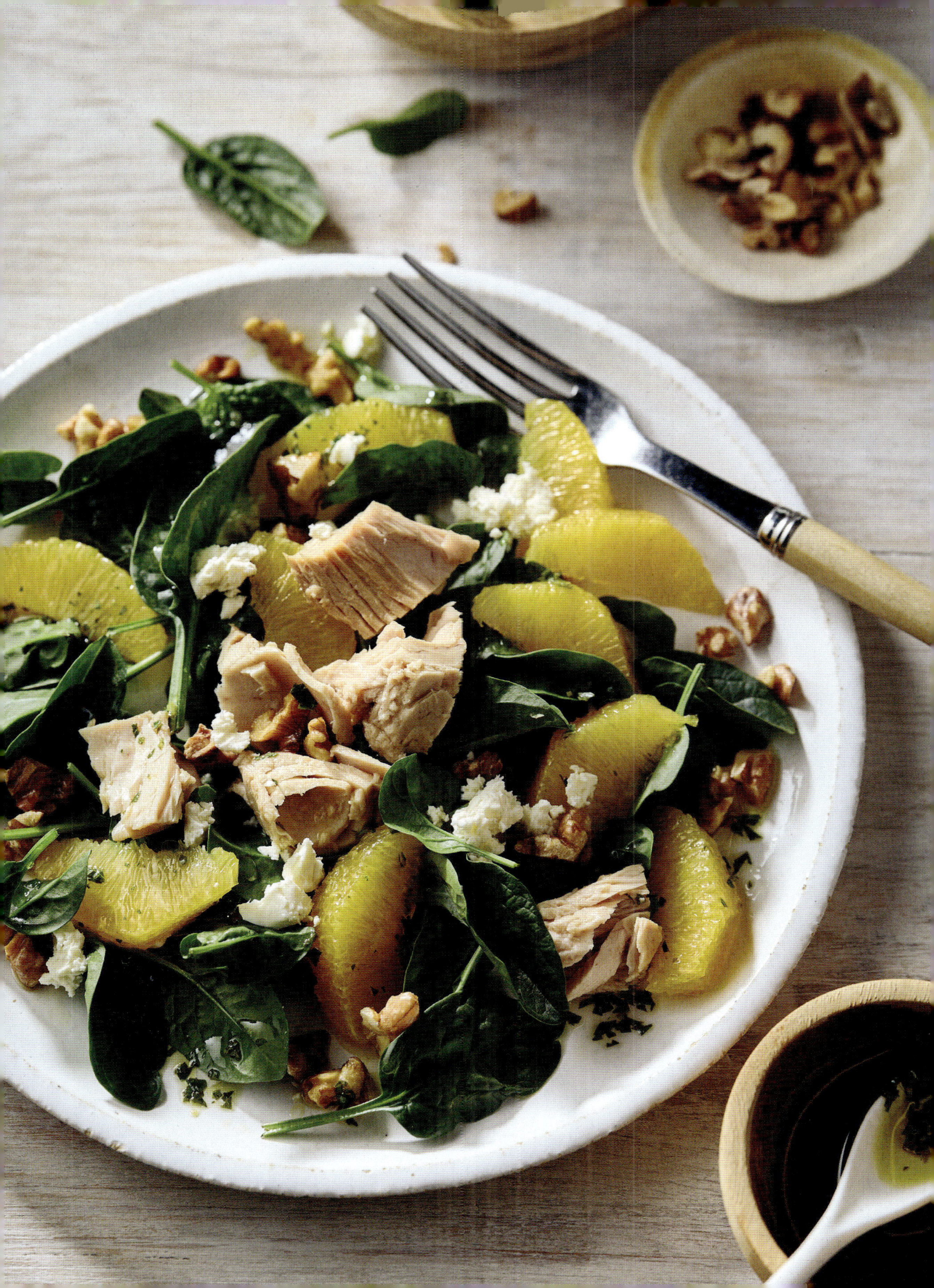

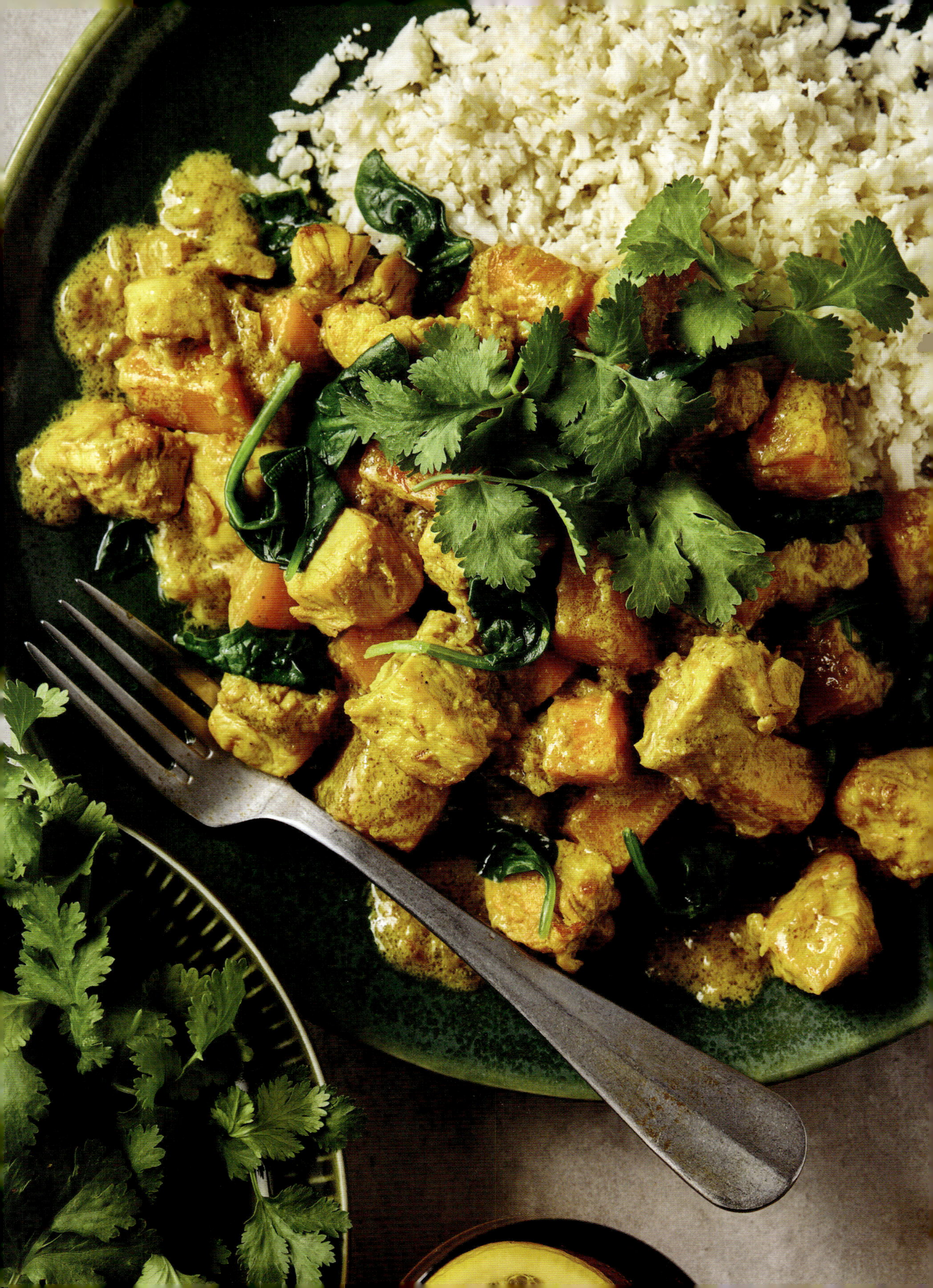

PUMPKIN CHICKEN CURRY

SERVES 2 • CARBS PER SERVE: 8 GRAMS

---

2 teaspoons extra-virgin olive oil

½ medium onion, diced

4 cloves garlic, minced

½ tablespoon fresh ginger, grated

250 grams skinless chicken breast, cubed

1½ teaspoons curry powder

200 grams peeled pumpkin, diced

200 ml canned coconut milk

1 cup baby spinach (optional)

salt and pepper

½ tablespoon chopped fresh coriander (optional)

cauliflower rice, to serve

1. Heat the olive oil in a saucepan on medium heat. Sauté the onion, garlic and ginger, until softened.

2. Add the chicken pieces and brown on all sides.

3. Stir in the curry powder and cook for 1 minute. Add pumpkin and coconut milk, bring to a gentle simmer, then cover and cook for 15–20 minutes, until the pumpkin and chicken are fork-tender.

4. Stir in spinach until just wilted. Season with salt and pepper, and scatter with fresh coriander (if using).

5. Serve with cauliflower rice or low-carb veggies.

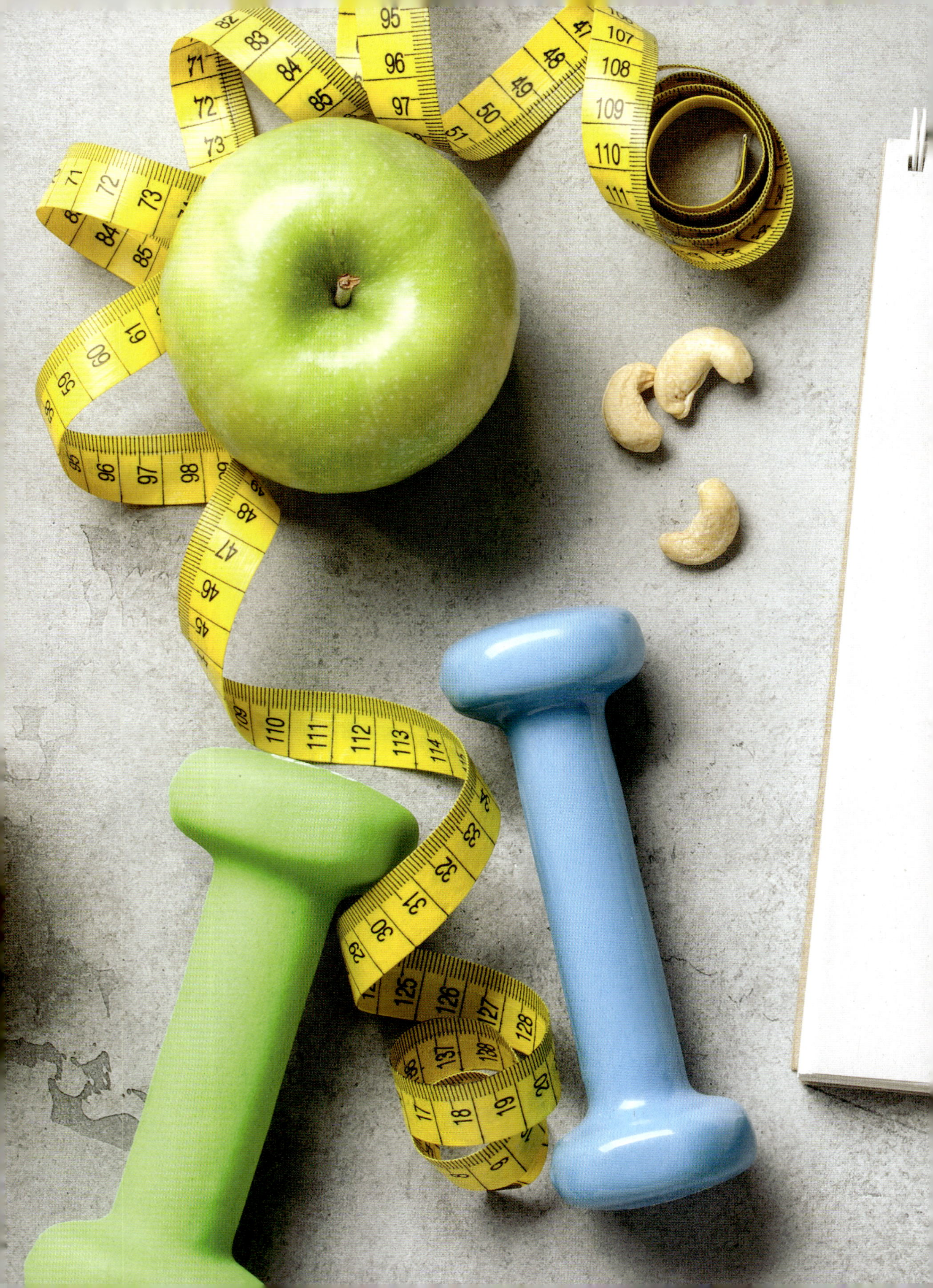

PHASE 3
(WEEKS 7–9):

Continued Weight Loss

We're aiming to intensify fat loss and hopefully reverse diabetes.

In this final phase, it's time to start thinking about the upcoming shift to maintaining your weight and health goals. Mid-morning and mid-afternoon snacks are no longer in the program. There are a few reasons for this. Having a break between each meal helps with blood sugar control because it reduces the amount of time any glucose can enter the bloodstream, really giving your body time to process and stabilise between meals.

This phase is about accelerated weight loss so you are having fewer calories. Avoiding snacking can really benefit blood glucose levels, supporting weight loss and making you more sensitive to insulin. I don't have patients do this in the early phases of the program because I'm very aware of hypoglycaemia.

The hypoglycaemia risk for someone with T2D following a ketogenic diet is generally highest at the start, particularly if you are still taking insulin or medications that lower blood glucose. As you lose weight and your carbohydrate intake drops, your insulin sensitivity improves and blood glucose stabilises, allowing many to reduce or discontinue these medications. The risk of hypoglycaemia is much lower and you are well and truly managing low-carb eating and ketosis.

If you want to still snack, however, choose from the following:

- 25 grams cheese
- ¼ cup cottage cheese with ½ teaspoon cinnamon
- 10:10 SDL protein bar
- 1 apple, 1 orange or 1 pear
- ½ cup blueberries or 1 cup strawberries
- 10 almonds, 15 pistachios or 5 walnuts
- 1 tablespoon hummus with ½ carrot
- 1 kiwifruit
- 2 stalks celery with 2 teaspoons almond butter

A few reminders

- For those of you on medications, stay on top of your check-ups.

- Continue to be aware of possible hypoglycaemia. Avoid this with close monitoring, medication reviews and prompt interventions. Don't get complacent.

- By now, you should be doing a combination of cardiovascular exercise as well as resistance training. Make sure you are looking at doing this like a job. Exercise is the elixir of life; it is non-negotiable. You need to be doing something daily. Where there's a will, there's a way.

- How are you feeling about your journey so far? Look back at your starting point – any pictures you took, measurements, weight, mood and skin conditions – and think about your sleep now, energy levels and success so far.

Are you still ...

- doing the 12/12 fast?
- walking after meals?
- stressing less?
- sleeping well?
- keeping track of your progress?

- doing your meal prep?
- exercising?
- managing medications?
- setting boundaries to make sure you are on track?

Remember – this is the biggest gift you can ever give yourself. You are changing the course of your life.

During these three weeks, we start to create lifelong habits. It takes about 66 days to create a lifelong habit, so embrace your new way of life and eating. Remember, what you did in the past was *not* normal eating because it created a disease called type 2 diabetes. Healthy eating is normal. Again, you can repeat meals and change proteins.

Supporting skin and preventing infections

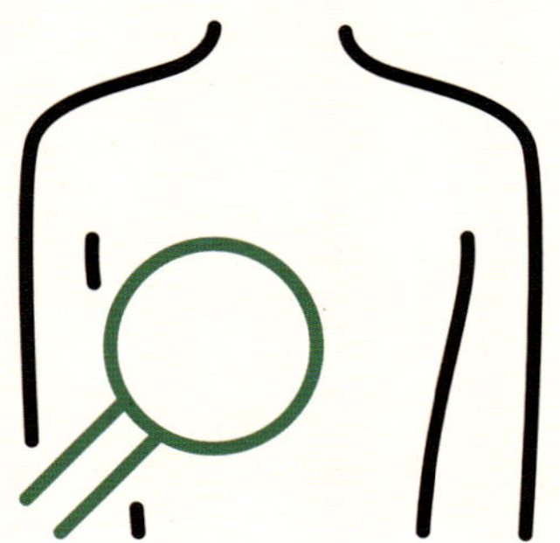

Focus: All about loving our skin while losing weight!

The program is still focused on accelerated weight loss but, as you all know, I like to tackle health holistically.

Taking care of and supporting your skin is essential.

Type 2 diabetes increases the risk of skin complications such as dryness, infections and poor wound healing, and can change the texture of the skin.

Diabetes can damage blood vessels, nerves and the immune system, leading to reduced circulation, impaired collagen production and a higher risk of skin infections. When the skin is dry and cracked, it's more vulnerable to infection, and slow-healing wounds can develop into serious complications if not managed.

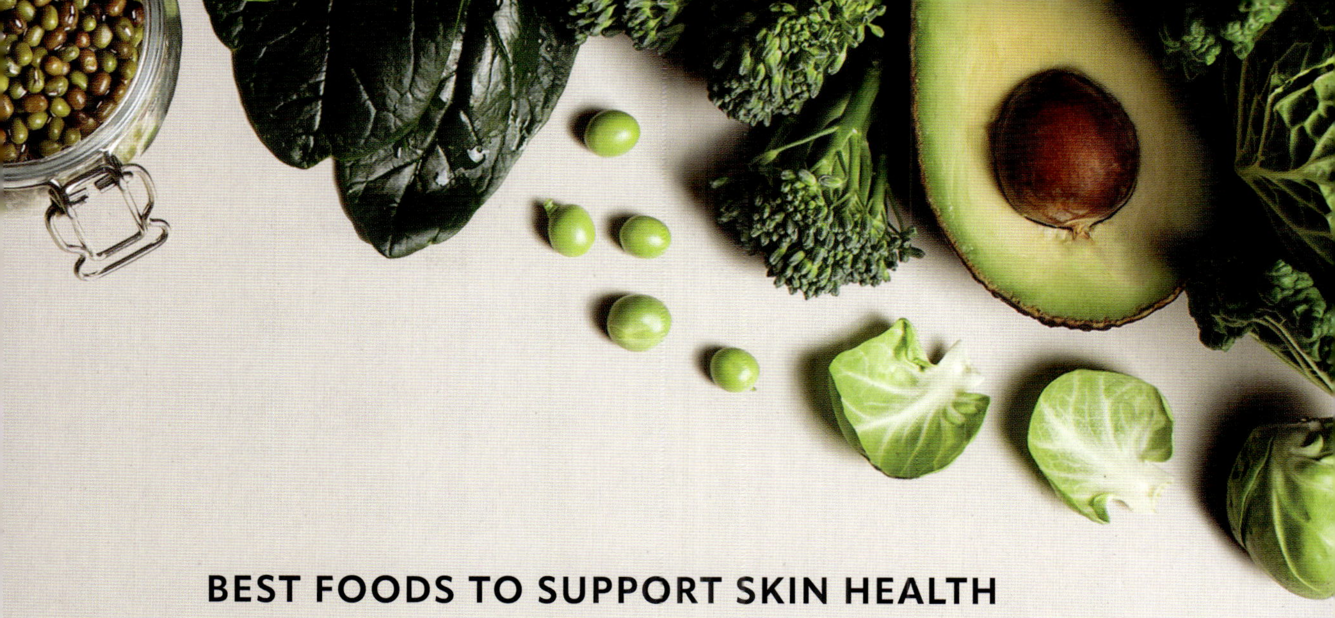

BEST FOODS TO SUPPORT SKIN HEALTH

Some foods are natural sources of collagen plus vitamins and minerals that support skin health. These include:

- fatty fish (salmon, sardines, mackerel)
- avocados
- nuts and seeds (walnuts, sunflower seeds, linseeds/flaxseeds)
- colourful vegetables (red and yellow capsicums, spinach, carrots)
- broccoli and leafy greens
- eggs and dairy
- green tea
- water-rich fruits and vegetables (watermelon, celery, cucumber).

If you have T2D, you should focus on a variety of omega-3 rich foods, low-GI vegetables, nuts, seeds and proper hydration to maintain strong, healthy skin and reduce the risk of complications. You could also consider topical skincare.

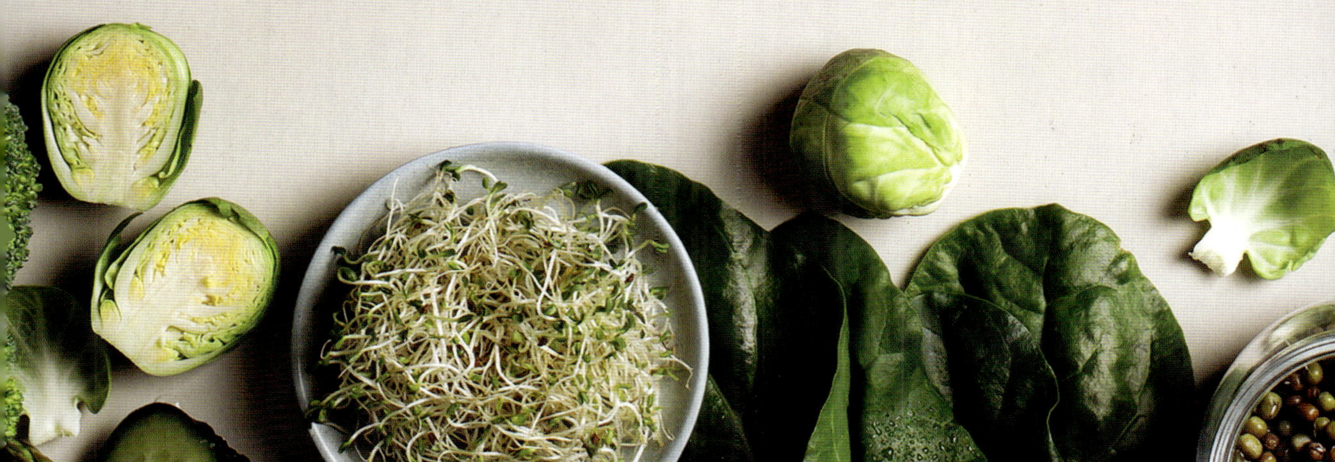

	BREAKFAST	MID-MORNING	LUNCH	MID-AFTERNOON	DINNER
MONDAY	Skin-healthy smoothie (page 357)	Nil	Sardine salad (page 292)	Nil	Broccoli fried rice with fish and egg (page 363)
TUESDAY	Greens and avocado omelette (page 366)	Nil	Cottage cheese wrap (page 268) with tomato, lettuce and cucumber	Nil	Salmon souvlaki and Greek salad (page 369)
WEDNESDAY	Diabetes-friendly chia pudding (page 270)	Nil	Avocado and salmon low-carb lunch bowl (page 289)	Nil	Shredded chicken noodle soup with konjac noodles (page 364)
THURSDAY	Skin-healthy smoothie (page 357)	Nil	Tofu rainbow salad (page 358)	Nil	Broccoli fried rice with fish and egg (page 363)
FRIDAY	Capsicum eggs (page 360)	Nil	Paprika chicken with capsicum, squash and quinoa (page 367)	Nil	Shredded chicken noodle soup with konjac noodles (page 364)
SATURDAY	Skin-glowing Greek yoghurt parfait (page 361)	Nil	Low-carb green goddess salad with chicken (page 321)	Nil	Prawn and bok choy broth (page 325)
SUNDAY	Skin-healthy smoothie (page 357)	Nil	Salmon health bowl (page 276)	Nil	Mackerel patties (page 319) and 1½ cups mixed steamed greens, garnished with fresh herbs, chilli and a drizzle of olive oil with juice of ½ lemon

BEVERAGES Water, plus optional coffee, tea, green tea, herbal tea, electrolytes

SKIN-HEALTHY SMOOTHIE

SERVES 1 • CARBS PER SERVE: 10 GRAMS

1 cup baby spinach

½ cup unsweetened almond milk

½ cup frozen strawberries

¼ avocado

1 tablespoon chia seeds, plus extra to serve

1 tablespoon hemp seeds or ground linseed (flaxseed)

1 serve collagen peptides or protein powder

juice of ¼ lemon

4–6 mint leaves, plus extra to serve

ice cubes, to make it like a frappe

Blend the spinach with almond milk until completely smooth. Add the strawberries, avocado, chia seeds, hemp seeds, collagen, lemon juice, mint and ice. Blend until creamy and pink–green. Pour, and garnish with extra seeds or mint.

Tip: If you're interested in my collagen, email contact@sarahdilorenzo.com

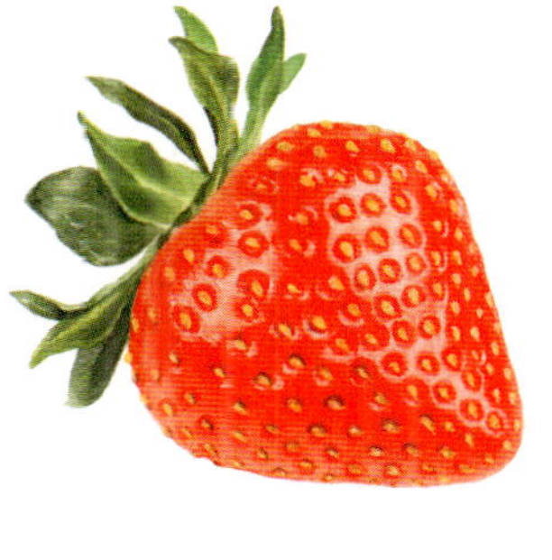
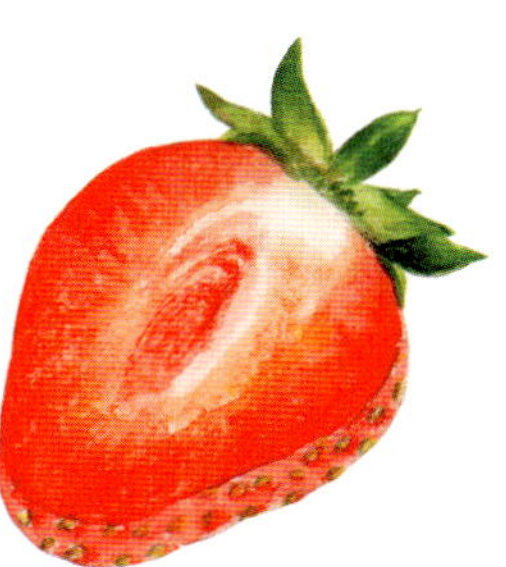

TOFU RAINBOW SALAD

SERVES 1 • CARBS PER SERVE: 9 GRAMS

100 grams firm tofu

½ cup baby spinach, roughly chopped

¼ medium red capsicum, thinly sliced

¼ small carrot, grated or julienned

¼ celery stalk, thinly sliced

¼ small Lebanese cucumber, sliced into half-moons

1 tablespoon chopped fresh herbs (parsley, basil, coriander or chives)

1 tablespoon extra-virgin olive oil

1 teaspoon lemon or lime juice

salt and pepper

pinch of garlic powder

chopped fresh coriander, to garnish

fresh chillies, to garnish (optional)

1 tablespoon crushed roasted almonds, to garnish

1. Pat the tofu dry, cut into cubes and pan-fry until golden brown on each side.

2. In a bowl, place the spinach and arrange the salad vegetables and fried tofu in piles on top. Scatter with chopped herbs, then the olive oil, lemon juice, salt and pepper to taste, and garlic powder. Toss salad together until well mixed.

3. Taste and adjust seasoning as needed. Garnish with fresh coriander and chillies (if using) and crushed almonds.

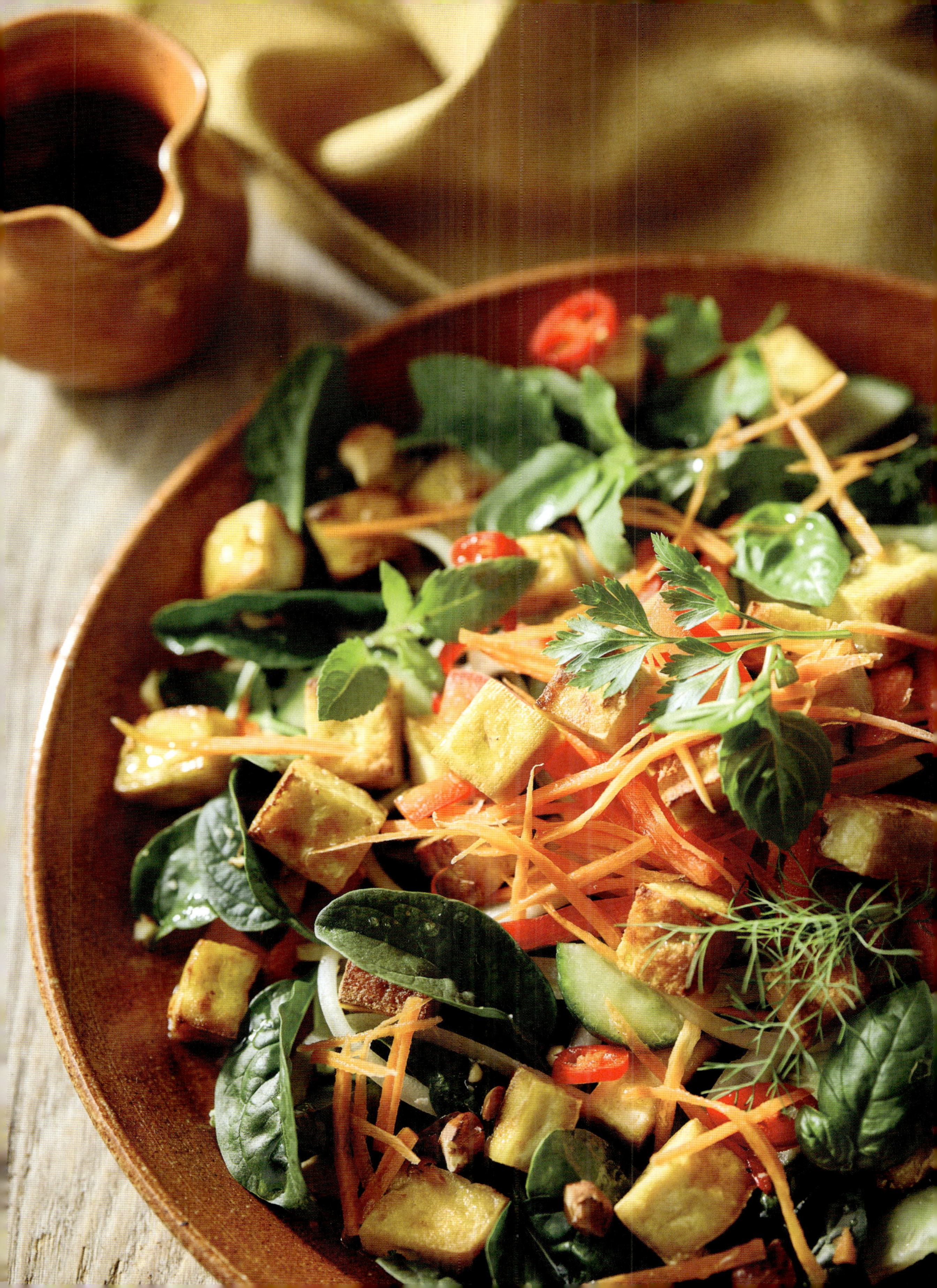

CAPSICUM EGGS

SERVES 1 • CARBS PER SERVE: 4 GRAMS

---

1 teaspoon extra-virgin olive oil

1 capsicum, cut crosswise to make two thick rings

2 eggs

salt and pepper

fresh parsley and chives, to garnish

2 teaspoons feta, to garnish (optional)

1. Heat the olive oil in a non-stick frying pan over medium heat. Place capsicum rings flat in the pan and cook for 1 minute.

2. Crack an egg into the centre of each capsicum ring. Cover and cook for 3–4 minutes, until the eggs are just set.

3. Season with salt and pepper, garnish with fresh herbs and feta (if using) and serve.

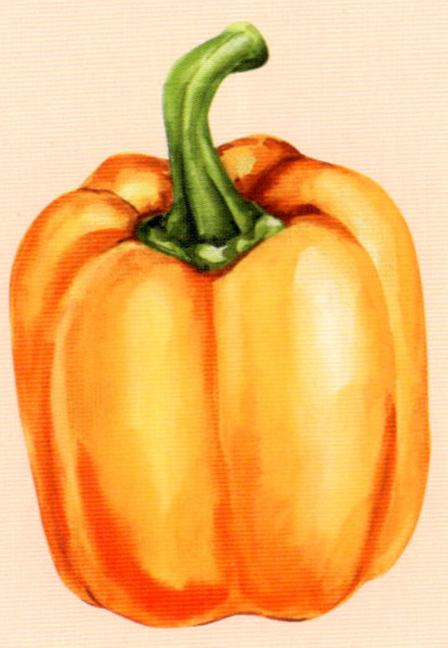

SKIN-GLOWING GREEK YOGHURT PARFAIT

SERVES 1 • CARBS PER SERVE: 8 GRAMS

⅔ cup full-fat Greek yoghurt

⅓ cup fresh or frozen raspberries

1 tablespoon chia seeds

1 tablespoon chopped almonds

1 tablespoon coconut cream

½ teaspoon cinnamon

Spoon the Greek yoghurt into a deep bowl or jar. Top with layers of berries, chia seeds and nuts. Add the coconut cream and cinnamon. Enjoy immediately!

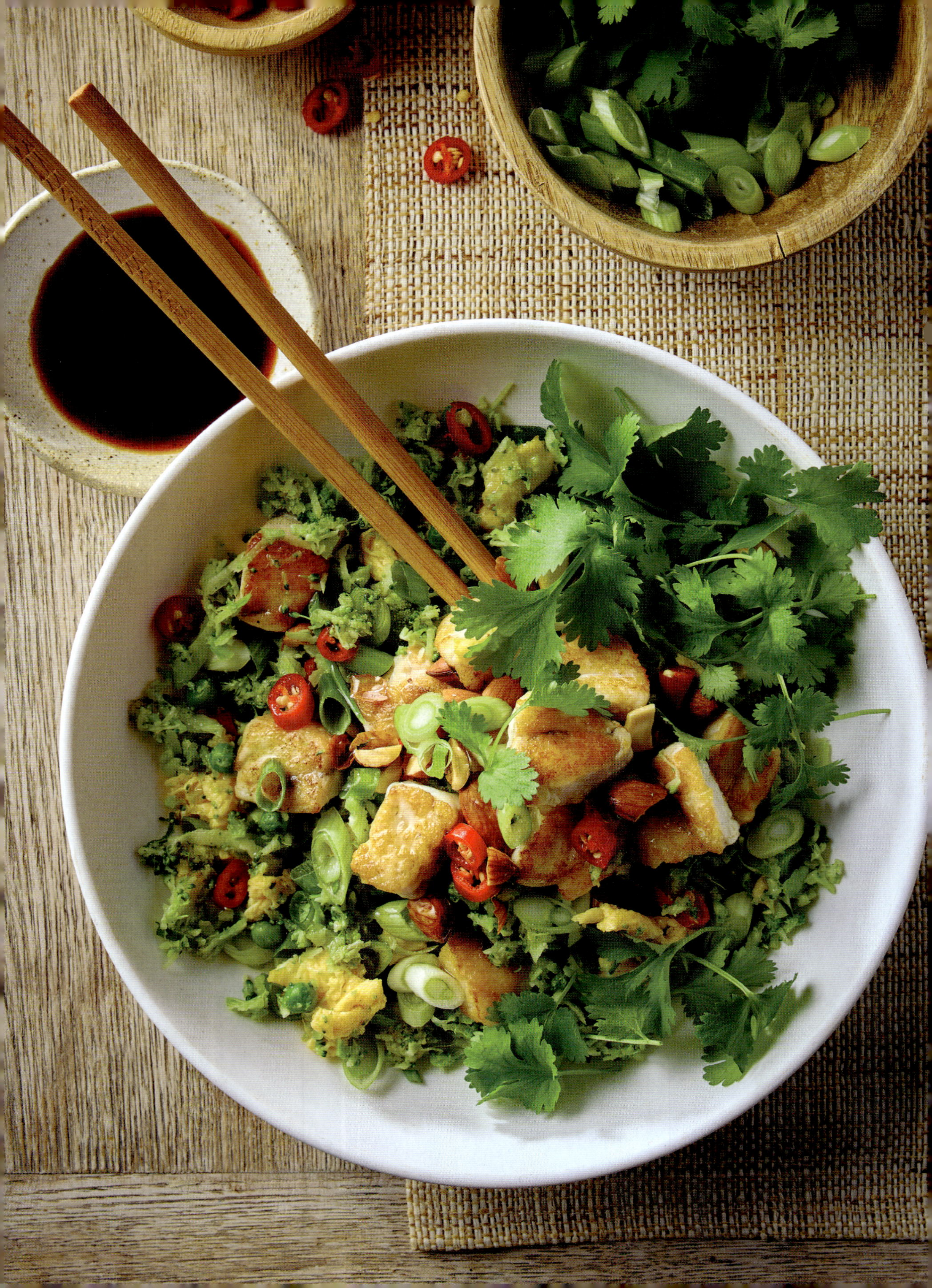

BROCCOLI FRIED RICE WITH FISH AND EGG

SERVES 1 • CARBS PER SERVE: 13 GRAMS

1 tablespoon extra-virgin olive oil

100 grams white fish fillet (e.g. barramundi or snapper), cut into pieces

2 cloves garlic, minced

2 teaspoons grated fresh ginger

½ small chilli, sliced

2 cups riced broccoli (about 1 medium, grated or food-processed)

¼ cup frozen peas

1 egg, lightly beaten

1 tablespoon tamari (or soy sauce)

2 spring onions, sliced, plus extra to garnish

1 tablespoon chopped roasted almonds, to garnish

fresh chilli slices, to garnish (optional)

1. Heat half the olive oil in a frying pan. Sear fish pieces for 2 minutes per side, or until just cooked. Remove and set aside.

2. In the same pan, add the remaining oil. Sauté the garlic, ginger and chilli for 30 seconds until fragrant. Add the riced broccoli and peas. Stir-fry for 3–4 minutes, until the broccoli is bright green and peas are hot.

3. Push the vegetables to one side, pour the egg into the empty side and scramble until just set. Then combine with the vegetable mixture.

4. Add the tamari and spring onions, plus the cooked fish pieces, and stir until everything is heated through.

5. Serve garnished with extra spring onion, almonds and chilli.

SHREDDED CHICKEN NOODLE SOUP WITH KONJAC NOODLES

SERVES 2 • CARBS PER SERVE: 5 GRAMS

1 chicken breast

2–3 cups chicken stock

2 cm fresh ginger, finely sliced or julienned

2 spring onions, sliced (white and green parts separated)

1 small red chilli, sliced (deseeded for mild)

1 cup sliced mushrooms (shiitake or button)

1 heaped teaspoon white or red miso paste

1 small bok choy, sliced

1 pack konjac noodles, rinsed and drained

1 tablespoon chopped fresh coriander

1 teaspoon sesame oil

1. Place the chicken breast in the stock in a saucepan on the stove. Bring to a gentle simmer and poach until just cooked, about 10–12 minutes. Remove the chicken and shred with a fork.

2. Add the ginger, white part of spring onion and chilli to the stock. Simmer for 2–3 minutes before adding the mushrooms. Cook for 3 minutes.

3. Remove some broth, stir through the miso paste to dissolve, then return to the pan.

4. Add bok choy and let wilt (about 1 minute). Add the konjac noodles and cook according to packet directions. Mix in the shredded chicken to warm through.

5. Serve in a deep bowl, topped with the green spring onion tops, fresh coriander and a drizzle of sesame oil.

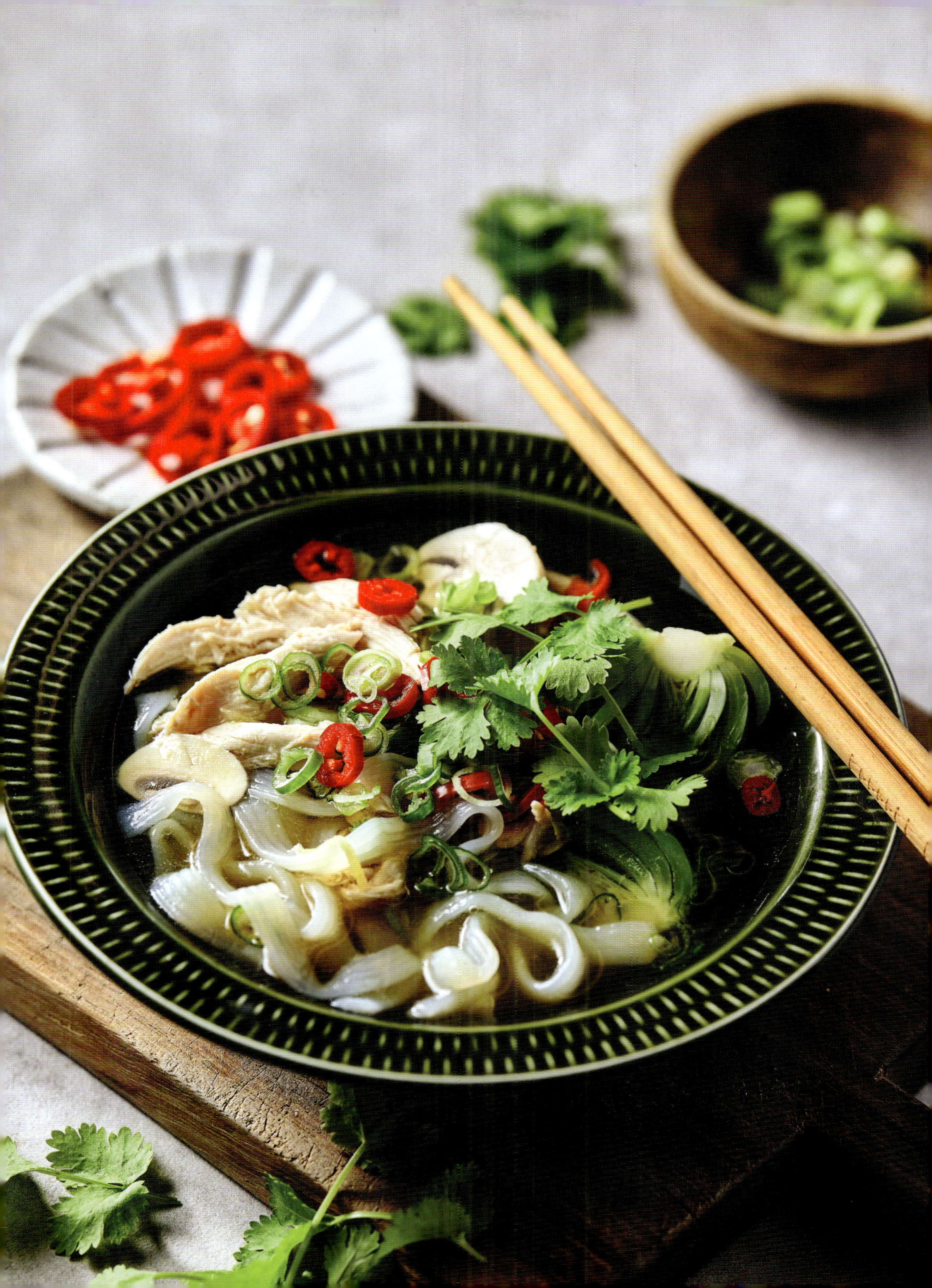

GREENS AND AVOCADO OMELETTE

SERVES 1 • CARBS PER SERVE: 4 GRAMS

---

1 teaspoon extra-virgin olive oil

⅓ cup diced mushrooms

⅓ cup baby spinach, chopped

¼ small tomato, diced (or 3 cherry tomatoes, sliced)

2 eggs

salt and pepper

1 tablespoon chopped mixed fresh herbs (parsley, chives, basil)

¼ avocado, sliced, to serve

1 tablespoon feta, to serve (optional)

chilli, to serve (optional)

1. Heat the olive oil in a non-stick frying pan over medium heat. Sauté the mushrooms for 2 minutes, until softened. Add spinach and tomato, then continue cooking for a couple of minutes.

2. Whisk the eggs in a bowl with salt and pepper to taste, then pour over the vegetable mixture. Scatter the mixed herbs over the top. Cook gently, lifting the edges to allow uncooked egg to flow underneath.

3. When set, fold the omelette in half. Serve with avocado slices on the side (or tucked inside), and add feta and chilli (if using).

PAPRIKA CHICKEN WITH CAPSICUM, SQUASH AND QUINOA

SERVES 1 • CARBS PER SERVE: 15 GRAMS

120 grams skinless chicken breast, cut into strips

1 teaspoon smoked paprika

salt and pepper

1 teaspoon extra-virgin olive oil

½ small capsicum, diced

1 yellow button squash

1 cup shredded lettuce leaves

¼ cup cooked quinoa

lemon wedge, to serve

fresh herbs (parsley or coriander), to serve

1. Toss the chicken strips with the smoked paprika, and salt and pepper to taste.

2. Heat the olive oil in a frying pan over medium heat. Add the chicken and cook for 6–8 minutes, until browned on each side. Remove and set aside.

3. In the same pan, sauté the capsicum and squash until just tender, about 3–5 minutes.

4. Arrange the lettuce on a plate and top with the quinoa, veggies and chicken. Serve with a squeeze of lemon juice and sprinkle of fresh herbs.

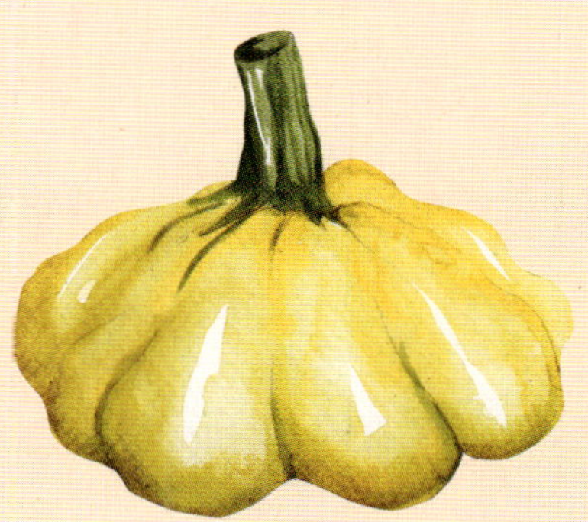

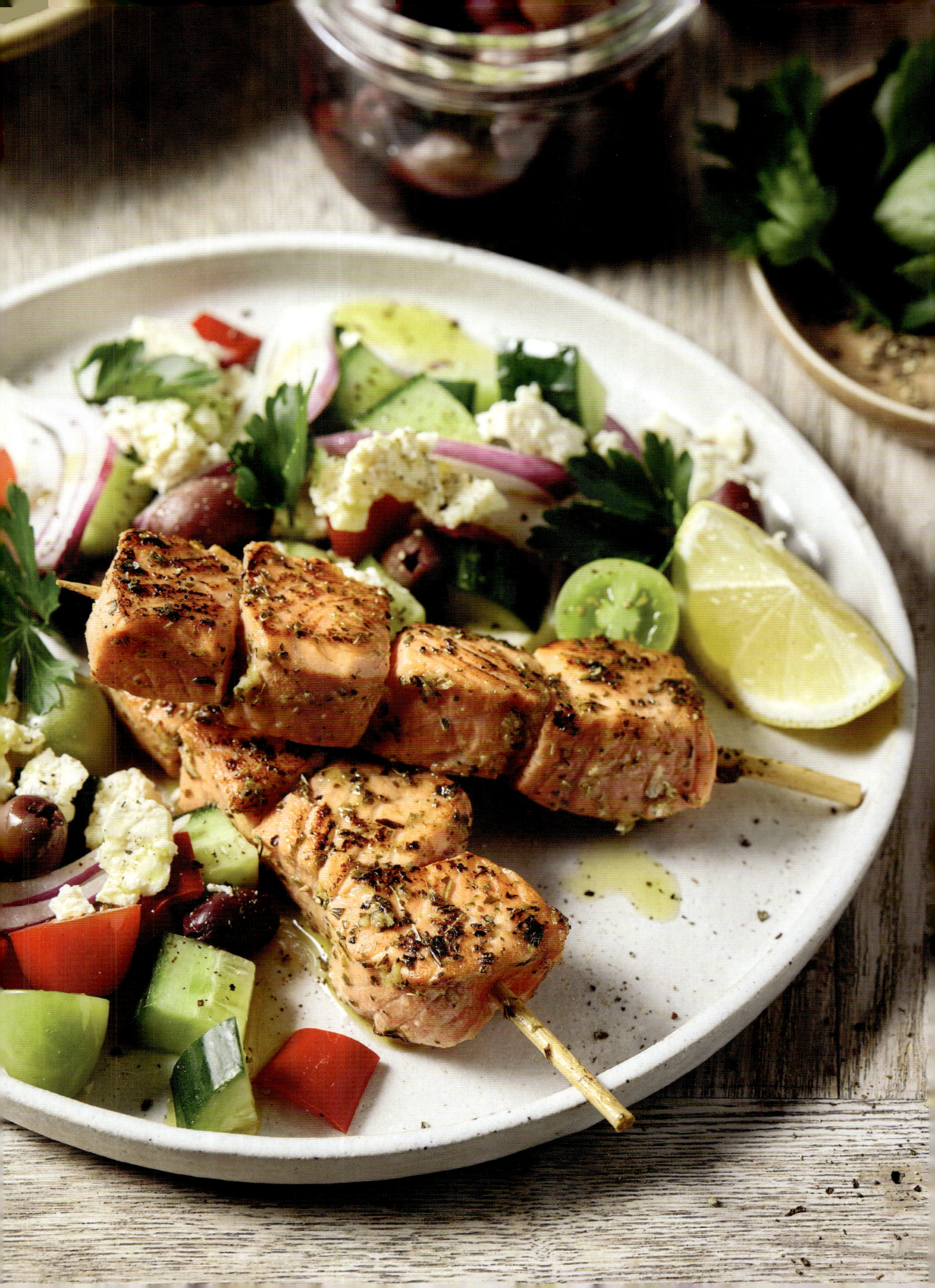

SALMON SOUVLAKI AND GREEK SALAD

SERVES 1 • CARBS PER SERVE: 8 GRAMS

1 tablespoon extra-virgin olive oil

1 tablespoon freshly squeezed lemon juice

½ teaspoon lemon zest

½ teaspoon dried oregano

2 cloves garlic, minced

salt and pepper

120 grams skinless salmon fillet, cut into large cubes

GREEK SALAD

½ cup diced Lebanese cucumber

½ cup halved cherry tomatoes

¼ small red capsicum, diced

2 tablespoons thinly sliced red onion

1–2 tablespoons Kalamata olives, pitted

30 grams feta cheese, crumbled

1 tablespoon extra-virgin olive oil

1 teaspoon red wine vinegar

pinch of dried oregano

salt and pepper

1. Combine the olive oil, lemon juice and zest, oregano, garlic, and salt and pepper to taste. Toss the salmon cubes in the marinade, and leave for at least 10 minutes.

2. Thread the marinated salmon onto two bamboo skewers. Grill or pan-sear for 2–3 minutes each side, until just cooked.

3. To make the salad, arrange the cucumber, tomatoes, capsicum and red onion in a bowl. Top with the olives and feta. Drizzle with olive oil, vinegar, oregano, and salt and pepper. Toss gently and serve.

Supporting mental health and cognition

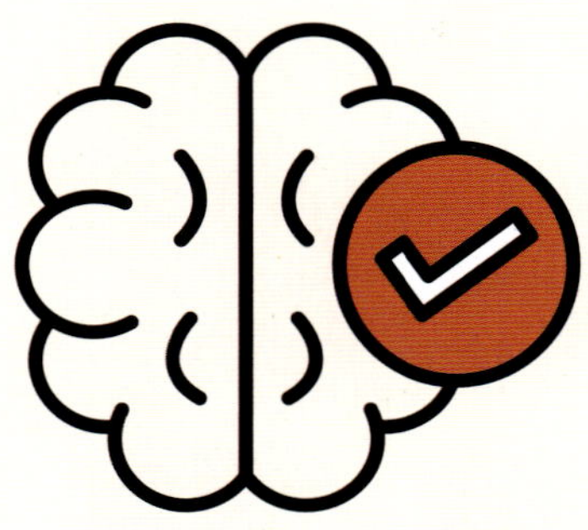

Focus: All about mental health – so critically important

Type 2 diabetes increases the risk of depression. The stress and emotional burden of it all can negatively affect your blood glucose control and overall health.

Living with diabetes means you need to be emotionally resilient and motivated.

When you have poor mental health, you're less inclined to adhere to treatment, lifestyle changes and eating well. This in turn can make your diabetes much worse.

Research shows that diabetes can accelerate brain aging, with faster declines in executive function, processing speed and memory. Insulin resistance in the brain can mean the brain utilises less glucose, and it has increased oxidative stress and neuronal damage. As a result, some people may have issues with memory, processing information and attention.

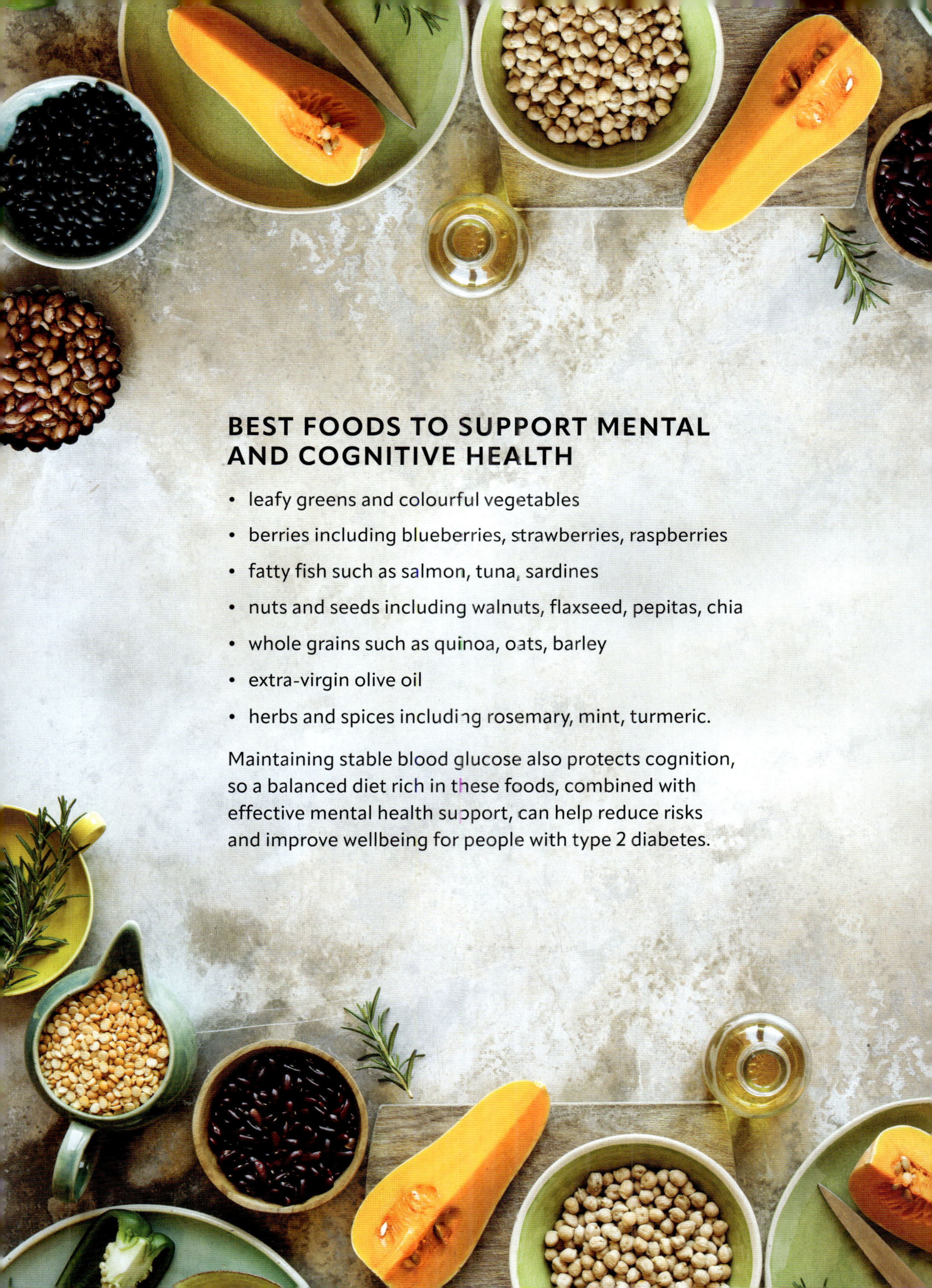

BEST FOODS TO SUPPORT MENTAL AND COGNITIVE HEALTH

- leafy greens and colourful vegetables
- berries including blueberries, strawberries, raspberries
- fatty fish such as salmon, tuna, sardines
- nuts and seeds including walnuts, flaxseed, pepitas, chia
- whole grains such as quinoa, oats, barley
- extra-virgin olive oil
- herbs and spices including rosemary, mint, turmeric.

Maintaining stable blood glucose also protects cognition, so a balanced diet rich in these foods, combined with effective mental health support, can help reduce risks and improve wellbeing for people with type 2 diabetes.

	BREAKFAST	MID-MORNING	LUNCH	MID-AFTERNOON	DINNER
MONDAY	Smoothie to boost mental health (page 373)	Nil	Tofu rainbow salad (page 358), garnished with sunflower seeds	Nil	Chicken turmeric vegetable curry (page 380)
TUESDAY	Oven-baked eggs with mackerel and spinach (page 377)	Nil	Grilled chicken breast salad (page 292)	Nil	Broccoli fried rice with fish and veg (page 363)
WEDNESDAY	Low-carb oat breakfast bowl (page 318)	Nil	Egg salad with turmeric (page 376)	Nil	Salmon souvlaki with Greek salad (page 369)
THURSDAY	Smoothie to boost mental health (page 373)	Nil	Chia bread (page 329) with 2 boiled eggs, ¼ avocado, 2 slices tomato, lettuce and chives	Nil	Chicken turmeric vegetable curry (page 380)
FRIDAY	Omelette with mushrooms, tomato and herbs (page 274)	Nil	Turkey and mixed veg bowl (page 339)	Nil	Steak with bean purée and green herb salad (page 379)
SATURDAY	Sarah's favourite breakfast (page 268)	Nil	Grilled chicken breast salad (page 292)	Nil	Beef mince cups with coriander (page 274)
SUNDAY	Smoothie to boost mental health (page 373)	Nil	Avocado and salmon low-carb lunch bowl (page 289)	Nil	Chicken and green vegetable broth with fresh herbs (page 374)

BEVERAGES Water, plus optional coffee, tea, green tea, herbal tea, electrolytes

SMOOTHIE TO BOOST MENTAL HEALTH

SERVES 1 • CARBS PER SERVE: 10 GRAMS

1 cup baby spinach

½ cup unsweetened almond milk or water

½ cup frozen mixed berries (blueberries, raspberries and blackberries)

8 fresh mint leaves

2 tablespoons walnuts

1 scoop whey protein isolate

1 tablespoon chia or linseeds (flaxseeds)

ice cubes

½ teaspoon vanilla extract (optional)

½ teaspoon ground cinnamon (optional)

1. Place the spinach and almond milk in a blender, then blend until smooth.

2. Add the berries, mint, walnuts, protein powder and seeds. Blend again until creamy.

3. Taste and add ice cubes or extra water for consistency, or a dash of vanilla or cinnamon for flavour (if using). Serve immediately.

CHICKEN AND GREEN VEGETABLE BROTH WITH FRESH HERBS

SERVES 2 • CARBS PER SERVE: 10.8 GRAMS

1 teaspoon extra-virgin olive oil

½ small onion, finely sliced

2 cloves garlic, minced

1 litre chicken stock

1 celery stalk, finely sliced

1 cup chopped asparagus

½ cup sugar snap peas

1 teaspoon white miso paste

200 grams cooked or poached chicken breast, shredded

1 large handful baby spinach

1 teaspoon lemon zest

1 tablespoon lemon juice

2 tablespoons chopped fresh parsley

1 tablespoon chopped fresh dill or basil (optional)

salt and pepper

fresh herbs, to garnish

cracked black pepper, to garnish

1. Heat the olive oil in a pot on medium heat. Add the onion and garlic and sauté until transparent.

2. Pour in the chicken stock and bring to a gentle boil. Add the celery, asparagus and peas. Reduce the heat and simmer for 10 minutes, until vegetables are tender.

3. Stir in the miso paste, shredded chicken, spinach and lemon zest. Simmer for another 3–5 minutes, until the spinach just wilts and chicken warms through.

4. Remove from heat. Stir through the lemon juice, parsley and dill (if using). Taste and adjust seasoning.

5. Ladle into bowls and enjoy warm. Garnish with extra herbs and cracked pepper.

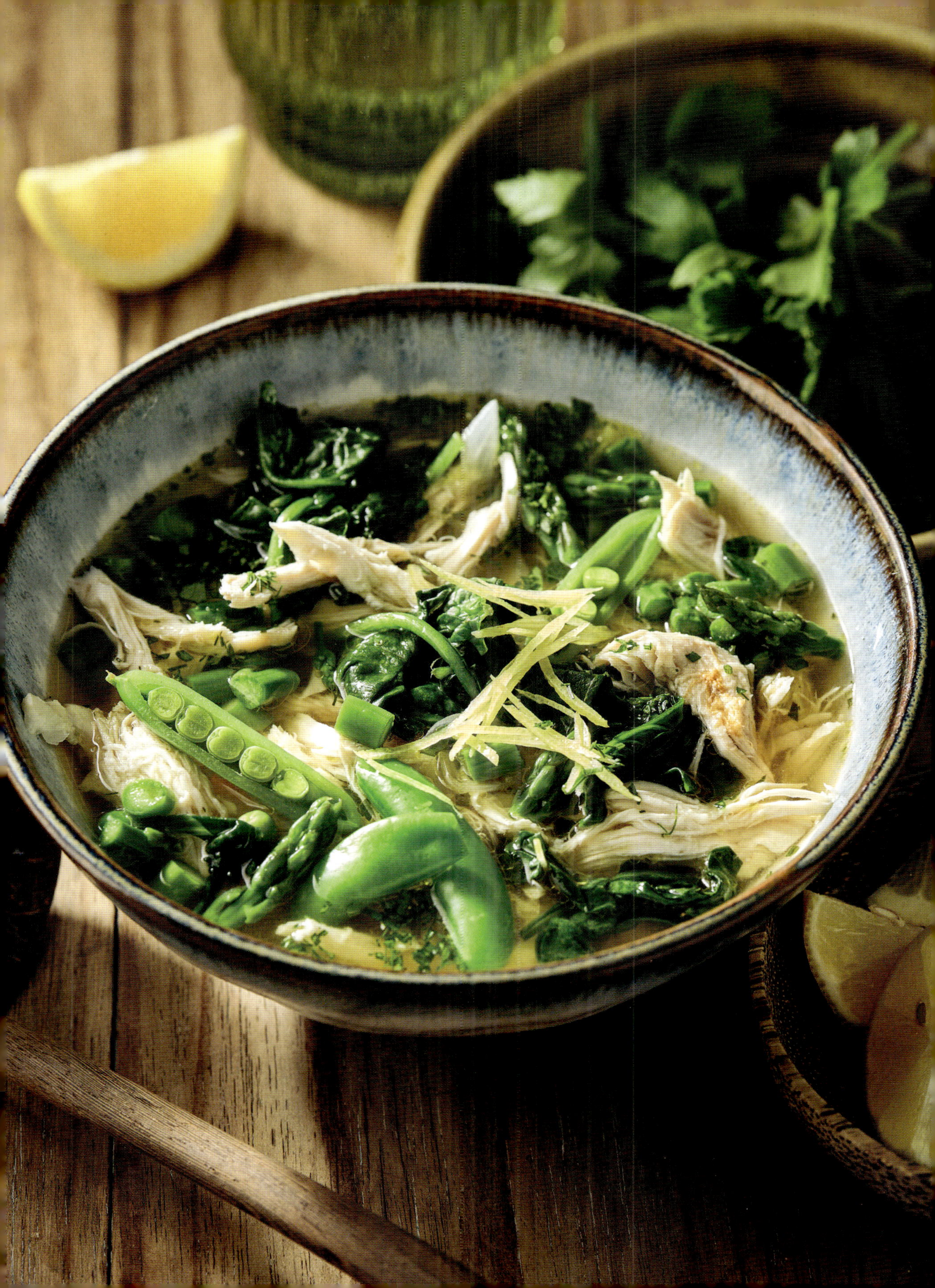

EGG SALAD WITH TURMERIC

SERVES 1 • CARBS PER SERVE: 4 GRAMS

---

2 tablespoons Greek yoghurt

¼ teaspoon ground turmeric

1 teaspoon Dijon mustard

1 tablespoon chopped fresh chives, parsley or dill, plus extra to garnish

½ teaspoon lemon zest

salt and pepper

2 eggs, hard-boiled and chopped

½ small celery stalk, finely diced

2–3 butter or iceberg lettuce leaves

1 teaspoon pepitas, to garnish

1. In a small bowl, combine the Greek yoghurt, turmeric, Dijon mustard, herbs, lemon zest, and salt and pepper to taste. Mix well.

2. Fold in the chopped eggs and celery until thoroughly coated.

3. Spoon the mixture into lettuce leaves. Garnish with extra herbs and pepitas sprinkled over the top.

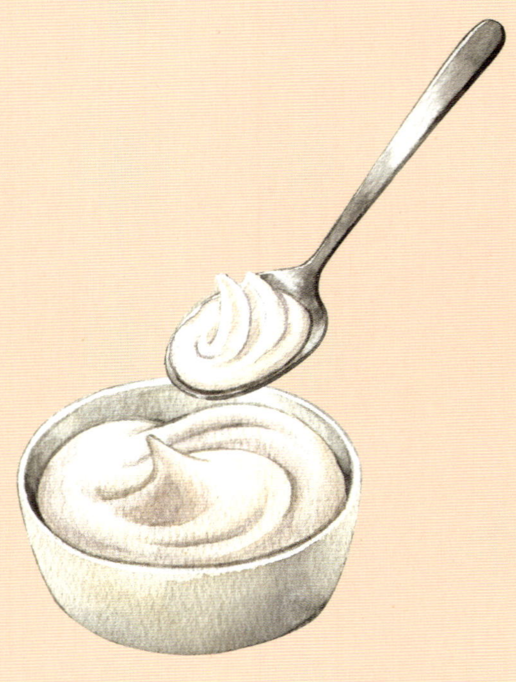

OVEN-BAKED EGGS WITH MACKEREL AND SPINACH

SERVES 1 • CARBS PER SERVE: 2 GRAMS

1 cup baby spinach

40 grams smoked mackerel, flaked

2 eggs

1 tablespoon Greek yoghurt

salt and pepper

2 tablespoons chopped fresh chives and dill, to garnish

1. Preheat the oven to 180°C.

2. Wilt the spinach and put in a small baking dish. Scatter mackerel flakes over the top. Break eggs into the dish then swirl in the yoghurt.

3. Bake uncovered for 12–15 minutes, until the eggs are cooked but yolks are still soft.

4. Season with salt and pepper to taste, and serve garnished with fresh chives and dill.

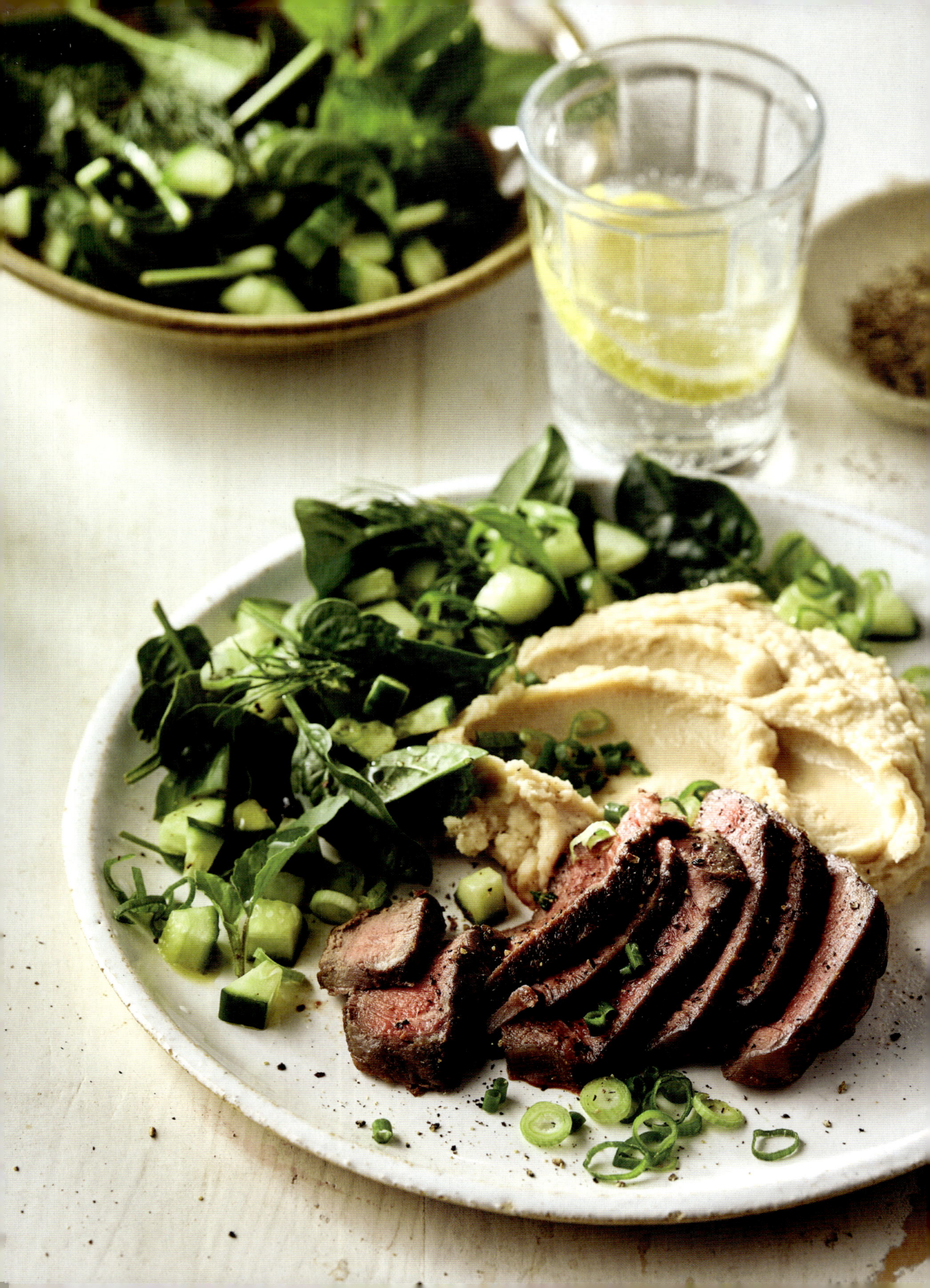

STEAK WITH BEAN PURÉE AND GREEN HERB SALAD

SERVES 1 • CARBS PER SERVE: 13 GRAMS

---

120 grams lean beef steak (sirloin, rump or scotch fillet)

½–1 teaspoon extra-virgin olive oil

salt and pepper

BEAN PURÉE

1 tablespoon extra-virgin olive oil

2 small cloves garlic, minced

½ cup canned cannellini or butter beans, drained and rinsed

2 teaspoons lemon juice

1–2 teaspoons water (optional, to thin)

salt and pepper

1 sprig fresh rosemary (optional)

GREEN HERB SALAD

1 cup baby spinach, rocket or mixed greens

¼ cup chopped Lebanese cucumber

2 tablespoons chopped fresh parsley, mint, dill, basil or chives

1 spring onion, sliced

1 tablespoon extra-virgin olive oil

2 teaspoons freshly squeezed lemon juice

salt and pepper

1. To make the bean purée, warm the olive oil in a small frying pan. Add the garlic and cook for 30 seconds. Add the beans, heat gently, then add the lemon juice, water, salt and pepper to taste, and rosemary (if using). Blend or mash.

2. Cook the steak by heating olive oil in a frying pan. Season the steak with salt and pepper to taste, then sear for 2–3 minutes on each side, or to your preferred doneness. Set aside to rest for a few minutes before slicing.

3. To make the herb salad, toss the spinach, cucumber, herbs and spring onion with the olive oil, lemon juice, and salt and pepper to taste.

4. To serve, spread the bean purée on a plate and top with slices of steak. Serve with the salad on the side.

CHICKEN TURMERIC VEGETABLE CURRY

SERVES 1 • CARBS PER SERVE: 18 GRAMS

1 tablespoon extra-virgin olive oil or coconut oil

1 clove garlic, minced

1 teaspoon grated fresh ginger

120 grams skinless chicken breast or thigh, diced

1 teaspoon ground turmeric

1 teaspoon curry powder

salt and pepper

½ red capsicum, diced

½ cup diced broccoli florets

½ cup chopped zucchini

½ cup chopped tomato

1 green chilli, sliced (or more to taste)

½ cup unsweetened coconut milk

1 tablespoon chopped fresh coriander, plus extra leaves to serve

lemon or lime wedge, to serve

1. Heat the olive oil in a non-stick frying pan. Sauté the garlic and ginger for 1 minute.

2. Add the chicken, turmeric, curry powder, and salt and pepper to taste. Cook for 2–3 minutes to colour the chicken.

3. Add all the vegetables and coconut milk. Simmer for 8–10 minutes, until the veggies and chicken are cooked.

4. Stir in the coriander, then taste and adjust seasoning. Serve with a squeeze of lemon or lime and some fresh coriander leaves.

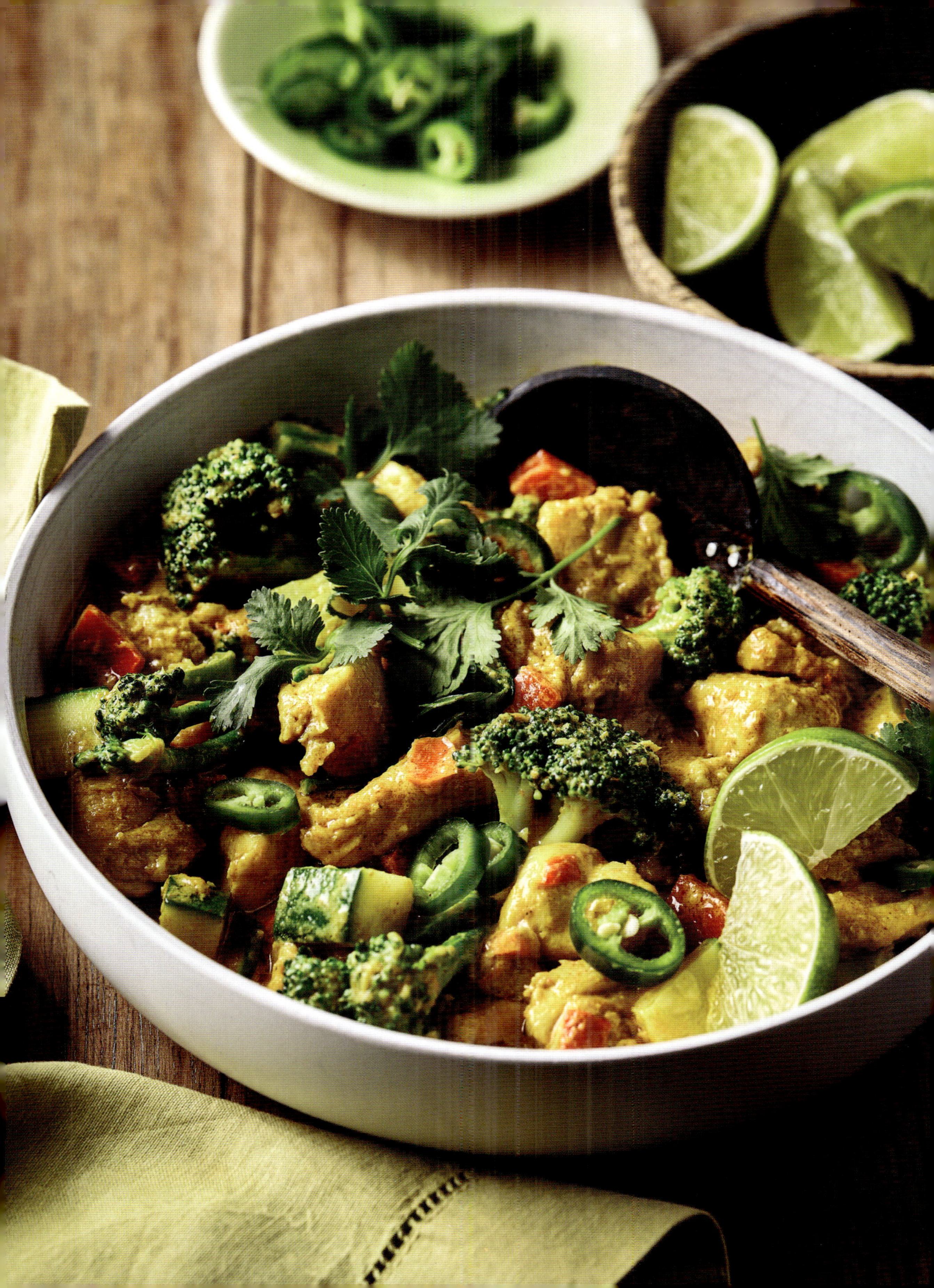

Supporting our immune system

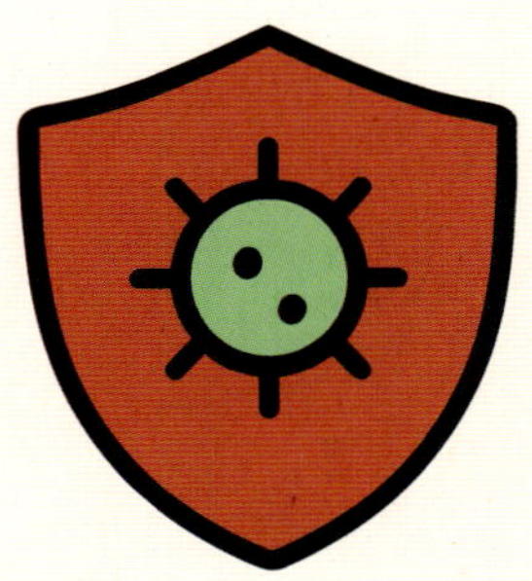

Focus: Finishing strong with a healthy immune system

Welcome to Week 9. You are so close to the finish line! I want you to think about how far you've come and what you have achieved so far. Think of the last 8 weeks as laying the foundation for what's ahead. A new normal.

This is the last week of accelerated weight loss.

If you do feel you need to snack, then refer back to the snack list (see Week 8). There is nothing wrong with snacking if you need to.

Supporting your immune system is incredibly important for people with type 2 diabetes. This is because high blood glucose and insulin resistance weaken the body's natural defence system and promote chronic inflammation.

This makes someone with diabetes more vulnerable to infections, slows healing and accelerates complications such as cardiovascular disease and kidney dysfunction. This is why in Week 9 I really wanted to address your immune system's health.

BEST FOODS TO SUPPORT THE IMMUNE SYSTEM

- **Green leafy vegetables** help protect immune cells from oxidative stress.

- **Berries and citrus** are rich in vitamin C, which improves white blood cell activity without spiking blood glucose due to their fibre content.

- **Fatty fish** contain omega-3 fatty acids, which lower inflammation and support immune cell signalling.

- **Yoghurt and fermented foods** contain probiotics that maintain healthy gut microbiota, enhancing immunity and glucose metabolism.

- **Garlic and ginger** contain bioactive compounds (allicin, gingerol) with strong antimicrobial and anti-inflammatory properties.

- **Nuts and seeds** are packed with nutrients vital for antibody formation and free radical protection.

- **Turmeric** (via the curcumin it contains) acts as a natural anti-inflammatory and antioxidant, supporting macrophage function and reducing cytokine imbalance. Always add black pepper to ensure the curcumin is absorbed.

- **Legumes and lentils** support tissue repair and gut health while stabilising blood glucose.

- **Extra-virgin olive oil** strengthens immunity by providing antioxidant protection, anti-inflammatory fats and gut microbiome support.

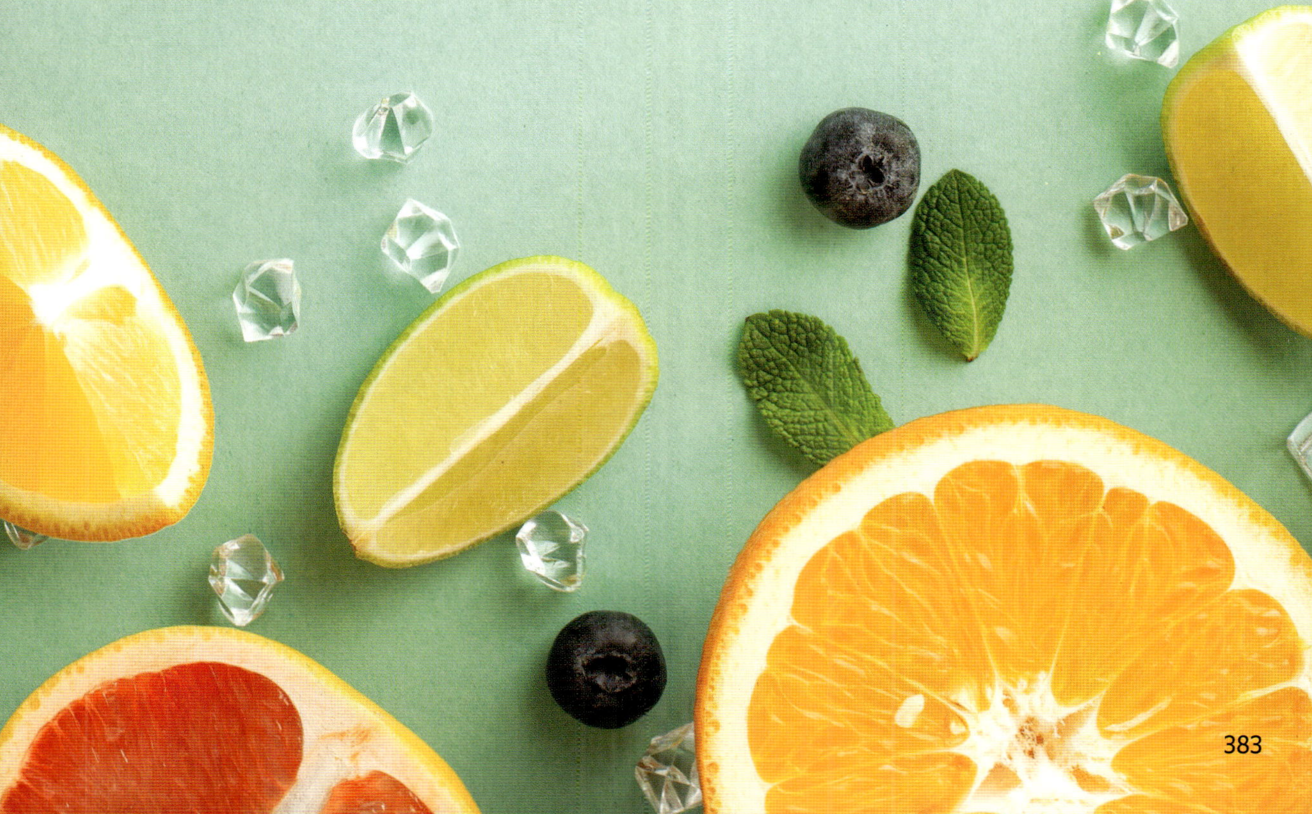

Reminders

- water intake
- exercise
- stress management
- goal setting
- walking after meals
- hydration
- continued blood glucose monitoring
- resistance training
- medication review and possible adjustment
- doing the 12/12 fasting
- order of eating
- hypoglycaemia prevention
- chewing each mouthful 20 times
- keeping track of your success
- calf raises after meals.

	BREAKFAST	**MID-MORNING**	**LUNCH**	**MID-AFTERNOON**	**DINNER**
MONDAY	Immune-boosting smoothie (page 388)	Nil	Immunity-boosting fermented salad (page 390) with 2 boiled eggs	Nil	Miso mushroom seafood soup (page 337)
TUESDAY	Low-carb oat breakfast bowl (page 318)	Nil	Mackerel patties (page 319) with Sarah's garden salad (page 275)	Nil	Prawn and bok choy broth (page 325)
WEDNESDAY	Turmeric scrambled eggs with spinach, avocado and cherry tomatoes (page 387)	Nil	Immunity-boosting fermented salad (page 390) with 120 grams shredded chicken	Nil	Tuna and white bean parsley mash with chilli and herbs (page 393)
THURSDAY	Immune-boosting smoothie (page 388)	Nil	Tuna and white bean parsley mash with chilli and herbs (page 393)	Nil	Chicken turmeric veg curry (page 380)
FRIDAY	Blueberry chia jam (page XX) with ⅔ cup Greek yoghurt and some fresh mint	Nil	Low-carb green goddess salad with chicken (page 321)	Nil	Immune-boosting garlic lemon fish with greens (page 394)
SATURDAY	High-protein, low-carb cinnamon pancakes with strawberries (page 286)	Nil	Immune-boosting garlic lemon fish with greens (page 394)	Nil	Shredded chicken noodle soup with konjac noodles (page 364)
SUNDAY	Immune-boosting smoothie (page 388)	Nil	Cottage cheese wrap (page 268) with salmon, avocado, pickles and onion	Nil	Gut-friendly green soup (page 303)
BEVERAGES Water, plus optional coffee, tea, green tea, herbal tea, electrolytes					

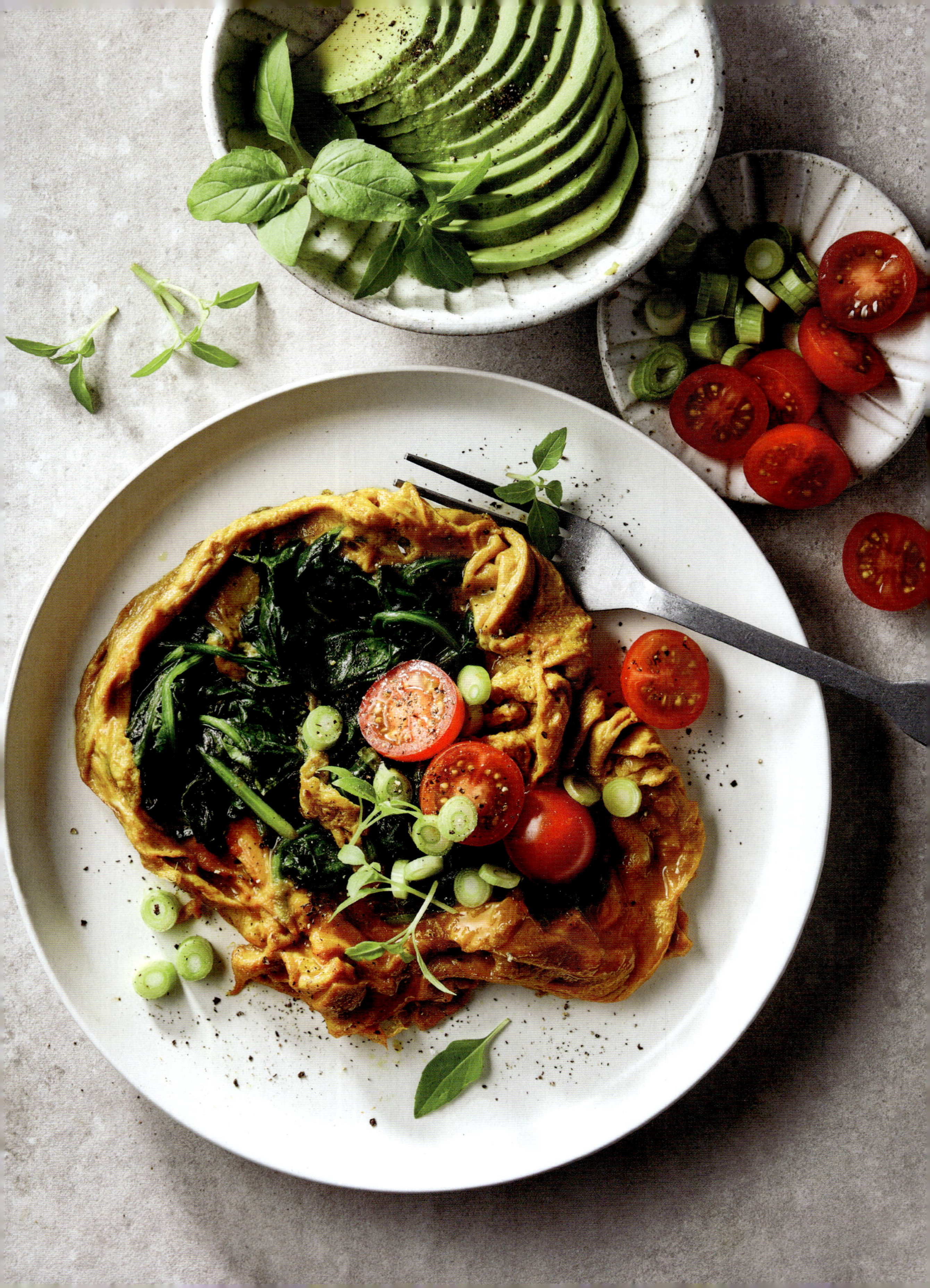

TURMERIC SCRAMBLED EGGS WITH SPINACH, AVOCADO AND CHERRY TOMATOES

SERVES 1 • CARBS PER SERVE: 4 GRAMS

2 eggs

1 teaspoon ground turmeric

salt and black pepper

1 tablespoon extra-virgin olive oil

1 cup baby spinach or kale

TOPPINGS

¼ avocado, sliced or diced

2–3 cherry tomatoes, halved or sliced

sliced spring onion

chopped fresh parsley, dill or coriander

1. Whisk the eggs with the turmeric, pepper and salt to taste.

2. Heat the olive oil in a non-stick frying pan over medium heat. Add spinach and cook until just wilted.

3. Pour in the egg mixture. Gently stir with a spatula until the eggs are softly set and creamy, about 2–3 minutes.

4. Serve topped with avocado, cherry tomatoes, spring onion and a sprinkle of fresh herbs. Add extra cracked pepper or a drizzle of olive oil if desired.

IMMUNE-BOOSTING SMOOTHIE

SERVES 1 • CARBS PER SERVE: 10 GRAMS

½ cup Greek yoghurt

½ cup unsweetened almond milk or water

½ cup baby spinach or kale

¼ cup mixed berries

1 teaspoon extra-virgin olive oil

1 teaspoon chia seeds

½ teaspoon grated fresh ginger

¼ teaspoon ground turmeric

pinch of black pepper

pinch of stevia powder

ice cubes (optional)

Put all the ingredients in a blender. Blend until smooth and creamy. Taste and adjust, adding more almond milk for thinness or extra yoghurt for creaminess. Serve immediately.

BLUEBERRY CHIA JAM

MAKES 12 TABLESPOONS • CARBS PER SERVE: 1.3 GRAMS

1 cup fresh or frozen blueberries

1–2 tablespoons water (as needed)

2 tablespoons chia seeds

2 teaspoons freshly squeezed lemon juice

1–2 teaspoons stevia powder

½ teaspoon vanilla extract (optional)

1. Place the blueberries in a small saucepan over medium-low heat. Add 1 tablespoon water if using fresh berries. Stirring often, cook gently for 5–7 minutes, until berries begin to burst and release their juice.

2. Lightly mash the berries with a fork or potato masher, leaving some chunks for texture. Stir in the chia seeds, lemon juice, stevia and vanilla (if using). Mix well. Let the mixture simmer for another 2–3 minutes, stirring occasionally. It will thicken as the chia seeds absorb liquid.

3. Remove from the heat and let it cool for 10–15 minutes; the jam will thicken further as it cools. Adjust consistency with a splash more water if needed.

4. Transfer the jam to a clean glass jar. Store in the fridge for up to 1 week.

Tip: Honey does work better with this recipe but is something to consider when you reach your goal weight.

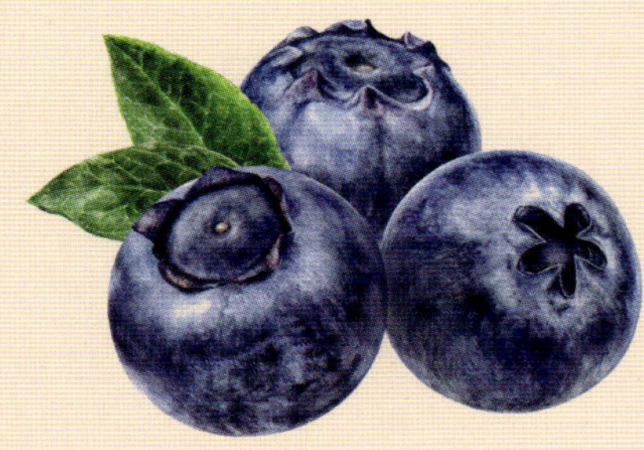

IMMUNE-BOOSTING FERMENTED SALAD

SERVES 2 • CARBS PER SERVE: 6 GRAMS

1 cup sauerkraut

½ cup kimchi or pickles

1 cup raw or lightly steamed broccoli florets

½ small red capsicum, diced

½ small avocado or ¼ large avocado, diced

1 tablespoon pepitas or sunflower seeds

fresh parsley or dill, to garnish

IMMUNE-BOOSTING DRESSING

2 cloves garlic, minced

1 tablespoon extra-virgin olive oil

1 teaspoon apple cider vinegar or lemon juice

½ teaspoon grated fresh ginger

¼ teaspoon ground turmeric

pinch of black pepper

1 tablespoon water (optional)

1. In a large bowl, combine the sauerkraut, kimchi, broccoli and capsicum.

2. To make the immune-boosting dressing, whisk all the ingredients together until emulsified.

3. Toss vegetables in the dressing, making sure everything is lightly coated. Fold through the avocado and seeds. Sprinkle herbs on top to serve.

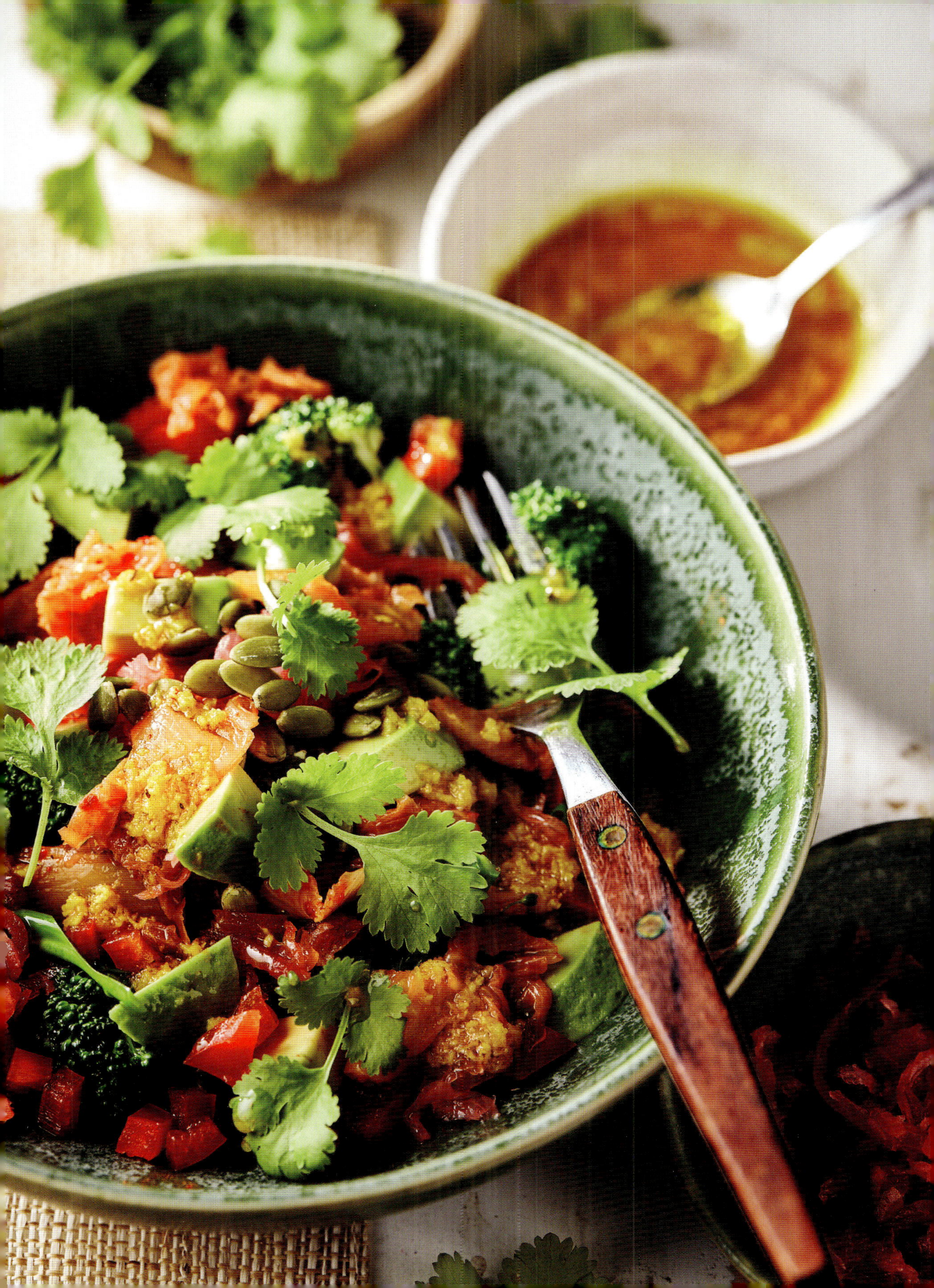

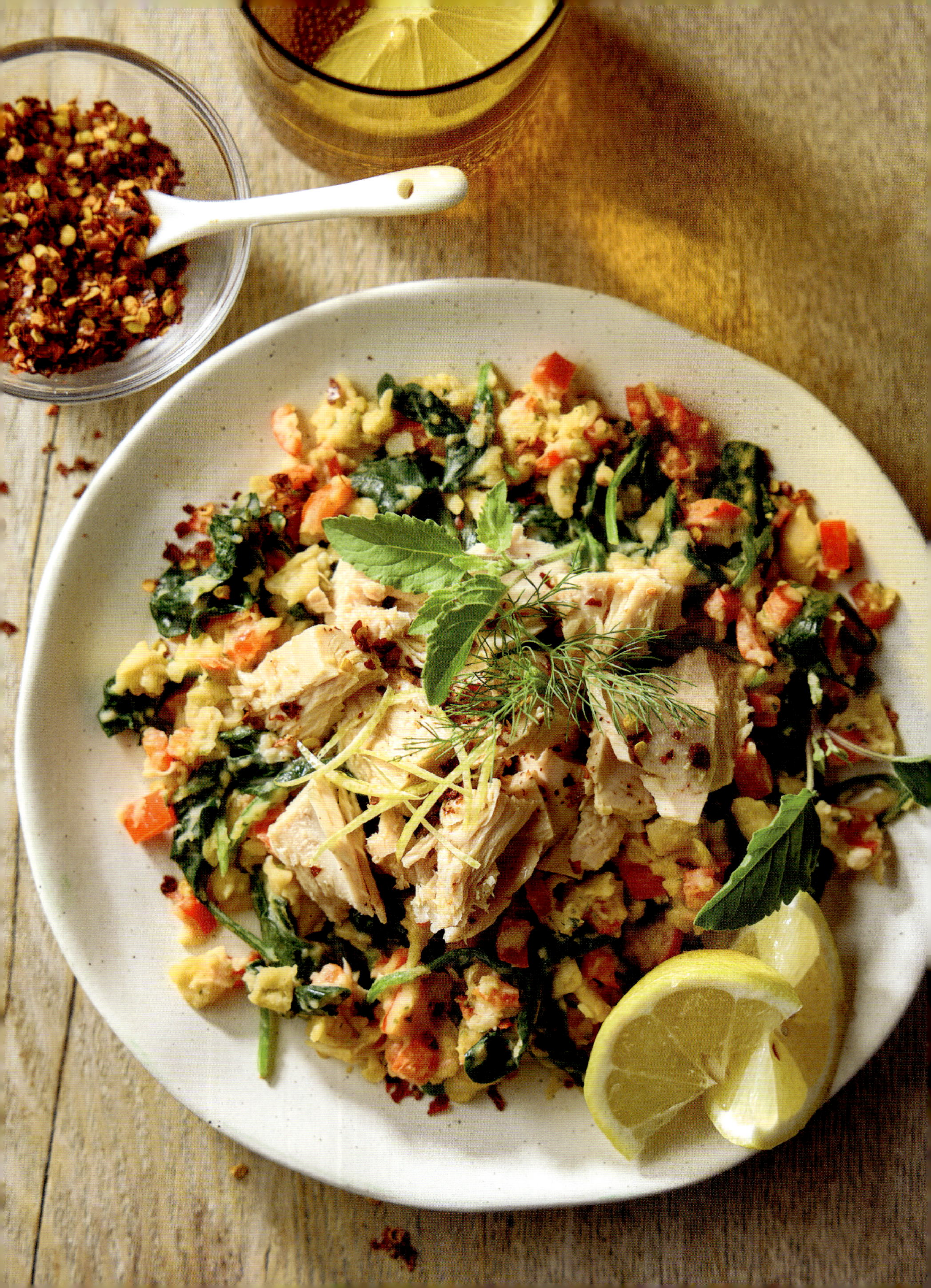

TUNA AND WHITE BEAN PARSLEY MASH WITH CHILLI AND HERBS

SERVES 2 • CARBS PER SERVE: 14 GRAMS

1 tablespoon extra-virgin olive oil

2 garlic cloves, minced

½ teaspoon dried parsley

½ red capsicum, diced

1 x 400-gram can cannellini beans, drained and rinsed

salt and pepper

80 grams baby spinach, chopped

1 x 185-gram can tuna in olive oil, drained

juice of ½ lemon

chilli flakes, to garnish

fresh dill and parsley, to garnish

lemon zest, to garnish

1. Heat the olive oil in a frying pan on medium heat. Add the garlic and dried parsley and heat briefly. Add the capsicum and sauté for a couple of minutes to soften.

2. Stir in the drained cannellini beans and heat through for 2 minutes, then roughly mash with a potato masher. Season with salt and pepper to taste, then fold in the spinach until just wilted.

3. In a small pan, gently warm the tuna and the lemon juice.

4. Serve the tuna over the mashed beans. Garnish with chilli flakes, fresh herbs and lemon zest.

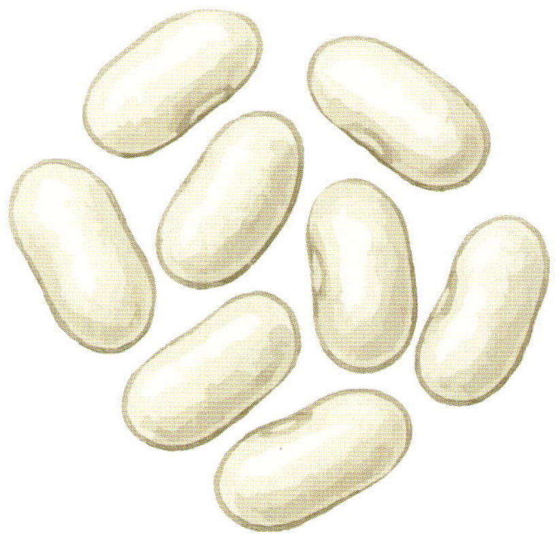

IMMUNE-BOOSTING GARLIC LEMON FISH WITH GREENS

SERVES 2 • CARBS PER SERVE: 5 GRAMS

2 tablespoons extra-virgin olive oil

1 tablespoon butter (optional)

6 large cloves garlic, finely sliced

1 teaspoon grated fresh ginger

½ teaspoon ground turmeric

pinch of black pepper

2 white fish fillets (cod, snapper or barramundi), about 180 grams each

salt

1 small zucchini, sliced

1 cup baby spinach or kale

juice and zest of ½ lemon

1 tablespoon chopped fresh parsley or dill

1 tablespoon crushed roasted almonds

fresh chilli (optional)

1. Heat the olive oil and butter (if using) in a large frying pan on a medium heat. Add the garlic and ginger and sauté for about 30 seconds, until transparent.

2. Sprinkle in the turmeric and black pepper, stirring to bloom the spices. Add the fish fillets, season lightly with salt, and pan-sear for 3–4 minutes each side, until cooked through.

3. Remove fish from heat and keep warm. In the same pan, add the zucchini and spinach, sautéing until the spinach is just wilted.

4. Squeeze fresh lemon juice over the vegetables, then return the fish to the pan to glaze lightly. Serve garnished with lemon zest, parsley, almonds and chilli (if using).

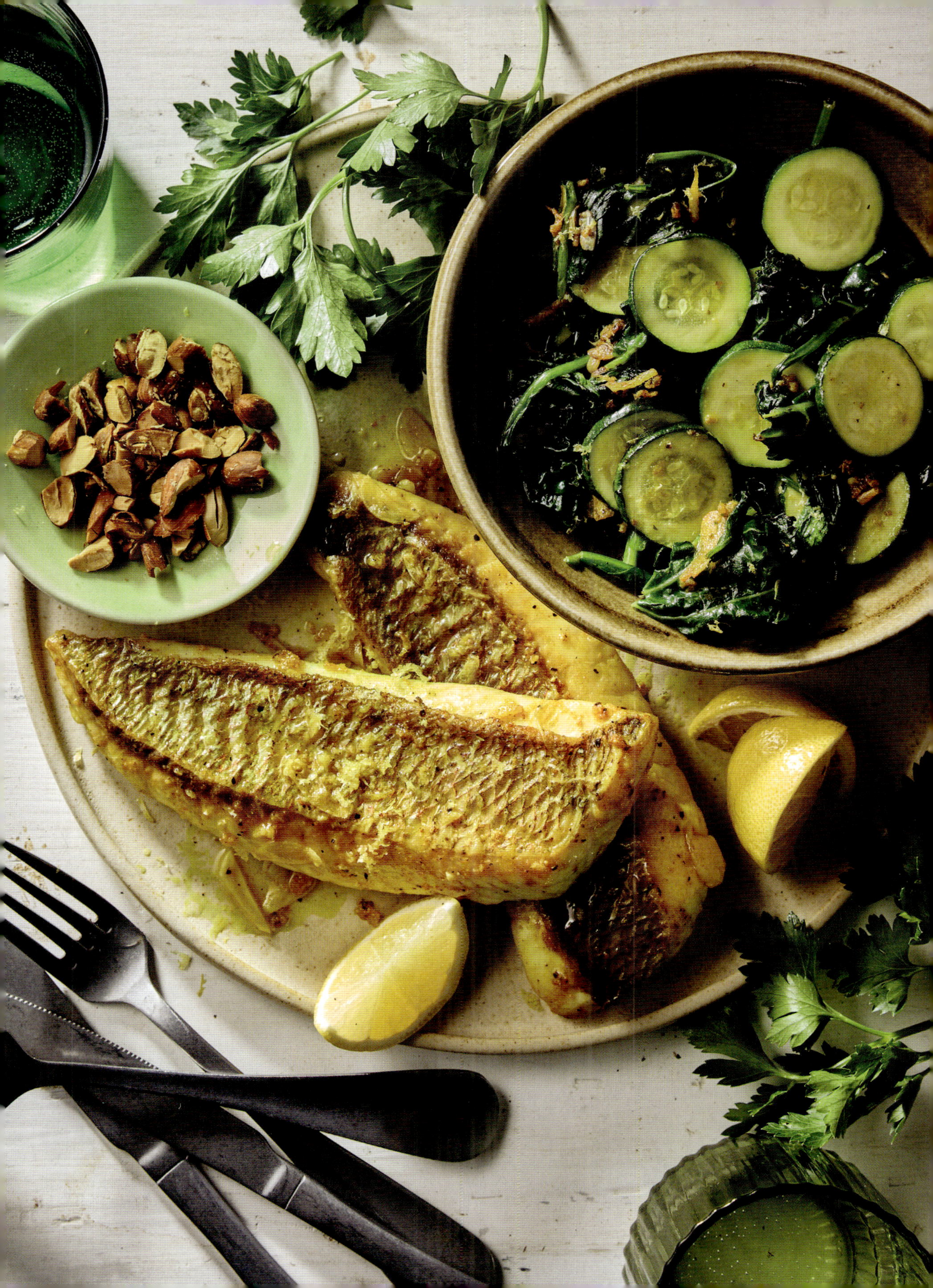

WHERE DO I GO FROM HERE?

Congratulations on finishing the 9-week program. YOU DID IT and it was so worth it!

Reflection: What did you achieve in the 9 weeks?

- Think about why you started this program in the first place.

- Realise that the rest of your life will be based on the foundations laid in this program.

- How you have been eating in the last 9 weeks is setting you up for your new normal.

- Are you still monitoring your weight and blood glucose and seeing your health care provider?

- Practising the order of eating, walking after meals and chewing your food thoroughly are your way of life now.

- Exercise is essential. Think of it like a prescription and something you do every day.

- Always manage your stress.

- Always be aware of managing hypoglycaemia.

- Aim for a balanced plate at meals with a rainbow of veggies, lean proteins and healthy fats.

- Aim to stick to 12/12 fasting protocol.

- Your long-term aim is to focus on low-carb living – eating protein, fat and low-GI carbs at meals.

CARB INTRODUCTION AND WHEN IN REMISSION

Moving forward, you should be living low-carb, but can increase your carbs to 80–100 grams per day from the 30–70 grams you've been on throughout the program. I would not recommend increasing it much past 100 grams per day.

The evidence shows that carb tolerance varies individually. Studies indicate that 75–110 grams/day is a 'sweet spot' for maintaining remission and avoiding relapse, balancing glycaemic control with getting enough nutrients and fibre. Some people remain in full remission at 80–120 grams total carbs/day, while others need to stay below 70 grams to keep glucose in the normal range. You need to find what works for you.

When you're in remission from type 2 diabetes, eating about 100 grams carbs/day should be both sustainable and metabolically healthy, as long as you maintain a stable weight, and normal HbA1c and insulin sensitivity. What is sustainable is what matters most. Both low and moderate carb intake can work if you can maintain your T2D remission and goal weight.

HOW DO YOU KNOW WHAT WORKS FOR YOU?

- Fasting glucose is under 5.5 mmol/L and post-meal spikes stay below 7.8 mmol/L.

- HbA1c remains under 5.7% (39 mmol/mol).

- Body weight and waist circumference remain stable or improving.

- Carbohydrates come from non-starchy vegetables, legumes in moderation, nuts, berries and fermented foods, not refined starches or sugars.

- If your fasting glucose starts to rise, post-meal readings exceed 8 mmol/L, or HbA1c drifts upward, temporarily lowering carbohydrate intake to about 50–75 grams/day may help regain stability.

- Stick to low-GI, fibre-rich foods, berries, yoghurt, legumes, whole grains, quinoa and small amounts of sweet potato.

- Make sure you eat protein with every meal.

Remember, never eat complex carbohydrates at night.

Seek out the support you need moving forward. Please join my Facebook community, The Sarah Di Lorenzo Community, for ongoing support as well. I am an active member there.

DAY ON A PLATE FOR TYPE 2 DIABETES REMISSION

When your T2D is in remission, your goal is to:

- maintain stable blood glucose
- reduce inflammation
- preserve weight loss
- follow a low-carb, whole-food balanced diet.

POST-PROGRAM DAILY OVERVIEW

NUTRIENT FOCUS	TYPICAL INTAKE
NET CARBS	40–100 grams (mostly from vegetables, legumes, yoghurt)
PROTEIN	1.2 grams per kilogram of body weight daily from eggs, fish, beans or lean meats
FAT	Mostly monounsaturated and omega-3 fats from olive oil, avocado, nuts and fish
FIBRE	Minimum of 30 grams, for blood glucose stability and gut support

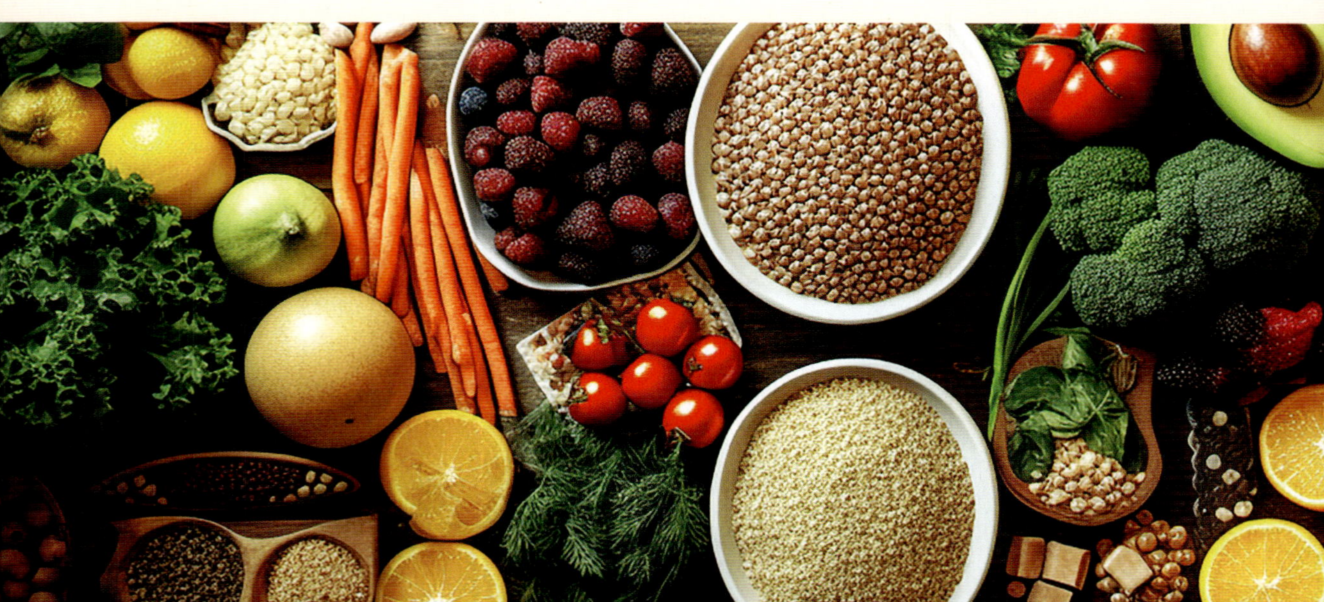

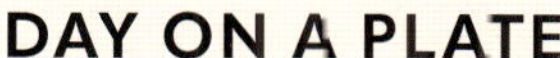

DAY ON A PLATE

BREAKFAST

Spinach and avocado egg bowl

2 eggs, poached or scrambled in olive oil

1 cup baby spinach, sautéed in a little olive oil

¼ avocado, sliced

1 teaspoon chia or flaxseed

Benefits: High in protein, magnesium and anti-inflammatory omega-3 fats. Eggs and spinach provide choline and antioxidants for insulin sensitivity.

MID-MORNING (OPTIONAL)

Options include:

- Small handful of mixed nuts (almonds, walnuts)
- Boiled egg
- 10:10 SDL protein bar
- Greek yoghurt (with a few blueberries)

Purpose: Keeps energy even without spiking glucose. Adds healthy fats and probiotics for gut health.

LUNCH

Tuna and white bean salad

1 small can tuna in olive oil

½ cup canned white beans, drained

¼ cup cooked quinoa

Mixed leafy greens, cucumber, onion and capsicum

Lemon–olive oil dressing with chopped garlic

Fresh herbs, roasted almonds and chilli to garnish

Benefits: Delivers protein, fibre and omega-3s to control post-meal glucose and support cardiovascular health.

MID-AFTERNOON (OPTIONAL)

Options include:

- Celery sticks with hummus
- Boiled egg with sea salt and dill
- 30 grams nuts and or seeds
- 1 apple
- 1 orange
- Pickles and cheese

Purpose: Keeps insulin response minimal while supporting satiety and nutrient intake.

DINNER

Garlic lemon fish with greens

1 fillet grilled or baked salmon, snapper or barramundi

Zucchini, spinach and broccoli sautéed with olive oil and garlic

Squeeze of lemon juice

Benefits: Rich in omega-3s, vitamin D and anti-inflammatory compounds that help maintain T2D remission and protect cardiovascular health.

EVENING

Chamomile tea or mint tea

Benefits: Promotes calm digestion and better sleep, often beneficial for fasting glucose regulation.

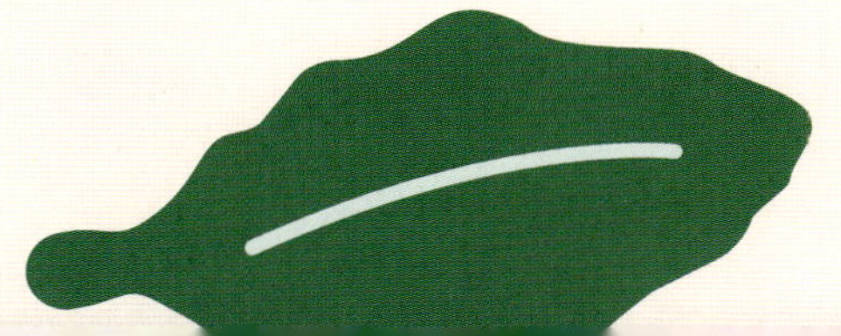

ACKNOWLEDGEMENTS

This part of any book I have ever written is so thought-provoking. It makes me think of who is in my life, who matters to me, how they make me feel and what they are like as a person.

Being an author means spending a lot of time alone researching, deep in thought, formatting, creating, mapping and being focused. When I have my designated writing days, I start at 4 a.m. and finish around 8 p.m. I have worked out when my brain is at its optimum and my productivity is high. The day flows with my circadian rhythms and aligned to this is my productivity. These days also mean I am off comms, and only doing essential tasks such as cooking my kids dinner and going for a run. Outside of that I am isolated. I really do love being an author but it also means I don't see those I love and cherish as much, so I'm going to acknowledge them all here.

I have to start with my beautiful three daughters: Charlotte, Coco and Chloe. Charlotte is now 23 and lives out of home, Coco is 21 and living with me still studying at university, and Chloe is in Year 11 and preparing herself for two big final years at school. Being a mum of three girls is a roller coaster. I'm in the mix of their careers and love lives, boyfriends coming and going, friendships, tears, joy and finding their way in life. For me, any spare time goes to them. But my three girls have always been there for me too.

My parents Nick and Terry watch all my TV segments, and always support my journey. I love their excitement, especially Mum's when I publish a new book – she is just so proud, as is my dad. They love sharing wonderful feedback from their friends who read my books and have success on my programs.

I also need to acknowledge my brother John Cassimatis, a successful chiropractor in Cairns. John has all my books in his clinic and shares them with his patients. John is a huge supporter of everything I do. My gorgeous sister Catherine Wisselink always calls to check in and is so supportive, while her father-in-law Jerry Wisselink cooks all my recipes, sends me photos and is just so wonderful.

My editors Rosie McDonald and Jess Cox. Love these two! We have an interesting story, all three of us attended the same primary school over the span of 20 years. First Rosie, then 10 years later me and around 10 years after that Jess. Here we are today, working as such a wonderful team. So grateful for all they do, their patience and expertise.

Another amazing human I am so grateful for is my agent, Lucie McGeoch. Lucie is one of a kind and one in a billion. She is there through it all, such a hard worker; she's supportive, enthusiastic, kind and authentic. It's so important to be surrounded by the right people in life and Lucie is that and so much more. I also want to acknowledge Michael Cassel here, always so supportive, enthusiastic and thoughtful.

Simon & Schuster have always been there for me with an amazing team. My publicist Jade Gould goes above and beyond for me as does the rest of the team there. So grateful again to be surrounded by such wonderful people.

My producer at Channel 7 Kaitlin Peek is someone else I just love and want to acknowledge. Kaitlin is so gorgeous, kind, supportive, caring and thoughtful. Kaitlin and I have worked together for almost 4 years, she is the other half of my TV segments. We are both hardworking Capricorns, always wanting to give everything 100%, so aligned and a great team.

I think about people who have made a difference in my life. I will forever be so grateful and never forget the people who believed in me when others did not. Two people immediately come to mind. The first is Dan Ruffino. Dan was the MD of Simon & Schuster, and it was because of him that I decided to go with S&S in the beginning. Dan understood me, saw my potential and backed me. Dan has been so positive, smart, funny, supportive and uplifting. The other person is Sarah Stinson. Like Dan, Sarah could see my messaging, work and potential, and has been just so supportive. I'm forever grateful.

Other amazing people who are incredibly supportive and who I just love so much are Monique Wright, Natalie Barr and Sally Bowrey. I just adore these amazing women!! All three have written a foreword for my previous books and are just amazing humans. I also want to acknowledge the staff at Channel 7 – they are always so supportive.

I want to acknowledge all the patients in my clinic. I get to meet thousands of people in my line of work, and because of my years of clinical experience I have the research underpinning the nutrition programs in my books.

To all of you who buy my books, thank you for your support. I'm so grateful and love that I can help you beyond my clinic. Helping all of you is what drives me to keep writing. I love hearing your success stories, emails, kindness and support.

To my friends, who I don't see as much as I should. Thank you for still being there when I come up for air. All relationships need effort to grow and be sustainable. In saying that, I'm so lucky to have such rock-solid female friends who are there forever. For this I am so grateful.

My Facebook community – The Sarah Di Lorenzo Community – you are incredible!!! All of you are so supportive, kind, caring and inspirational. I acknowledge each and every one of you for not only being supportive and protective of me, but also living your best lives from following my work. Love you all so much.

Finally, to my darling Gigi Di Lorenzo, the most loyal, loving, kind cuddly ragdoll cat of mine. When I write, she is next to me all the time, sitting on the printer or my keyboard, between the keyboard and me, or on the window ledge. Gigi is always by my side. The unconditional love of an animal is priceless. Gigi, you are in my heart now and forever.

ABOUT THE AUTHOR

Sarah Di Lorenzo is a qualified clinical nutritionist who has dedicated her career to overhauling the health of people of all ages. She is the bestselling author of *The 10:10 Plan*, *The 10:10 Recipe Book*, *The 10:10 Kickstart*, *The 10:10 Simple Recipe Book*, *The Gut Repair Plan*, *My Mediterranean Life*, *The Liver Repair Plan* and *The Power of Protein*. As well as running a successful clinic in Sydney, Sarah is a regular public speaker and media nutritionist, well known as the resident nutritionist on Channel 7's *Weekend Sunrise* and *Sunrise*.

Sarah is also an entrepreneur who has launched a very successful protein bar business called 1010SDL. She has also recently also launched her podcast series *10:10 Be Well* covering all aspects of wellness.

Sarah has a weekly column at *The Nightly* and has a regular column at *New Idea* Magazine.

A single mother of three daughters, Sarah is also a keen exerciser and firmly believes in the benefits of a healthy lifestyle.